T0226133

Effective Treatments in Psychiatry

Effective Treatments in Psychiatry

Peter Tyrer

Imperial College London

Kenneth R. Silk

University of Michigan

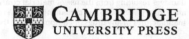

CAMBRIDGE
UNIVERSITY PRESS

CAMBRIDGE
UNIVERSITY PRESS

University Printing House, Cambridge CB2 8BS, United Kingdom

One Liberty Plaza, 20th Floor, New York, NY 10006, USA

477 Williamstown Road, Port Melbourne, VIC 3207, Australia

314-321, 3rd Floor, Plot 3, Splendor Forum, Jasola District Centre, New Delhi - 110025, India

79 Anson Road, #06-04/06, Singapore 079906

Cambridge University Press is part of the University of Cambridge.

It furthers the University's mission by disseminating knowledge in the pursuit of education, learning and research at the highest international levels of excellence.

www.cambridge.org
Information on this title: www.cambridge.org/9780521124652

First published 2011

A catalogue record for this publication is available from the British Library

Library of Congress Cataloging in Publication data
Tyrer, Peter J.
Effective treatments in psychiatry / Peter Tyrer, Kenneth R. Silk.
  p. ; cm. – (Cambridge pocket clinicians)
Includes bibliographical references.
ISBN 978-0-521-12465-2 (pbk.)
1. Psychiatry – Handbooks, manuals, etc.   2. Mental illness – Treatment – Handbooks, manuals, etc. I. Silk, Kenneth R., 1944– II. Title.   III. Series: Cambridge pocket clinicians.
[DNLM : 1. Mental Disorders – therapy – Handbooks.   2. Psychiatry – methods – Handbooks.
  WM 34]
RC456.T97   2011
616.89–dc23

2011015547

ISBN 978-0-521-12465-2 Paperback

Contents

Preface

Progress in psychiatry, and indeed in all parts of medicine, moves like the sea in a time of global warming. We, on the shores of evidence, note the often dramatic ebb and flow of the tides but also can identify a gradual rise in the sea of knowledge. The problem in interpreting the rise is that it is much less perceptible than the tidal changes. In the last few years the growth of evidence-based medicine has been tremendous and is now moving at a breakneck pace compared with 20 years ago. Indeed, the number of randomized trials, systematic reviews and meta-analyses is now so large that we are not able to keep up with apparent advances and will have to work out a new set of priorities to keep our information in order

(Bastian et al., 2010). We in psychiatry have contributed greatly to this expansion, and although at one level we can be pleased with this progress, all too often in retrospect it can be seen as a spring tide of advance that is followed by an ebb of disillusion. The most obvious example of this is the increasing concern that trials promoted by the pharmaceutical industry tend to overstate the benefits of candidate drugs still under patent, and when all the evidence is collected independently, including that from unpublished trials, the level of advance is seen to be infinitesimally small (e.g. Whittington et al., 2004).

Since the publication of the *Cambridge Textbook of Effective Treatments in Psychiatry* in 2008 there has been much agitation in the seas of psychiatry while evidence levels have not changed greatly. But they have altered sufficiently to justify a shorter book that brings practitioners up to date with latest developments, be they ephemeral or lasting, and also makes the book easier to handle ("pocket size" as our publishers suggest). For those who want to know more details about the data that lead to the evidence presented here, the longer book is still needed, but this version, combined with essential references and an evidence-based table after each chapter, can serve as an aide-memoire. The chapters are set out in the same order as in the original textbook but there are no preliminary sections on treatments in general or on classification issues. The evidence level for each intervention follows the format given in the Appendix.

We thank all our authors for helping us to bring their chapters up to date and for reviewing and approving the shortened version lest we leave out essential information. We greatly appreciate the secretarial and other assistance of Jemma Reilly Ayton and Ellie Flynn. We also thank Cambridge University Press for staying with this endeavour and for helping us bring this version to press. Our hope is that this book will help both tide watchers and depth measurers and add benefit to patients through better clinical practice.

This book is an updated and shortened version of the more complete *Cambridge Textbook of Effective Treatments in Psychiatry* published in 2008. The process of arriving at the final version of the chapters published in this text was as follows: Either Dr Tyrer or Dr Silk reviewed each chapter from the original book that has been published here in this text. The chapters then were shortened so that they were each of approximately 2000 words in text length (not including references and the summary table). During the shortening process, updated information and references known to Drs Tyrer and Silk were added. The shortened chapter was then sent on to the original authors for their critique and additional input to ensure that the final version of the chapter contained the most recent information (up to the second half of 2010). The chapter was then sent back and forth between the book editor and the lead author until a final chapter length and content was agreed upon.

Thus although either Dr. Tyrer or Dr. Silk had significant input into the shortening of each chapter, the content and the timeliness of the data in the chapter was the product of the individuals whose names appear under each chapter heading.

Peter Tyrer
Kenneth R. Silk

Organic disorders

Delirium

Based on "Delirium" by Laura Gage and David K. Conn in Effective Treatments in Psychiatry, Cambridge University Press, 2008

Introduction

Delirium needs treatment for both its causes and manifestations, as, if ignored, it is associated with excessive periods of hospitalization or early mortality. The common causes include infection, drug intoxication, renal or hepatic insufficiency, vascular disease affecting the brain, and (often forgotten) electrolyte disturbance. The main interventions are environmental and pharmacological and the symptoms on which they are focused are agitation, overactivity, restlessness, and other behavioural disturbance, and psychotic symptoms such as hallucinations, delusions, and paranoid reconstruction of the world. As might be expected, randomized controlled trials are very difficult to carry out in this population as the manifestations of delirium are acute and cannot be ignored, and most of the evidence of efficacy of interventions is based on less convincing models.

Non-pharmacological interventions

Delirium is very common in hospitalized patients, particularly after surgery and other interventions, and providing a consistent environment with the right level of stimulation has long been thought to avoid or reduce manifestations of delirium. Only one randomized trial has been carried out of 31 patients following open heart surgery in an intensive care unit (Budd & Brown, 1974). Patients randomized to a specific reorientation procedure, focusing on time, place, person, and physical status, given by intensive care nurses, showed fewer symptoms of delirium, had significantly fewer postoperative complications, and were discharged from hospital an average of 4 days earlier compared with a control group of patients who did not receive this intervention but who had standard care. Other non-randomized studies have supported these findings (Chatham, 1978; Williams et al., 1985; Milisen et al., 2001).

A review by Cole et al. (1996) concluded that systematic interventions to stabilize the environment and offer support were more effective with older surgical patients compared with patients on medical units. A recent Cochrane Review of multidisciplinary team interventions in patients with chronic cognitive impairment concluded that although nine controlled trials were identified for possible inclusion in the review, only one (Budd & Brown, 1974) met the inclusion criteria. Despite the presumptive evidence from other studies they concluded that delirium is currently managed empirically and that there was no evidence in the literature to support changes to current practice (Britton & Russell, 2004).

Despite the relative absence of good data supporting controlled environmental interventions the American Psychiatric Association still recommend them because of wide clinical experience and, perhaps more importantly, their lack of adverse effects (American Psychiatric Association, 1999). This has increased in importance as the technology of intensive care has improved and environments become less homely. Patients with delirium can become overstimulated by the excessive noise in such units. Similarly, if stimulation is too low delirium can also become more likely.

Pharmacological interventions

Typical antipsychotic drugs

Only one randomized controlled trial has compared typical antipsychotics in delirium. Breitbart et al. (1996) compared the effectiveness of chlorpromazine, haloperidol, and lorazepam in hospitalized patients with AIDS. All included met diagnostic criteria for delirium and scored 13 or more on the delirium rating scale (DRS). Two hundred and forty-four patients were included and 30 of these subsequently developed delirium and were randomized to one of the three study medications.

The efficacy of intervention was similar for haloperidol and chlorpromazine and improvement was noted within the first 24 hours. Those patients allocated to lorazepam developed major side effects but the mean daily dosage of the drug (4.6 mg) was much higher than the usual dosage. As there was no placebo control arm, haloperidol or chlorpromazine may not have performed better than no intervention. All other studies in the published literature are small and have weak methodology so no conclusions can be drawn. A combination of benzodiazepines and haloperidol was compared in a naturalistic study by Menza et al. (1988). It was noted that those who received the haloperidol and benzodiazepines had fewer extrapyramidal symptoms than those who received haloperidol alone (with haloperidol given intravenously).

Atypical antipsychotic drugs

Olanzapine

Olanzapine has been compared with haloperidol in a randomized controlled trial involving 73 patients. Patients satisfying DSM-IV criteria for delirium were randomized to haloperidol or olanzapine and the results showed no difference in the reduction of delirium over time. However, intravenous haloperidol as a rescue drug was used in 36% of those taking olanzapine on the first day of delirium and 18% of patients on the second day; this clearly contaminated interpretation of the findings. No other controlled trials have been carried out with olanzapine but reports suggest that it is efficacious and with few extrapyramidal effects (Sipahimalani & Masand, 1998).

Risperidone

A randomized double-blind trial of risperidone and haloperidol in the treatment of delirium (Han & Kim, 2004) showed no difference between the two drugs but only 24 patients entered the trial. However, those treated with haloperidol had a 75% response compared with 42% on risperidone. Rather better results have been understandably found in open studies (Horikawa et al., 2003; Parellada et al., 2004). It is difficult to make any firm conclusions about risperidone on the basis of these data.

Quetiapine, ziprasidone, and remoxipride

Open studies have suggested that these three drugs may have some value in the treatment of delirium (Robertson et al., 1996; Schwartz & Masand, 2000; Kim et al., 2003) but no definite conclusions can be drawn from them.

Cholinesterase inhibitors

As these drugs are commonly used in the treatment of dementia and behavioural disturbance (see following chapters) it is not surprising that they, mainly donezepil and rivastigmine, have been used in the treatment of delirium. One small trial with 15 patients treated with rivastigmine (1.5 mg increasing to 3.0 mg/day) showed shorter duration of delirium compared with placebo (Overshott et al., 2010), but another larger trial of rivastigmine 4.5 mg daily versus placebo (Gamberini et al., 2009) showed no benefit for the active drug.

Benzodiazepines

Although benzodiazepines reduce the risk of extrapyramidal symptoms (Menza et al., 1998) they sometimes promote cognitive impairment. This problem has only been marked in the study by Breitbart et al. (1996), which used high doses. Nevertheless, a recent Cochrane Review concluded "no adequately controlled trials could be found to support the use of benzodiazepines in the treatment of non-alcohol withdrawal-related delirium among hospitalized patients, and at this time benzodiazepines cannot be recommended for the control of this condition" (Lonergan et al., 2009).

Mianserin

This atypical antidepressant drug has been compared with haloperidol in 40 patients diagnosed with delirium using DSM-IV criteria (Nakamura et al., 1997). Again there was no difference in the improvement between the groups with 7 out of 10 patients improving on these treatments. Mianserin was given in a dose of between 10 mg and 60 mg a day and caused oversedation in two patients.

Electroconvulsive therapy

This treatment has been given in the past for delirium but is highly unlikely to be given nowadays. Nevertheless, an old study based on retrospective chart review suggested that patients receiving ECT together with conventional treatment had a shorter duration of delirium symptoms than those just receiving the treatment without ECT (Dudley & Williams, 1972).

Guidelines

The American Psychiatric Association Practice Guidelines for the Treatment of Patients with Delirium (American Psychiatric Association, 1999) supports the use of antipsychotics as the main pharmacological treatment of choice in delirium. Haloperidol has been identified as the most appropriate and it is suggested that the dosage should be started at 1–2 mg every 2 to 4 hours as needed (with half of this dosage in the elderly) and, when problems become more severe, the

Table 1.1 Evidence base for interventions in delirium

Treatment	Form of treatment	Psychiatric disorder	Level of evidence to test efficacy	Comments
Environmental manipulation of those at risk	Reorientation procedures	Delirium	Ib	One randomized trial gave results supportive of this intervention
Typical antipsychotic drugs	Haloperidol in oral, intramuscular or intravenous form	Delirium of all types including hypoactive delirium	Ib	Effective, but the extrapyramidal and sedative effects may preclude use
	Chlorpromazine			
Atypical antipsychotic drugs	Risperidone	Delirium with or without dementia	Ib	Limited evidence, most favouring risperidone
	Quetiapine		III	
	Remoxipride		III	
Atypical antipsychotic drugs	Olanzapine	Delirium of all types	III	Alleged similar efficacy to haloperidol but studies inadequate to confirm
Benzodiazepines	Lorazepam	Delirium of all types but specifically effective in alcohol withdrawal delirium (see p. 52)	Ib	Probably effective in lower dosage, but adds to cognitive impairment in higher dosage
Benzodiazepines and antipsychotic drugs	Haloperidol and lorazepam	Delirium	III	A favoured combination, but no good evidence in support

Table 1.1 (cont.)

Treatment	Form of treatment	Psychiatric disorder	Level of evidence to test efficacy	Comments
Benzodiazepines and opioids	Diazepam, flunitrazepam, and pethidine	Prevention of postoperative delirium	IIb	Some evidence of efficacy but needs replication
5-HT$_3$ receptor antagonists	Odansetron	Postoperative delirium	III	Only tested in open study
Cholinesterase inhibitors	Donepezil Rivastigmine	Mixed delirium	Ib	Two randomized trials of rivastigmine in delirium, one positive (small trial) and the other negative (large trial)
Tetracyclic antidepressants	Mianserin	Delirium of all types	IIa	May be equivalent in efficacy to haloperidol but limited evidence
Psychostimulants	Methylphenidate	Hypoactive delirium	III	One study (before–after) with limited conclusions
Electroconvulsive therapy (ECT)	Bilateral	Delirium tremens in particular	III	Case reports only

drug can be given by intravenous injection of 10 mg followed by intravenous infusion of up to 5–10 mg per hour. However, this is based on only one case series and has come under criticism (Tauscher et al., 2000).

The National Institute for Health and Clinical Excellence has also developed a guideline for prevention and treatment and the recommendations for prevention of delirium for patients at risk are to 'ensure that people at risk of delirium are cared for by a team of healthcare professionals who are familiar with the person at risk' (National Clinical Guidance Centre for Acute and Chronic Conditions, 2010).

For those diagnosed with delirium the recommendations are to '(i) identify and manage the possible underlying cause or combination of causes and (ii) ensure effective communication and reorientation and provide reassurance for people diagnosed with delirium', with family, friends, and carers when available, who may be able to help with this. If these non-pharmacological approaches are ineffective, the guideline suggests the practitioner should "consider giving short-term (for 1 week or less) haloperidol or olanzapine". This guideline is not fundamentally different from the American one and does not alter the basic recommendations.

Summary

Delirium is an acute psychiatric event and it is understandable that there are few randomized controlled trials comparing forms of treatment, and none which includes placebo control. This complicates interpretation of management but there is a large body of data that supports (i) sensitive environmental adjustment and reorientation (for prevention and initial management) and (ii) pharmacological intervention with antipsychotic drugs (for delirium unresponsive to environmental interventions). The other drugs considered for the treatment of delirium are not to be used without very careful consideration after first-line treatments have failed (Table 1.1).

2

Management of behavioural and psychological symptoms of dementia and acquired brain injury

Based on "Management of behavioural and psychological symptoms of dementia and acquired brain injury" by Joel Sadavoy, Krista L. Lanctôt and Shoumitro Deb in Effective Treatments in Psychiatry, Cambridge University Press, 2008

Introduction

Some might find the title and terminology of this chapter a little unusual, but it comes from the guidelines of the International Psychogeriatric Association (1998, 2002) which brought together this group of symptoms under the heading of Behavioural and Psychological Symptoms in Dementia (BPSD). Although it is not a diagnostic term it is nonetheless useful when it comes to managing individual patients, as it is the symptoms and manifest behaviour that the clinician is called upon to treat irrespective of their diagnostic background. As often these behaviours are acute in presentation, drug treatment is used most frequently in their management.

These disturbances are very common and occur almost always at some point in a long dementing illness. Rubin et al. (1988) describes seven types of these behavioural problems – memory disturbance, physical violence and hitting, incontinence, catastrophic reactions, suspiciousness, and accusatory behaviour. These are clearly disturbing symptoms and can often lead to major problems in hospitals, care homes, and the community. Because the delineation of these symptoms is not ideal and it has only recently been formalized in this way the evidence base for interventions is relatively small. These treatments are discussed first in the setting of dementia and then in acquired brain injury.

Pharmacotherapy for BPSD

Antipsychotic drugs

These are the most commonly used medications for the control of these symptoms. Typical antipsychotic drugs have been evaluated in 17 randomized controlled trials (Lanctôt et al., 1998; De Deyn et al., 1999). When these data have been subject to meta-analysis the drug–placebo difference is small, only amounting to about 20% (Lanctôt et al., 1998).

The atypical antipsychotic drugs, risperidone, olanzapine and quetiapine, have also been used and seven randomized trials reported. There is consistent evidence that the atypical drugs are superior to placebo in relieving symptoms. Of concern is evidence that atypicals in this population of elderly demented patients increase the risk of cerebrovascular adverse events (De Deyn et al., 2005) and mortality (Schneider et al., 1990) compared with placebo, and typical antipsychotic drugs have comparable rates

(Herrmann et al., 2004a). In view of these adverse effects, and those of extrapyramidal side effects with typical antipsychotic drugs, the use of this group of agents should be limited.

Antidepressants

There is some support for using selective serotonin reuptake inhibitors (SSRIs), but not typical antidepressants, in the treatment of BPSD. The benefits of these drugs were similar to those of antipsychotic drugs in one study (e.g. Pollock et al., 2002) and trazodone has also shown some benefit (Sultzer et al., 1997). Buspirone has limited or low effectiveness (Stanislav et al., 1994) and although it became a popular alternative to the benzodiazepines it has never proved to be of great value. Because of the problems of orthostatic hypotension with typical antidepressant drugs these are used less frequently.

Cognitive enhancers

The evidence for efficacy of these drugs in BPSD is somewhat weak. Studies with donepezil, galantanine, rivastigmine, and memantine show small positive effects at most (Cochrane reviews). While apathy may respond to cholinesterase inhibitors, a recent independently funded study showed no evidence of efficacy for agitation (Howard et al., 2007), although memantine may target this symptom (Wilcock et al., 2008).

Anticonvulsants and mood stabilizers

Carbamazepine, valproate, and gabapentin have all been tested in randomized controlled trials against placebo (Tariot et al., 1994; 1998; Lonergan et al., 2004) and showed benefits in reducing aggression and agitation in dementia, although unfortunately these tend to be at higher dosage when adverse effects are more prominent (Tariot et al., 1994; 2001; Moretti et al., 2003). Agitation and aggression are said to be reduced. Unfortunately at the high doses necessary to reduce symptoms there are adverse effects such as thrombocytopaenia (So & Wong, 2002) and sedation and related effects with valproate (Lonergan et al., 2004), which means these drugs cannot really be recommended and should only be used in selected circumstances. Lithium has provided limited open studies of evidence that cannot be used to reach formal conclusions.

Benzodiazepines

While this group of drugs is a natural choice for the treatment of anxiety and agitation because of their common use in general psychiatry, there is little evidence to support their regular use. For rapid effects, intramuscular lorazepam may be given (Meehan et al., 2002). As now is well known, benzodiazepines may cause dependence in regular dosage (Tyrer et al., 1981) and if prolonged treatment is being given it should be withdrawn gradually to avoid withdrawal symptoms (Oude-Voshaar et al., 2006). In this population withdrawal seizures may be a problem and so the importance of gradual taper cannot be over-emphasized.

Beta-blockers

There is some evidence from single randomized controlled trials (Herrmann et al., 2004a; Peskind et al., 2005) that pindolol and propranolol have some benefit in reducing aggression, agitation, and anxiety but this only takes place at higher dosages at which the effects are probably unrelated to direct beta-blockade.

Psychological management of non-cognitive symptoms of dementia

Because pharmacological ways of dealing with agitation, anxiety, and other related symptoms is relatively ineffective there has been growing interest in psychological methods of treatment. Psychodynamic forms of treatment have been used for many years but have never been formally tested in research designs. Reminiscence therapy includes a range of treatments that recall past events and experiences in the demented patient's life and may help them to adjust to the changed setting in which they find themselves. Although these are attractive interventions comprehensive reviews have yielded equivocal results with no clear evidence of efficacy (Pusey, 2000; Spector et al., 2003). When given in group form there is similarly no good evidence of efficacy (Spector et al., 2003).

Group therapies

There is no good evidence that group therapy is effective for this range of symptoms although it is very popular. The most widely used is reality orientation therapy but this is badly defined and a recent review suggests only transient benefits from this approach (Scott & Clare, 2003).

Validation therapy

This is a similar approach to reminiscence therapy which addresses the need for the demented patient to be reminded of their personal identity. Such validation groups include not only reminiscence, but add active support from therapists and activities such as discussion and singing (Morton & Bleathman, 1991). Again, no clear conclusions can be drawn from the relatively poor studies that have been carried out in terms of evaluation.

Other approaches

There is some very limited support for the value of bright light therapy for agitation in dementia, although this seems to alter the timing of behaviour disturbance rather than improve its manifestations (Ancoli-Israel et al., 2003). Improved milieu therapy in residential placements, including staff training plus token economy or stimulation programmes, social and other reinforcers for returning dawdlers, training wandering residents to recognize hazardous areas by visual cues, and linking behaviour to a learnt visual stimulus (such as a large orange disc) that signals acceptable or unacceptable actions, may all be of value (Laundreville et al., 1998).

Pharmacotherapy in the treatment of behaviour disturbance in acquired brain injury

This section presents a systematic review of the research published in the English language on the effectiveness of drugs for the treatment of neurobehavioural disorders in patients with acquired brain injury (ABI), but as the evidence is based mainly on case studies we cannot conclude with any confidence that drugs are effective or ineffective in the treatment of behaviour disorders in patients with acquired brain injury.

Lithium

Although there is no conclusive evidence to support lithium's effectiveness in these disorders, the information elsewhere in this book gives some support to its anti-aggressive action (see Chapter 36). It is however, important to recognize that bipolar affective disorder may manifest as neurobehavioural symptoms in some patients with ABI. As lithium is an effective prophylactic treatment for bipolar affective disorder, it is likely to improve agitation and other behavioural problems in those brain-injured patients who have bipolar disorder. The adverse effects of lithium should be borne in mind and appropriate investigations should be carried out at regular intervals for those who are treated with it.

Antipsychotics

Few studies have examined the effectiveness of antipsychotic drugs in this disorder and the two that have been studied most, thioridazine and droperidol, have now been withdrawn from use. Clozapine may reduce aggression but can lead to epileptic seizures.

Antidepressants

Several small studies suggest that behavioural symptoms can be improved after antidepressants but that improvement in most cases could be interpreted as affective in nature. This is not surprising considering the fact that antidepressants are primarily indicated for the treatment of depression. It is possible that depression and other affective disorders that are not uncommon following TBI (Deb et al., 1999) may be important causes of agitation and aggression. In this context it is worth noting that in clinical practice it is not always easy to differentiate between "abulic", "apathy" and "depressive" symptoms among patients with acquired brain injury.

Psychostimulants

Based on a few controlled trials that included small cohorts, it appears that the evidence is equivocal for the effectiveness of psychostimulants in improving target behaviours in ABI patients. These drugs seem to be particularly effective in treating symptoms such as slowness of behaviour and lack of initiative and attention. There is also some evidence to suggest that these drugs might also be useful in the treatment of anger outbursts. The use of psychostimulants has to be monitored very closely because of the potential

Table 2.1 Evidence base for treatment of behavioural and related symptoms in conjunction with dementia and acquired brain injury

Treatment	Form of treatment	Psychiatric disorder	Level of evidence	Comments
Typical antipsychotic drugs (e.g. haloperidol)	Oral or intramuscular	BPSD	Ia	Large studies showing relative but small superiority over placebo (around 20%) but compromised by extrapyramidal and other adverse effects at higher doses (which are often necessary to show efficacy)
Atypical antipsychotic drugs (e.g. risperidone)	Oral	BSPD	Ia	Generally similar in efficacy to typical antipsychotic drugs with fewer extrapyramidal effects but some evidence of an increase in cerebrovascular complications with twice the mortality rate of placebo
Selective serotonin reuptake inhibitors (SSRIs) (e.g. citalopram)	Oral	BPSD	Ia	Reasonable level of evidence of equivalent efficacy to antipsychotic drugs with citalopram showing strongest evidence, which appears to be largely independent of depressive symptoms
Tricyclic antidepressants (amitriptyline)	Oral	BPSD	IIa	Less evidence than for SSRIs and concern over cardiotoxicity and other adverse effects
Trazodone	Oral	BPSD	Ib	Some evidence of efficacy for aggressive and challenging behaviour
Buspirone	Oral	BPSD	III	Limited evidence of relatively little value
Venlafaxine	Oral	BPSD	III	Open studies but no controlled ones suggesting some value

Table 2.1 (cont.)

Treatment	Form of treatment	Psychiatric disorder	Level of evidence	Comments
Mirtazapine	Oral	BPSD	III	Open studies but no controlled ones suggesting some value
Cholinesterase inhibitors (e.g. rivastigmine)	Oral	BPSD in Alzheimer's disease and Lewy body dementia	Ia	General evidence of efficacy at all stages of dementia, with possibly less evidence in severely advanced cases
Anticonvulsants (e.g. carbamazepine)	Oral	BPSD	Ib	Carmazepine shows best evidence for efficacy, with no adequate evidence for gabapentin and weak support for sodium valproate offset by risk of thrombocytopaenia
Benzodiazepines (e.g. diazepam)	Oral or intramuscular injection	BPSD	Ia	Generally similar, or slightly inferior, in efficacy to antipsychotic drugs with sedating adverse effects
Beta-blocking drugs (e.g. propranolol)	Oral	BPSD	Ib	Some improvement in aggression but only with large doses
Oestrogens	Oral	BPSD	Ib	Some evidence of efficacy from controlled trials
Psychostimulants (e.g. methylphenidate)	Oral	BPSD	IIb	Some limited evidence from small studies
Individual psychotherapy	Individual	BPSD	IV	Strong belief of efficacy in some quarters but no real evidence

			Evidence level	
Reminiscence therapy	Individual or group	BPSD	Ib	One randomized trial showed very slight evidence of efficacy
Group therapy (including reality orientation)	Group	BPSD	Ib	Some evidence from controlled trials of effectiveness but doubts about sustainability
Validation therapy	Group	BPSD	III	No controlled studies but often highly supported by therapists
Light therapy	Individual	BPSD	IIb	Small controlled studies only with uncertain methodology
Walking therapy	Group	BPSD	IIb	May be of value but studies limited
Lithium salts	Oral	Traumatic brain injury	Ib	Of some value but effect size not clear

adverse events associated with their use. In the UK, psychostimulant drugs have only been licensed for the treatment of attention deficit hyperactivity disorder (ADHD) in children (http://www.nice.org.uk). Some patients following ABI may develop symptoms similar to that of ADHD. It is also possible that some children and young adults with ADHD are prone to sustain ABI. However, their diagnosis may remain undetected in adult life. Therefore, it is possible that the psychostimulants may indirectly improve neurobehavioural symptoms by treating the underlying ADHD in these ABI patients.

Anticonvulsants

There is only anecdotal evidence based on case reports that carbamazepine, sodium valproate, divalproex sodium, and lamotrigine can reduce aggressive behaviour and agitation as well as treat symptoms of affective disorder in these patients.

Dopaminergic drugs

Although there are two randomized double-blind, placebo-controlled, crossover trials of dopaminergic drugs (Schneider et al., 1999; Meythaler et al., 2002) these only included 10 and 35 patients, respectively. The first trial showed no difference between amantadine and placebo; the second suggested more rapid functional improvement among patients treated with amantadine than the placebo. This provides equivocal evidence of the effectiveness of psychostimulants in patients with acquired brain injury.

Beta-blockers

There is weak evidence not amounting to anything that could be regarded as a recommendation that beta-blocking drugs in high dosage (e.g. propranolol equivalents of 400–500 mg/day) might have a beneficial effect on agitation.

Conclusion

The treatment of behavioural and psychological symptoms associated with dementia and acquired brain injury is currently in an area where individual clinical skills count as much as the evidence base of treatment which is relatively limited. The summary in Table 2.1 shows no clear leaders in terms of preferred treatment and it is likely that most clinicians would use a judicious mix of several of these at different times. There is an urgent need to carry out more studies with larger numbers in this group of patients, particularly those with acquired brain injury.

3

Dementia: pharmacological and non-pharmacological treatments and guideline review

Based on "Dementia: Pharmacological and non-pharmacological treatments and guideline review" by Martine Simard and Elizabeth L. Sampson in Effective Treatments in Psychiatry, Cambridge University Press, 2008

Introduction

The treatment of dementia, or more accurately, the prevention of the progress of dementia, constitute a very active and important set of interventions that have advanced enormously when one considers that little was available 20 years ago. Both drug and psychological treatments have been tested formally in recent years, but it is the advances in drug treatment, particularly with anticholinesterase inhibitors, that have been the most striking. Many other drug and psychological treatments have been tried also and there is now a growing evidence base.

Acetylcholinesterase (AChE) inhibitors

These drugs increase the concentration of acetylcholine (ACh) available for neurotransmission by inhibiting the main enzymes responsible for its breakdown. Donepezil, rivastigmine, and galantamine are drugs in this group that have all been well tested in randomized controlled trials.

19

Donepezil

Donepezil has been tested in both Alzheimer's disease and vascular dementia and meta-analyses of more than 20 studies have demonstrated benefits over placebo for improvement in cognitive function, behavioural problems, and activities of daily living.

The detailed data are presented in the original chapter in full in *Effective Treatments in Psychiatry* (Cambridge University Press) but in summary 15 and 24 weeks of treatment with donepezil (5 and 10 mg/day) is superior to placebo in arresting cognitive decline (e.g. Rogers et al., 1998a; 1998b) but these benefits disappear after a 6-week placebo washout period (Doody et al., 2001).

Patients who originally received placebo in the double-blind study showed a larger decline in cognitive functioning after 1, 2, and 3 years of donepezil treatment than did those who had taken donepezil from the beginning of the double-blind studies (Doody et al., 2001). Adverse effects, mainly insomnia, nausea, and diarrhoea, were dose-related and generally mild and transient (Rogers et al., 1998a; 1998b; Doody et al., 2001). Other studies have in general confirmed these general findings of a small but significant difference in favour of donepezil (Winblad et al., 2001; 2009; AD2000 Collaborative Group, 2004). Following 2 years of treatment, no benefits were registered with donepezil 5 and 10 mg/day compared with placebo in institutionalization and progression of disability, and also no significant differences were seen between donepezil and placebo in behavioural and psychological symptoms, carer psychopathology, formal care costs, unpaid caregiver time, adverse events or deaths, or between 5 mg and 10 mg donepezil (AD2000 Collaborative Group, 2004).

Rivastigmine

Three randomized controlled trials and several quasi-randomized and open-label studies with rivastigmine in a dose of 3–12 mg daily have also shown significant improvement in cognitive function compared with placebo as well as improvement in activities of daily living. A Cochrane Review analysing data on 3660 participants demonstrated that rivastigmine (6 to 12 mg daily) was associated with a 2.1 point improvement in cognitive function (on the Alzheimer's Disease Assessment scale – Cognitive score) compared with placebo (weighted mean difference −2.09, 95% confidence interval −2.65 to −1.54, on an intention-to-treat basis) and a 2.2 point improvement in activities of daily living assessed on the Progressive Deterioration Scale (weighted mean difference −2.15, 95% confidence interval −3.16 to −1.13, on an intention-to-treat basis) at 26 weeks. These differences represent definite clinical improvement but overall is still modest. There were higher levels of nausea, vomiting, diarrhoea, anorexia, headache, syncope, abdominal pain, and dizziness among patients taking high-dose rivastigmine than among those taking placebo which were statistically significant (Birks et al., 2000).

Memantine

Memantine is not an anticholinesterase inhibitor but acts on the glutamatergic neurotransmitter system that is heavily concerned with memory. Four randomized controlled trials have been carried out with memantine in Alzheimer's disease (AD) and other dementias. For example, the Swedish multicentre 12-week R-DB-PC trial of Winblad et al. (2001) involved 166 patients with severe dementia, later separated clinically between AD (n=79) or vascular dementia (VaD)/mixed dementia (n=87) sub-groups. The patients received either memantine 5 mg/day during the first week and 10 mg/day during the next 11 weeks, or matching placebo tablets. Minimal improvement was found in 52% and much improvement in 21% of patients treated with memantine, compared

with 45% improvement in the patients treated with placebo, and this was irrespective of the type of dementia.

McShane et al. (2006) undertook a Cochrane meta-analysis of the evidence and concluded that memantine was generally well tolerated in patients with Alzheimer's disease, and pooled data in those with moderate to severe dementia indicated a beneficial effect at 6 months on cognition (2.97 points on the 100-point Severe Impairment Battery, 95% CI 1.68 to 4.26, P <0.00001), activities of daily living (ADL) (1.27 points on the 54-point Alzheimer's Disease Cooperative Study-ADLsev, 95% CI 0.44 to 2.09, $P = 0.003$), and behaviour (2.76 points on the Neuropsychiatric Iventory, 95% CI 0.88 to 4.63, $P = 0.004$). These data again indicate some, but only modest, clinical gains from treatment with memantine.

Galantamine

Galantamine has also been well tested in 10 randomized placebo-controlled trials at a dose of 8–16 mg daily. A Cochrane synthesis of the evidence from these trials totalling 6805 subjects demonstrated that treatment with galantamine led to a significantly greater improvement in cognitive performance at all dosing levels with greater effect over 6 months compared to 3 months. For example, the mean treatment gain *t* for 24 mg/ day over 6 months was a 3.1-point reduction in ADAS-Cog. Functional and neuropsychiatric outcomes were reported only in a small proportion of trials; all showed significant treatment effect in some individual trials at least. Galantamine's adverse effects appeared similar to those of other cholinesterase inhibitors and to be dose-related (Loy & Schneider, 2006).

Comparisons between individual drugs

A meta-analysis of pooled data compared the effect of galantamine, rivastigmine, and donepezil on safety (drop-outs due to adverse events) and selected cognitive outcomes: the ADAS-Cog and the Clinician Interview-Based Impression of Change (CIBIC) plus Carer Interview (Ritchie et al., 2004). All three drugs showed greater benefit on ADAS-Cog scores compared to placebo, with a dose-related effect observed for donepezil and rivastigmine of approximately 3 points on the ADAS-Cog. Galantamine showed a similar benefit at all dose levels. Donepezil and galantamine were associated with improvement on the Clinical Global Improvment scale, but in this case the effect was not dose-related, possibly because the scale is relatively insensitive to change. There

was evidence for increased dropout rates with galantamine and rivastigmine compared with donepezil.

Donepezil, rivastigmine, and galantamine have been approved for the treatment of dementia in several countries but memantine only in the United States. Memantine may be similar to the other drugs but there have been many fewer studies of this drug and so the evidence base is not nearly so large. Economic analyses have suggested that while all cholinesterase inhibitors reduce the need for full-time care, only galantamine and donepezil are associated with an overall reduction of costs (Caro et al., 2003). Because of somewhat less value of economic benefit in those with more severe dementia, the NICE guidelines for treatment originally recommended that only those with moderate dementia should be treated with these drugs in the National Health Service; although this decision has not been reversed it has been modified (http:// www.nice.org.uk/CG42) (as of March 2011).

Differences in responses between dementia subtypes

In general the drug effects in patients with vascular dementia and dementia with Lewy bodies are similar to those in patients with Alzheimer's disease. Randomized trials of donepezil

(Malouf & Birks, 2004), rivastigmine (Kumar et al., 2000) (benefit shown most with a high dose of 6–12 mg/day), galantamine (Erkinjuntti et al., 2002), and memantine (Orgogozo et al., 2002) have demonstrated this benefit in vascular dementia and very similar results have been found in dementia with Lewy bodies (McKeith et al., 2000), although there have been very few formal trials on this disorder.

Other treatments

There have been suggestions that vitamin E, an antioxidant, may protect against dementia. A single randomized controlled trial (Sano et al., 1997) compared vitamin E in the form of alpha-tocopherol against selegiline, a combination of both drugs, and placebo in 169 patients with dementia. There was no difference in cognitive function but subsidiary post hoc analyses suggested there might be some benefit in preventing the onset of dementia with vitamin E. There is really insufficient evidence on the basis of this trial to suggest that vitamin E is effective in the treatment of dementia. Selegiline is a monoamine oxidase beta inhibitor that may be of value in dementia because it increases dopamine synthesis but its value is limited despite some evidence of benefits on cognitive function (Birks & Flicker, 2003). Some benefits have

also been claimed for nonsteroidal anti-inflammatory drugs (NSAIDs) such as aspirin and indomethacin but evidence is derived mainly from epidemiological studies (Szekely et al., 2004). The largest randomized controlled trial of rofecoxib, naproxen, and placebo showed no significant difference in cognitive functioning between the active treatments and placebo. In this instance the epidemiological findings are contradicted by the randomized controlled trials and so on current evidence NSAIDs cannot be recommended for the treatment of Alzheimer's disease.

Epidemiological data has suggested that the use of oestrogen and hormone replacement therapy may decrease the risk of developing Alzheimer's disease (relative risk 0.56, 95% CI 0.46 to 0.68) (Hogervorst et al., 2000). However these observational studies and the intervention trials included in the systematic review have been criticized for not controlling for important confounders such as age and education. The most recent evidence from the Women's Health Initiative Memory Study found that oestrogen did not reduce the incidence of dementia and may adversely affect global cognitive function.

Gingko biloba, an interesting tree that is intermediate in phylogenetic development between the flowering plants and the ferns, has been claimed to be of value in dementia. One systematic review of 33 double-blind, placebo-controlled RCTs, few of which used intention-to-treat analysis, showed some benefit (Birks et al., 2002), but a major study since has not confirmed this finding (McCarney et al., 2008), and so the treatment, despite a further positive review (Weinmann et al., 2010) remains controversial.

Psychological treatments (see also Chapter 2)

Cognitive rehabilitation and cognitive training

These treatments have developed from those used in the treatment of acquired brain injury and include individual and group therapeutic approaches. They overlap considerably; cognitive training concentrates on improving cognitive performance whereas cognitive rehabilitation is more individualized and has a wider range of preferred outcomes. A systematic review (Clare et al., 2003) concluded that no observable benefits have been found with either of these approaches. More recently, another review concluded that some of these interventions showed preliminary efficacy, but still require further investigation before they can be prescribed on a current basis for patients with Alzheimer's disease (Grandmaison & Simard, 2003).

Reminiscence therapy

This involves a structured and guided process of reflection on an individual person's life. It usually takes place in groups, sometimes with additional aids such as video material or pictures. This is based on the long-standing evidence that old memories are protected to a much greater extent than recent ones in dementia. The principles of reminiscence therapy are widely used in dementia services but have not been well studied in research. One systematic review (Woods et al., 2005) gives some support for reminiscence therapy improving cognition compared with control treatment but the effect size is small.

Reality orientation therapy

Reality orientation therapy varies from a simple calendar board to a formal teaching approach where patients take part in exercises. The evidence base for this is limited. One systematic review (Spector et al., 2000) of six randomized trials suggested small benefits to those receiving reality orientation therapy but there was considerable overlap between this and other forms of cognitive stimulation and this review was withdrawn in February 2003. At present the benefits of reality orientation therapy in dementia are not strong enough for this treatment to be recommended.

Table 3.1 Summary of evidence base for drug treatments of cognitive deficits in dementia

Treatment	Form of treatment	Type of dementia	Level of evidence for efficacy	Comments
Acetylcholinesterase (AChE) inhibitors (Cholinesterase inhibitors)	Donepezil 5–10 mg	Mild to moderate	Ia	Improvements in cognition demonstrated for first 9–12 months of treatment
	Rivastigmine 6–12 mg	Alzheimer's disease	Ia	Results as for donepezil but possibly longer period of efficacy in published studies
	Galantamine 16–24 mg	Ditto	Ia	As for rivastigmine
N-methyl-D-aspartate antagonists	Memantine	Mild to moderate Alzheimer's	Ia	Similar efficacy to AChEs
AChEs	Donepezil 5–10 mg	Vascular dementia	Ia	Effective at least till 24 weeks
	Rivastigmine 6–12 mg	Ditto	Ia	Effective at least till 24 weeks
	Galantamine 24 mg	Ditto	Ia	Probably effective until 1 year
N-methyl-D-aspartate antagonists	Memantine 20 mg	Vascular dementia	Ia	Effective until at least 9 months
AChEs	Donepezil 5–10 mg	Full range of severity of Lewy body dementia	Ib	Effective up to one year
	Rivastigmine 6–12 mg		Ib	Effective up to 6 months
	Galantamine 24 mg		III	May specifically improve behaviour

Table 3.1 (cont.)

Treatment	Form of treatment	Type of dementia	Level of evidence for efficacy	Comments
Vitamin E	Alpha-tocopherol (2000 IU daily)	Alzheimer's disease	Ib	Little change in cognition but delay in death, severity of dementia, and daily living
Oestrogen		Alzheimer's disease	Ib	No evidence of value
Gingko biloba	Leaf extract	Alzheimer's disease	Ib	No clear evidence of efficacy in large trials
Monoamine oxidase B inhibitor	Selegiline 10 mg	Alzheimer's disease	Ib	Small but significant improvement at 4 months – needs confirmation

Summary

Guidelines in the UK, US, and Canada all agree that donepezil, galantamine, and rivastigmine are beneficial for improving cognitive function in all forms of dementia but memantine is given only qualified approval (American Psychiatric Association (APA), 1997). In the UK, the long-standing guidance from NICE, first published in 2004, recommended that only moderate or severe dementia could be treated cost-effectively with donepezil, galantamine, and rivastigmine, with memantine not given approval except in trial situations, but in October 2010 this decision was reviewed and it is likely that cholinesterase inhibitors will be prescribed in the NHS for mild dementia also.

We therefore have a strong evidence base (Table 3.1) for many treatments of dementia, but we must remember that the effect sizes of treatments are small and there is much more to be done.

4

Pharmacological treatment of psychosis and depression in the elderly

Based on "Pharmacological treatment of psychosis and depression in older adults" by Mark Rapoport, Cara Brown and Craig Ritchie in Effective Treatments in Psychiatry, Cambridge University Press, 2008

Introduction

The delusions and hallucinations which represent the most abnormal manifestations of neurological disorder strike everyone as odd as they are out of keeping with the patient's normal behaviour. Predictably treatment of these disorders is mainly with antipsychotic drugs but the evidence for their effectiveness in this population is limited and it must be kept in mind that drug treatment should be reserved for the treatment of psychosis that is disruptive to patients' functioning, and/or causing distress to patients and/or caregivers, not of symptoms alone. Most of the evidence available has been obtained in patients with Alzheimer's and Parkinson's Disease. Depression is also discussed in this chapter as it is a very common accompaniment to all forms of dementia and Parkinson's disease. It is protean in its manifestations and often missed in practice, and is important because it is potentially treatable.

Treating psychosis in dementia

The prevalence of psychosis in Alzheimer's disease (AD) has been estimated to be as high as 34% in clinic populations and between 7% and 20% in the community (Schneider & Dagerman, 2004), and antipsychotic drugs are given to approximately one in four patients in nursing homes with dementia within a year of arrival (Bronskill et al., 2004).

Typical antipsychotic drugs are demonstrably effective in the treatment of psychosis and related disruptive behaviours but the effect size is small (Schneider et al., 1990). The use of these drugs is compromised by the relatively high incidence of tardive dyskinesia in this population with 23%–60% developing this syndrome after 3 years of treatment (Jeste et al., 1995; Caligiuri et al., 2000), as tardive dyskinesia is generally more common in older people.

Two studies have investigated the impact of discontinuation of antipsychotics in patients with dementia on chronic typical antipsychotics whose behavioural disturbance was well controlled. One group of 34 patients with dementia in long-term care were randomized to either continue with their antipsychotics or to have them discontinued for a 6-month study period (van Reekum et al., 2002). The primary finding was that the group whose antipsychotics were continued had more behavioural disturbances than those in the discontinuation group. A similar study was conducted in 82 patients with AD in long-term care (Ballard et al., 2004). It was found that the baseline level of behavioural disturbances predicted outcome depending on the treatment received. In particular, those with low levels of baseline neurobehavioural disturbance had a better outcome if switched to placebo, whereas patients with a higher level of disturbance at baseline had significant problems when their antipsychotics were discontinued. Reassessment and discontinuation after a period of behavioural stability is suggested (Herrmann & Lanctôt, 2007).

Although atypical antipsychotic drugs have become much more popular in this population, and the trials have been much larger, the same findings are found as with typical antipsychotic drugs (De Deyn et al., 1999). Most comparisons of these drugs have been against placebo, where both risperidone (Brodaty et al., 2003) and olanzapine (Street et al., 2000) show clear but modest positive effects in favour of the active drug. In these studies olanzapine and risperidone were basically similar in efficacy (Fontaine et al., 2003; Gareri et al., 2004). A major concern with these studies is the higher incidence of cerebrovascular accidents and mortality with atypical antipsychotics compared with placebo (Herrmann & Lanctôt, 2006).

Of interest, a recent retrospective epidemiological study found that olanzapine and risperidone were not associated with an increased risk of stroke compared to typical antipsychotics among patients 65 and over (Herrmann et al., 2004b). Given the increased risk of extrapyramidal symptoms, cerebrovascular events, and mortality with typicals, the best evidence is for atypicals to be given in low doses when psychosis is severe or potentially harmful (Hermann et al., 2004).

Cholinesterase inhibitors, normally used for the treatment of cognitive impairment in Alzheimer's disease, have also been used for the treatment of behaviour disturbance in these patients, but in one large trial no benefit of donepezil was found compared with placebo (Howard et al., 2007), and most of these trials have not selected for patients with behavioural disturbance. There is also no good evidence that anticonvulsants are effective in the treatment of psychosis in dementia. Antidepressants may have a place. A recent randomized controlled trial for hospitalized patients with psychosis and/or behavioural disturbances in the context of dementia showed citalopram, but not perphenazine, to be associated with significantly greater improvement in psychosis and other disturbances than placebo (Pollock et al., 2002).

Treating psychosis in Parkinson's disease

Psychotic symptoms are common in Parkinson's disease (PD), occurring in one in six patients in the community (Aarsland et al., 1999). Unfortunately, psychotic symptoms are a well-recognized complication of the dopaminergic drugs used for the treatment of parkinsonism, particularly levodopa, but are much less common in drugs such as amantadine and selegiline. As typical antipsychotic drugs also induce Parkinsonism these are generally avoided.

Clozapine has also been found to be effective in at least two randomized placebo-controlled trials for the treatment of psychosis in PD without worsening of motor symptoms (Parkinson Study Group, 1999; Pollak et al., 2004). These trials each had 60 patients and used a dosage of less than 50 mg/day. Open-label extensions of these studies for 12 weeks showed that the improvement was sustained but disappeared when the drug was stopped (Pollak et al., 2004). Somnolence is common, and while agranulocytosis is rare, these adverse effects warrant careful clinical attention especially in treating older patients with Parkinson's disease. Clozapine also has a tendency to lower the seizure threshold. The somnolence and necessity of frequent labwork associated with clozapine often lead clinicians to consider the newer antipsychotics first. However, a careful trial of clozapine should be considered in patients with distressing symptoms of psychosis, particularly given the concerns about the newer agents discussed below.

Quetiapine has been used fairly widely in the treatment of Parkinson's disease for patients with psychosis and seems to be tolerated well but there are few randomized trials of its efficacy in this population, with mixed results, with generally negative conclusions (Kurlan et al., 2007; Rabey et al., 2007; Friedman, 2010).

Given the existing evidence, it is difficult to make firm recommendations on pharmacological treatment of psychosis in Parkinson's disease. Informed consent and monitoring of adverse effects is clearly warranted. Typical antipsychotics almost uniformly increase extrapyramidal and related symptoms, there is little supportive data with quetiapine, many reports of increased symptoms with olanzapine, and inconsistent reports of increased symptoms with risperidone. At present, the bulk of the evidence for efficacy rests with clozapine, although careful monitoring of sedation and hematological indices is warranted. Clinicians using other atypicals should be advised to use low doses and monitor extrapyramidal symptoms carefully, and work in close conjunction with the neurological treatment team, as doses of dopaminergic agents may need to be adjusted.

Treatment of depression

Dementia

Although depression is common in dementia, following stroke, and in Parkinson's disease, it is often missed against the background of neurological impairment. The classification of BPSD (behavioural and psychological symptoms of dementia) arose as an attempt to understand both the aetiology and management of behavioural and psychological symptoms in the context of dementia. One such symptom is depression. The array and timing of BPSD symptoms varies greatly between individuals with the same subtype of dementia, between subtypes, and even within individuals during the course of their illness. There is no typical picture of BPSD symptoms in Alzheimer's disease – nor is there any characteristic presentation of depression. However, it is generally considered that depression developing in milder illness presents in a similar fashion to that observed in non-demented individuals, whereas in more severe dementia, the presentation of depression is characterized by predominantly behavioural problems, for example aggression. It is important to recognize clinically that challenging behaviours may be secondary to lowered mood so that appropriate treatment can be instigated. Much of the evidence suggests that antidepressants are helpful in these conditions. In Alzheimer's disease there is conflicting evidence of the benefits of sertraline compared with placebo with both early positive (Lyketsos et al., 2003) and more recent negative (Rosenberg et al., 2010) findings, and some slight evidence that the typical antidepressants are less effective in this condition because of greater rates of dropout (Taragano et al., 1997). There still have been no good studies of antidepressants in vascular dementia or Lewy body dementia even though this is recognized now to be an important source of affective symptoms (McKeith et al., 2006).

Depression following stroke

Between 20% and 40% of patients develop depression at some point after having strokes (Vataja et al., 2002) and again this may fail to be recognized by clinicians who are concentrating on the neurological deficits. There are different models which explain the frequently observed association between depression and stroke. Firstly, depression may precede and be a risk factor for stroke. Secondly, depression may be a symptom of stroke due to the area and extent of cortical damage. Thirdly, depression may occur as an affective response to the physical sequelae of stroke and finally, the two conditions (both being reasonably common in late life) may co-exist in the same individual entirely through chance (Stewart, 2002).

There is good evidence that citalopram and fluoxetine improve post-stroke depression (Andersen et al., 1994; Fruehwald et al., 2003) and also some lesser evidence that antidepressants given after the development of a stroke may improve outcome both of depression and stroke recovery (Dam et al., 1996). These early studies have not been complimented by more recent, larger or longer duration studies. There is also some evidence that antidepressants reduce mortality long after the discontinuation of therapy.

Although depression is common in Parkinson's disease the effect of antidepressants is equivocal and a recent Cochrane Review (Ghazi-Noori et al., 2003) showed no clear evidence of benefit of antidepressants. However, the three trials included in this review only included one placebo-controlled trial. More recent work suggests that the dopaminergic drug, pramipexole, improves mood in patients with Parkinson's disease and depression (Bxarone et al., 2010) and there may

Table 4.1 Summary of evidence base for treatments of psychosis in dementia, Parkinson's disease, and traumatic brain injury

Treatment	Form of treatment	Psychiatric disorder	Level of evidence for efficacy	Comments
Typical antipsychotic drugs (initiation)	Haloperidol or equivalent	Psychosis in dementia	Ia	Lower dosage needed initially than for younger patients; high risk of extrapyramidal symptoms
Typical antipsychotic drugs (discontinuation)	Haloperidol or equivalent	Psychosis in dementia	Ib	Worse outcome in those with high baseline disturbance on drug withdrawal
Atypical antipsychotic drugs	Risperidone	Psychosis in dementia, also with concomitant aggression	Ib	1–2 mg/daily was effective, worse EPS with 2 mg daily. Risk factor: risk of stroke and mortality
Atypical antipsychotic drugs	Olanzapine	Psychosis in dementia	Ib	2.5–10 mg/day effective, 15 mg ineffective. Risk factor: risk of stroke and mortality
Atypical antipsychotic drugs	Quetiapine	Psychosis in dementia	III	Small studies only
Acetylcholinesterase inhibitors (AChEI)	Rivastigmine, donepezil metrifonate	Behavioural symptoms in dementia	III	Some evidence of effectiveness but few trials
Selective serotonin reuptake inhibitors (SSRIs)	Citalopram	Psychosis in dementia	IIa	Greater efficacy of citalopram than perphenazine but mechanism unclear

Table 4.1 (cont.)

Treatment	Form of treatment	Psychiatric disorder	Level of evidence for efficacy	Comments
Atypical antipsychotics	Clozapine	Psychosis in Parkinson's disease	Ib	Good response but careful blood monitoring needed
Atypical antipsychotics	Risperidone/ olanzapine	Psychosis in Parkinson's disease	Ib	Motor side effects may preclude continued treatment except in Lewy body dementia
Atypical antipsychotics	Quetiapine	Psychosis in Parkinson's disease	III	Few controlled studies, mixed results but motor symptoms not worsened
Antidepressants	Citalopram, fluoxetine	Depression following stroke	Ib	Evidence of effectiveness seems good but is uncertain as few independent studies
Traumatic brain injury	Atypical antipsychotics	Psychosis in traumatic brain injury	IV	Little evidence of treatment indications

be particular benefit from traditional tricyclic antidepressants (nortriptyline) compared to SSRIs (paroxetine) (Menza et al., 2009).

Conclusions

The evidence suggests that drug treatment for psychotic symptoms and depression in the elderly with comorbid neurological disorders is generally less effective than in that in younger people or those who do not have neurological disease, mainly because the risks are greater and the benefits less (Table 4.1). The most positive aspect of treatment is the benefit of antidepressants in stroke but longer-term follow-up studies are needed to confirm this.

Alcohol

Alcohol

5

Psychological treatments of alcohol use disorders

Based on "Psychological treatments of alcohol use disorders" by Deirdre Conroy, Kirk J. Brower, Jane Marshall and Mike Crawford in Effective Treatments in Psychiatry, Cambridge University Press, 2008

Introduction

Treatment for alcohol dependence is usually composed of three phases: management of the alcohol withdrawal syndrome, motivation for and initiation of abstinence, and prevention of relapse. Both pharmacological and psychosocial interventions are used in the prevention of relapse, either separately or in combination. These interventions do not operate in a clinical vacuum, and their effectiveness is associated with a number of variables including premorbid client/patient characteristics,

severity of alcohol dependence, therapist characteristics, and the process of treatment delivery. Treatment outcomes are likely to be different in different countries. For instance, European outcomes have historically been less favourable than outcomes in the USA. Although severe alcohol problems are chronic and intermittent, randomized studies have not been designed to study long-term treatment perspectives. Most studies assess treatment interventions between 1 and 3 months' duration with 1-year follow-up.

Summary of details

This chapter will summarize psychological treatments. Psychological treatments include psychosocial and behavioural treatments and involve a professional relationship between a therapist and a patient who work together to accomplish specific improvements in behaviour, thinking, mood regulation, and self-esteem. These treatments constitute the primary professional interventions for alcohol dependence, whereas pharmacotherapy and other interventions are generally thought of as adjunctive to psychological treatment. Treatment goals that include sobriety or moderate drinking depend on a thorough assessment of the patient's drinking history and severity of problems, drinking diagnosis (abuse vs. dependence), co-occurring medical and psychiatric disorders, readiness to change, and psychosocial stressors and supports. Screening for and assessment of at risk drinking, alcohol abuse, and alcohol dependence should be an essential part of standard health care in all relevant clinical settings.

The behavioural and psychosocial interventions are essentially "talking therapies", based on conceptual models of addiction which can be delivered on a one-to-one basis, in a group setting, or as part of a couple/ family therapy approach. Elements of effective treatments are aimed at building motivation, enabling behavioural change and modifying the social context. It can sometimes be difficult to distinguish between some of these interventions, so it is important for definitions of treatments as well as the severity of the alcohol use disorder in the target group to be defined clearly both in systematic reviews and meta-analyses.

Brief interventions

Overall the evidence indicates that **screening and brief interventions** (SBI) are effective in reducing excessive alcohol consumption to safer levels (Moyer et al., 2002). **Brief interventions** (BIs) are designed to be conducted by health professionals who typically do not specialize in addiction treatment such as in general medical and other primary care settings. BIs generally consist of four or fewer visits that range from a few minutes to an hour in duration. BIs are used to prevent alcohol-related problems in heavy drinkers at risk of developing those problems and for acute intervention for patients with established alcohol use disorders. The goals vary from moderate drinking to abstinence. For patients with moderate to severe alcohol problems or dependence, the goals are abstinence and acceptance of an addiction specialty referral when indicated (Graham & Fleming, 1998). BIs may differ in intensity from a single 5-minute session of simple advice to stop drinking to multiple sessions lasting up to 60 minutes each. BIs also differ in terms of the therapeutic techniques utilized and can include motivational interviewing. A number of published articles and manuals on techniques have been developed to guide clinicians at providing BIs (US DHHS, 2003). In the USA, insurance companies do not usually reimburse for BIs.

The content of brief interventions for alcohol misuse varies but generally includes features incorporated in the acronym "FRAMES": Feedback about the adverse effects of alcohol, an emphasis on personal Responsibility for changing drinking behaviour, Advice about reducing or abstaining from alcohol consumption, a Menu of options for further help to meet treatment goals, an Empathic stance towards the patient, and an emphasis on Self-efficacy (Miller & Sanchez, 1993).

Reviews and meta-analyses (Wilk et al., 1997; Miller & Wilbourne, 2002; Moyer et al., 2002; Vasilaki et al., 2006) reveal that BIs are better than no treatment and are cost-effective (Fleming et al., 2002). Some studies suggest that the effect of brief intervention can be sustained over time, but this appears to be somewhat dependent upon regular follow-up. There is strong evidence for its effectiveness in primary care settings and less evidence in general hospital and emergency room settings, trauma settings, and obstetric clinics.

Motivational enhancement therapy (MET)

MET is based upon motivational interviewing (MI) (Miller & Rollnick, 1991). In MET, the clinician seeks to create a non-judgemental and respectful atmosphere while employing persuasive strategies for motivating patients to change their (drinking) behaviours. It is often applied to people with high levels of anger or resistance to treatment. It differs from behavioural therapies which prescribe how the patient should make changes by teaching new skills and reinforcing recovery-sustaining behaviours. Instead, MET encourages patients to utilize their own skills and resources for change. Once the patient has expressed motivation for change, set an appropriate goal for change (such as abstinence), and formulated a plan for making that change, the major work of MET is completed. MET leaves the patient with the responsibility to effect his or her own change. It was found to be effective in 12 of 17 studies (Miller & Wilbourne, 2002). Project MATCH outcome for MET was equivalent to outcome for

CBT or twelve-step facilitation therapy (TSF) (Project MATCH Research Group, 1997). For patients with good prognosis, MET is more cost-effective than CBT or TSF (Holder et al., 2000). MET appears equally effective in either individual or group format (John et al., 2003). Burke and colleagues' (2003) meta-analysis of 15 trials of MET revealed that those receiving MET reduced drinking by an average of 20 drinks per week (effect size 0.82).

Cognitive behavioural therapy (CBT)

CBT constitutes a group of therapies based on social learning theory that has been given various names depending on the investigators who developed them and differences in emphasis. They include relapse prevention strategies, coping skills therapy, social skills training, cognitive behavioural coping-skills training, and communication skills training. It is employed both for abstinence-based treatment of alcohol dependence and for moderation-based treatment to reduce alcohol consumption and related problems such as harm reduction (Marlatt & Witkiewitz, 2002). The focus of CBT is to identify and improve any deficits in skills or maladaptive thoughts that the patient may have which could lead to a lapse to drinking. It teaches people who misuse alcohol to focus on improving problem solving and avoiding "alcohol cues" which lead to resumption of drinking following abstinence periods (Morgenstern & Longabaugh, 2000). Patients are encouraged to learn new behaviours and thought patterns that will help them cope with stress and problems other than by relying on alcohol. There are a number of CBT manuals (Monti et al., 1989; Kadden et al., 1994). It is used extensively in both the USA and the UK, especially in relapse prevention group therapy.

Several comprehensive reviews support the efficacy of CBT for treating alcohol use disorders (Holder et al., 1991; Irvin et al., 1999). It is effective in individual and group formats, in inpatient as well as outpatient settings, and is effective when compared with other active treatments. Irvin at al. (1999) calculated an effect size of 0.37 based on 10 studies. It may be better than other forms of treatment when a rapid reduction in consumption is needed, for those with low levels of anger, and aftercare patients with low levels of dependence. Low levels of psychiatric severity weaken the effectiveness of CBT when compared with twelve-step facilitation therapy (TSF). Cognitive therapy alone does not appear as effective as CBT. There is little evidence that variants of CBT are superior to one another or to other active treatments such as TSF,

MET, or interactional therapy. But there is good evidence in many studies that CBT effectively increases coping skills, and this is linked to better outcome.

Twelve-step facilitation therapy (TSF)

TSF is designed to familiarize patients with, and to encourage attendance at, twelve-step meetings, especially Alcoholics Anonymous (AA) (Nowinski et al., 1994). TSF differs from AA in that TSF is a professionally delivered treatment designed mostly to introduce the patient to AA concepts and facilitate attendance at AA meetings, but it does not re-create the structure or strategies of AA itself. The evidence base for AA *per se* is reviewed in Chapter 8 in this volume. TSF is not viewed as a complex therapy because it does not employ multiple components and strategies to target a large number of different problem areas associated with alcoholism. The evidence for TSF efficacy, therefore, focuses both on attendance at AA as well as drinking behaviours. It is based upon a disease model of alcohol dependence, that it is not the patient's fault that she/he developed alcoholism and that she/he is powerless over alcohol; nonetheless it is the patient's responsibility to take an active role in recovery, and this implies participation in twelve-step groups. It is the most common specialized treatment for alcoholism in the USA. It has been found effective in extending time to relapse and abstinence for the post-treatment year (Ouimette et al., 1997; Project MATCH, 1997).

Behavioural therapies (BT)

BT are therapies that emphasize positive reinforcement and these have been shown to be effective (Holder et al., 1991). Two major types of behavioural treatments are **contingency management** (CM) and **cue exposure therapy** (CET). CM is based on operant conditioning theory, and while there is evidence for its effectiveness, very few controlled studies have been done (Kadden & Conney, 2005). CET has more evidence than CM, but there are issues related to the types and frequency of cues given.

Behavioural couples therapy (BCT), **behavioural marital therapy** (BMT), **and other family-based interventions** (FBI) refer to treatment approaches that include the partner or spouse of the patient in the therapy. It has roots in both social learning theory and family system models and combines efforts to develop better self-control with the spouse's support of their partner's efforts to reduce alcohol consumption. Overall, studies of BCT/BMT have found reduced alcohol consumption and partner violence,

Table 5.1 Effectiveness of psychological treatments of alcohol use disorders

Treatment	Form of treatment	Psychiatric disorder/ target audience	Level of evidence for efficacy	Comments
Brief interventions	Various very short psychosocial interventions	Mild to moderate alcohol misuse	Ia	Decreases alcohol consumption and alcohol-related problems such as injuries and drunk driving
Motivational enhancement therapy (MET)	Specific psychosocial intervention to increase motivation and includes motivational interviewing	Alcohol dependence	Ia	Decreases alcohol consumption and days of heavy consumption. Increases attendance at treatment programmes, especially in people with high levels of anger
Cognitive behavioural therapy	Includes many different types of CBT	Alcohol dependence	Ia	Decreases alcohol consumption and increases harm avoidance. Can be delivered as individual or group treatment. There are many different types of CBT but there may be different impact with different subtypes of patients depending upon global psychopathology, sociopathy, psychiatric severity, and anger
Twelve-step facilitation therapy (TSF)	Includes but not limited to Alcoholics Anonymous	Alcohol dependence	Ia	Project MATCH. Most likely to lead to abstinence first year post treatment. Increases time to first relapse. Increased abstinence at 1 and 3 years.

Behaviour therapy	Includes contingency management and cue exposure therapy	Alcohol dependence	IIb	Decreases daily drinking including number of heavy drinking days, drinks per day, and overall frequency of drinking
Behaviour couples/ behaviour marital therapy	Various types of these treatments	Alcohol dependence	Ib	Improves drinking outcome. Decreases domestic violence and verbal abuse. Increases marital functioning. Increases retention in treatment
Family-based interventions	Various types of these treatments	Alcohol dependence	Ib	Probably need long-term treatment to be effective to prevent relapse. Increases motivation for treatment and level of engagement over time. Decreases drinking
Network therapy	Involves significant others	Alcohol dependence	Ib	Reduction in overall alcohol consumption
Interactional group therapy	Group therapy	Alcohol dependence	IIb	Comparable to CBT
Psychodynamic psychotherapy	Individual psychotherapy	Alcohol dependence	IV	No evidence for effectiveness

and improved marital functioning and treatment retention (McCrady et al., 1999; Miller & Wilbourne, 2002). BMT has also been shown to be more cost-effective than individual therapy for reducing substance use, reducing legal, family and social problems, and for sustaining abstinence.

Reviews of **family-based interventions** (FBI) have concluded that family involvement and interventions are effective treatments for alcohol use disorders (Health Technology Board for Scotland, 2002; Liddle, 2004) and for engaging unwilling patients to seek treatment or reduce drinking (Barber & Gilbertson, 1997). **Network therapy** involves both patients and friends in the treatment with people in the network becoming part of the treatment team. In the UK, a similar therapy is known as **social**

behaviour and network therapy. Both have been shown to improve drinking outcome.

Interactional group therapy is longer-term (12 months) and focuses on real-time communications and interactions among group members (Brown & Yalom, 1977). There is some evidence that this is comparable to CBT group therapy.

Psychodynamic psychotherapy is based on the idea that alcohol use is a form of self-medication to alleviate anxiety and emotional distress. It is widely practised in the USA, primarily by therapists who do not specialize in the treatment of alcohol. There is no evidence for this treatment because the appropriate studies have not been performed (Holder et al., 1991). Interventions discussed in this chapter are summarized in Table 5.1.

6

Pharmacotherapy of alcohol misuse, dependence, and withdrawal

Based on "Pharmacotherapy of alcohol misuse, dependence, and withdrawal"
by George A. Kenna, Kostas Agath and Robert Swift in Effective Treatments in
Psychiatry, Cambridge University Press, 2008

Introduction

This chapter summarizes the evidence base of the pharmacotherapy of alcohol misuse, dependence, and withdrawal. It uses the terms "harmful use of alcohol", "alcohol dependence", and "alcohol withdrawal", which reflect relevant diagnostic categories from the ICD-10.

Harmful use of alcohol

Harmful use of alcohol, an ICD-10 diagnosis, refers to physical and/or mental damage due to a pattern of alcohol use in the absence of a diagnosis of another specific form of alcohol disorder (such as dependence). It has no direct DSM-IV equivalent. The diagnosis depends upon accurate reporting of alcohol-related physical or mental health problems. Harmful alcohol use (problem drinking) is believed to play a role in behavioural patterns associated with amounts of alcohol use considered hazardous leading to decreased worker productivity, increased unintentional injuries, aggression and violence against others, and child and spouse abuse. An individual may periodically abuse alcohol at harmful levels but may yet not be alcohol-dependent.

47

There is no firm quantitative definition for harmful alcohol use in the US. Risk of occupational injuries increases with the frequency of five or more drinks per occasion (one standard drink in the US: 12 ounces of beer, 5 ounces of wine, or 1.5 ounces of 80-proof spirits; National Institute on Alcohol Abuse and Alcoholism (NIAAA), 2000a) with a more than fivefold increase in risk (Zwerling et al.,1996) compared to people who drink one or two drinks. Heavy drinking is alcohol consumption exceeding 14 drinks per week for men (or more than four drinks per drinking occasion), more than seven drinks per week for women (or more than three drinks per occasion), and greater than seven drinks per week for all adults 65 years and older (NIAAA, 2000a). Heavy alcohol use has also been defined as drinking five or more drinks at the same time on at least five separate occasions during the previous month.

In the UK no official guidelines exist for the pharmacological treatment of harmful alcohol use. Appropriate pharmacological treatment depends upon the health problem related to the harmful use. The use of naltrexone (NTX) for non-dependent problem drinkers is limited. While NTX was better than placebo in reducing heavy drinking frequency, it did not significantly reduce number of drinking days. Other studies do not support NTX's effectiveness though some studies report fewer drinking days, fewer heavy drinking days, and less craving (Rubio et al., 2002). At present, there is insufficient evidence to support daily or targeted use of NTX for harmful alcohol use.

Alcohol dependence

The pharmacological treatments of alcohol dependence focus on relapse prevention once detoxification is complete. They are used adjunctive to psychosocial treatments (Slattery et al., 2003; Lingford-Hughes et al., 2004).

Disulfiram

Despite some inconsistency in findings, there is consensus that oral disulfiram reduces the number of drinking days (Garbutt et al., 1999), and supervision of compliance with disulfiram leads to a better outcome (Slattery et al., 2003). Disulfiram treatment is usually initiated after psychosocial treatment has failed.

Disulfiram reinforces an individual's desire to stop drinking by providing a disincentive associated with an increase in acetaldehyde resulting in palpitations, hypotension, flushing, nausea, and vomiting when patients consume alcohol. The primary issue predicting success with disulfiram is that candidates must be committed to total abstinence from alcohol. It is often used for special high-risk situations (e.g. weddings, graduations). Unfortunately, because of unblinding due to the drug's intended action, good double-blind RCTs proving effectiveness remain lacking.

Acamprosate (ACAM)

Based on European results, Garbutt et al. (1999) concluded that the proof for efficacy of acamprosate (ACAM) was strong. A series of meta-analyses and systematic reviews demonstrated that when used adjunctive to psychosocial interventions, ACAM improves drinking outcomes such as the length and rate of abstinence (Miller & Wilbourne, 2002; Slattery et al., 2003; Mann et al., 2003). This effect is doubtful if ACAM is not initiated quickly after detoxification (Chick et al., 2000). There is evidence that the effect of ACAM on abstinence lasts up to 1 year after treatment is stopped but has no effect on non-drinking days (Whitworth et al., 1996). The addition of NTX to ACAM compared to placebo enhances outcome (Kiefer et al., 2003). Though ACAM was approved for use in the US, its success seems limited to European trials as recent US trials failed to demonstrate significance for

primary outcome measures (Anton et al., 2006; Mason et al., 2006). While there have been negative studies reported, most studies suggest that ACAM is safe and well tolerated for the promotion of alcohol abstinence.

ACAM appears especially useful for a therapeutic regimen targeted at promoting abstinence. There are few contraindications for treatment. There is little consistent information about patient characteristics that predict improvement while taking ACAM. Candidates for ACAM should be committed to abstinence and begin the medication after being abstinent from alcohol (Mason et al., 2006).

The crucial issue surrounding ACAM use is delineating the most specific alcohol subtype it should be used for. Results from the COMBINE (The Combined Pharmacotherapies and Behavioural Interventions) study suggest that it has no significant effect on drinking versus placebo, either by itself or with any combination of the other treatments in the study. Despite the negative results for ACAM in COMBINE, a randomized controlled study of 160 patients found that combining NTX and ACAM was more effective than either placebo or ACAM alone, but was not significantly more effective than NTX alone (Kiefer et al., 2003).

Acamprosate is approved by the US Food and Drug Administration (FDA) for maintenance of abstinence in alcohol-dependent individuals who are abstinent at treatment initiation. A meta-analysis showed a significant effect of ACAM to improve the abstinence rate and treatment retention compared to placebo (Bouza et al., 2004).

Naltrexone (NTX)

Evidence supports the use of NTX as an adjunct to psychosocial interventions (Miller & Wilbourne, 2002; Slattery et al., 2003; Anton et al., 2006), with higher abstinence rates in short-term treatment (Srisurapanont & Jarusuraisin, 2003) and as a deterrent to progressing from a lapse to a full-blown relapse (Garbutt et al., 1999). NTX is as efficacious as disulfiram and probably more efficacious than ACAM (Kranzler & Van Kirk, 2001; Kranzler et al., 2003; Srisurapanont & Jarusuraisin, 2003). The addition of ACAM to NTX does not enhance outcome (Kiefer et al., 2003).

Studies indicate that NTX is most effective in patients with strong craving, poor cognitive status at study entry, and high compliance (Volpicelli et al., 1997). A systematic review of all data published up to 1997 concluded that NTX produced a consistent decrease in relapse rate to heavy drinking and in drinking frequency, though it did not enhance absolute abstinence rates (Garbutt et al., 1999). NTX reduces craving. The COMBINE study supports the effectiveness of NTX in that each of the groups of patients receiving NTX in conjunction with medical management (MM) had a higher percentage of days abstinent than those receiving placebo+MM without NTX or a combined behavioural intervention. NTX also reduced the risk of heavy drinking and has been approved for use in the first 90 days of abstinence when the risk of relapse is highest. Naltrexone injection appears to be significantly more effective in those who are abstinent when starting treatment, and in men (Garbutt et al., 2005).

Antidepressants

The SSRIs and other antidepressants seem not to be effective solely for alcohol dependence treatment (Garbutt et al., 1999; Miller & Wilbourne, 2002). In the presence of depression, however, SSRIs could improve mood (but not drinking outcome) when treating alcohol dependence (Lingford-Hughes et al., 2004).

Anticonvulsants

Though more commonly used to treat alcohol withdrawal, some anticonvulsants have also been shown to reduce alcohol use (see Leggio et al.,

2008 for a review). Carbamazepine is reported to reduce alcohol consumption in alcohol-dependent subjects; there is similar data for divalproex. More data exist for topiramate which is reported to significantly reduce the number of drinks per day and drinks per drinking day, and results in significantly fewer drinking days, more days of abstinence, and less craving than placebo.

Buspirone

Three studies reported a positive effect on reducing drinking or craving though data are contradictory. It appears most useful with comorbid anxiety disorder.

Alcohol withdrawal

Introduction

For many alcohol-dependent individuals with significant physical dependence, a cluster of withdrawal symptoms known as "alcohol withdrawal syndrome" (AWS) may occur upon cessation or reduction of alcohol consumption or after reaching a level of such significant tolerance that some individuals cannot consume enough alcohol to delay withdrawal. Depending directly on the degree of physical dependence, this syndrome can range from creating significant discomfort to mild tremor to alcohol withdrawal-related delirium (AWD), hallucinosis, seizures, and potentially death (Bayard et al., 2004). Though most alcohol-dependent persons do not fit the stereotypical image of an alcoholic, individuals who are nutritionally compromised, dehydrated, or have other organ deficiencies are at more risk for withdrawal. Repeated withdrawal episodes may contribute to the development of alcohol dependence and to negative consequences associated with excessive alcohol consumption. Predictors for AWS complications include duration of alcohol consumption, total number of prior detoxifications from alcohol, and previous withdrawal-related seizures and episodes of AWD (Asplund et al., 2004). The incidence of seizures in alcohol-dependent individuals waiting for detoxification ranges from 1% to 15% (Chan, 1985).

The pharmacological treatment of alcohol withdrawal aims to reduce the severity of non-specific features (elevated blood pressure, high pulse, tremor, agitation, anxiety, depression), while avoiding the occurrence of specific features (seizures, delirium tremens). The distinction between specific and non-specific symptoms is reflected in the differential efficacy of the various pharmacological agents employed for the treatment of alcohol withdrawal.

Pharmacotherapy

Benzodiazepines

Several reviews agree that benzodiazepines reduce both the specific and non-specific symptoms of alcohol withdrawal and are the treatment of choice for alcohol withdrawal syndrome (Mayo-Smith, 1997; Lingford-Hughes et al., 2004), the only recommended monotherapy for it. The results of a meta-analysis on treatments for alcohol withdrawal indicated a statistically significant decrease of 4.9 cases of delirium for every 100 patients treated with benzodiazepines (Mayo-Smith, 1997). Long-acting benzodiazepines such as chlordiazepoxide and diazepam and short-acting agents such as lorazepam and oxazepam represent the most efficacious pharmacotherapies for treatment of acute alcohol withdrawal (Kosten & O'Connor, 2003). They are effective in preventing both first seizures and subsequent seizures during withdrawal. Longer-acting benzodiazepines may provide for easier weaning as they gradually self-taper upon metabolism and excretion and thus cause fewer rebound effects and withdrawal seizures upon discontinuation. Shorter-acting agents that do not undergo hepatic metabolism, such as lorazepam or oxazepam, require more frequent dosing but may be more appropriate for alcoholics with liver disease and the elderly (Lejoyeux et al., 1998).

Benzodiazepines are frequently administered in a fixed-schedule tapering regime though "symptom-triggered" regimens based on CIWA-AR scores are used more often. Several studies confirm that symptom-triggered regimens when compared to fixed-dose regimens result in a shorter duration of necessary therapy and less total medication.

Apart from benzodiazepines, a few other agents were found to be superior to placebo in treating non-specific symptoms of alcohol withdrawal syndrome, although there is no consensus about their place in treatment because of either non-proven efficacy in treating specific symptoms or because of dangerous side effects.

Anticonvulsants

The anticonvulsant agent carbamazepine, widely used in Europe for AWS, effectively decreases the severity of withdrawal symptoms, is comparable to the benzodiazepines in terms of adverse events, and is as equally effective as lorazepam at decreasing alcohol withdrawal symptoms. Carbamazepine may be superior to lorazepam in preventing rebound withdrawal symptoms and reducing post-treatment drinking (see Leggio et al., 2008 for review).

Table 6.1 Effectiveness of pharmacotherapy treatments for alcohol misuse, dependence and withdrawal

Treatment	Form of treatment	Psychiatric disorder	Level of evidence for efficacy	Comments
Pharmacotherapy	Disulfiram	Alcohol dependence	Ib	Despite widespread belief in its effectiveness, true double-blind studies are lacking. Controlled studies reveal inconsistent results. Appears to work best in those who are truly motivated to cease drinking
Pharmacotherapy	Acamprosate	Alcohol dependence	Ia	Probably is most effective when instituted shortly after completion of detoxification. It does increase length of time of abstinence
Pharmacotherapy	Naltrexone	Alcohol dependence	Ia	A decrease in relapse rate in heavy drinkers and a decrease in drinking frequency especially in addition to psychosocial interventions. No absolute improvement in abstinence rates
Pharmacotherapy	Antidepressants	Alcohol dependence	III	Perhaps some mild impact with comorbid anxiety or depression
Pharmacotherapy	Mood stabilizers (esp. topiramate)	Alcohol dependence	Ib	Decreased drinking per day, decreased days drinking, decreased craving, and increased days of abstinence. Also an effect on smoking and cocaine use
Pharmacotherapy	Ondansetron	Alcohol dependence	IIa	May be useful in subtype of early age onset drinking group. An RTC has been completed, waiting for published results
Pharmacotherapy	Buspirone	Alcohol dependence	Ia	Results are contradictory. May be useful in subtypes with comorbid anxiety disorders

Table 6.1 (cont.)

Treatment	Form of treatment	Psychiatric disorder	Level of evidence for efficacy	Comments
Pharmacotherapy	Benzodiazepines	Alcohol withdrawal	Ia	Clearly most useful in alcohol withdrawal. Dosing schedules appear to favour symptom-triggered approach. Longer-acting may be more effective here
Pharmacotherapy	Anticonvulsants (carbamazepine, gabapentin)	Alcohol withdrawal	Ib	May be useful in withdrawal particularly in cases of mild to moderate withdrawal

Adjunctive treatments

Alcohol-dependent clients are deficient in thiamine and have a higher risk for developing Wernicke's encephalopathy (Cook et al., 1998). Rapid correction of brain thiamine should be achieved by parenteral supplementation since absorption of the oral thiamine by the gastrointestinal tract is minimal. Interventions discussed in this chapter are summarized in Table 6.1.

7

Educational interventions for alcohol use disorders

Based on "Educational interventions for alcohol use disorders" by Robert Patton, Kirk J. Brower, Shannon Bellefleur and Mike Crawford in Effective Treatments in Psychiatry, Cambridge University Press, 2008

Introduction

Education is inherent in most alcohol-related treatment interventions. Brief interventions provide educational feedback to patients about normative patterns of drinking. CBT teaches patients how to identify high-risk situations and provides coping skills to prevent relapse. Twelve-step facilitation therapy involves educating patients about the disease model of alcoholism and what to expect in meetings of Alcoholics Anonymous.

Educational interventions are designed to increase knowledge about alcohol in order to change an individual's attitude and behaviour.

Providing information about health risks and brief advice emphasizing strategies to reduce consumption are the only interventions that have been recommended for both hazardous and harmful consumption of alcohol. While education may be usefully employed as part of more complex (brief) interventions, we consider it here as a "stand-alone" treatment.

Psychoeducation, like psychotherapy, is designed to reduce drinking and improve psychological functioning. It can be either self-administered (Mains & Scogin, 2003) or provided by paraprofessionals (or professionals) or educators without formal training in psychotherapy.

Educational approaches may involve as little as one session (Apodaca & Miller, 2003). Contact with the educator can occur in-person or by telephone, postal mail or computer. Thus, it is cost-efficient and can be used in stepped-care models of treatment for alcohol use disorders (Sobell & Sobell, 2000).

General advice and information

Harmful use of alcohol often persists for a long time before help is requested, and the value of educational interventions might be considered optimal in this group. There is some evidence that supports this. A randomized controlled trial comparing advice via a booklet and general advice delivered by a family practitioner to a no-intervention control found significantly greater reduction in indicators of alcohol consumption in the intervention group (Wallace et al., 1988). A large multinational and multicultural randomized trial of misusers who were non-dependent compared the effects of screening plus 5 minutes of brief advice with screening plus 15 minutes of counselling or "screening alone". The study found that 5 minutes of brief advice was as effective as 15 minutes of counselling. Men, but not women, who

received either active intervention reported drinking 25% less alcohol daily compared to those who received screening alone (Babor & Grant, 1992).

The effectiveness of educational interventions has been reviewed repeatedly (Mullen et al., 1997; Moyer et al., 2002) with similar conclusions that brief educational interventions directed toward those drinking excessively result in reductions in alcohol consumption. There is little additional benefit for extended interventions. But brief interventions may have lesser impact as the severity of the alcohol-related problems increases (Moyer et al., 2002), and it is believed that the effectiveness may not last beyond 12 months.

Educational interventions are popular in the USA, and most mainstream bookstores have moderately sized sections devoted to self-help and recovery books. Surveys of internet-based and mail-delivered educational interventions indicate a high degree of acceptance by users (Kypri et al., 2005).

Bibliotherapy

Bibliotherapy has been defined as the use of self-help materials or "any therapeutic intervention that was presented in a written format, designed to be read and implemented by the client" (Apodaca & Miller, 2003). More simply, bibliotherapy refers to "the therapeutic use of written materials to effect behavioural change" (Walitzer & O'Connors, 1999). Examples of bibliotherapy include the *Big Book of Alcoholics Anonymous*, though this can include listening to lectures, watching movies, and utilizing computer-assisted and website formats. Thus, bibliotherapy refers to a broad category of heterogeneous interventions.

Bibliotherapy for alcohol misuse was originally developed as an adjunct to psychological treatments. Apodaca and Miller (2003) conducted a meta-analysis of 22 randomized trials on the effectiveness of bibliotherapy for problem drinking. All studies involved the distribution of self-help reading materials and did not involve more than one face-to-face session with a professional. The conclusion was that bibliotherapy compared to no treatment has a small beneficial effect (weighted mean effect size = 0.31), but that it is not more effective than extensive interventions. It appears more effective for self-referred drinkers and that self-help materials that included specific behavioural strategies (such as setting drinking goals, monitoring drinking habits, and solving problems without alcohol) are more effective than those

containing general information and advice to reduce drinking only (Spivak et al., 1994). It is recommended for at risk and problem drinkers but not for patients with severe alcohol dependence.

Other educational interventions

School-based education efforts for public and college students

Studies which examined the impact of public education campaigns have generally reported no impact on levels of alcohol consumption (Raistrick et al., 1999). A review of the effectiveness of school-based alcohol education concluded that it has a positive effect on knowledge and attitudes but cautions that just 6/59 studies demonstrated a reduction in consumption (Anderson et al., 2009). Randomized trials of school-based educational interventions aimed at preventing alcohol and drug misuse have demonstrated changes in attitudes to alcohol but little impact on actual consumption patterns (Palinkas et al., 1996). A quasi-randomized Australian study of students provided with an intervention of teaching combined with skills training and use of videos and workbooks delivered over a 2-year period found changes in knowledge and attitudes to alcohol with students receiving this teaching reporting 31% less alcohol consumption than those who did not (McBride et al., 2004).

Among college students, educational programmes which only provide information in the absence of motivational or skills-building strategies are not effective (Larimer & Cronce, 2002). College students typically overestimate how much other students drink and attempts to correct this misperception is called normative education. Heavy drinking college students when provided with normative education material had significantly fewer heavy drinking episodes at the 6-week follow-up assessment than a group who received educational materials without the normalizing education information.

Other groups and other interventions

Education has long been a mainstay intervention for convicted drunk drivers. In a group of repeat drunk drivers, education in combination with psychotherapy was more effective than education alone, which was more effective than probation alone (Wells-Parker et al., 1995). Group psychoeducation performed as well as CBT in improving alcohol outcomes in 88 adolescents with mixed diagnoses of alcohol abuse or dependence and/or marijuana abuse or dependence

(Kaminer et al., 2002), but it was inferior to standard outpatient alcoholism treatment for the outcome of abstinence in a study of male alcoholic veterans (Davis et al., 2002).

Strengthening Families Programme (SFP)

The Strengthening Families Programme is designed to reduce adolescent substance misuse by increasing parenting skills and helping young people to develop their confidence and life skills. The intervention involves parents and young people meeting separately and together in interactive groups using educational materials, themed discussions, and role-play. A systematic review of educational programmes to prevent alcohol misuse among young people (aged 25 and under) concluded that the SFP showed promise as an effective prevention initiative (Foxcroft et al., 2003).

Internet and computer-based education, educational lectures, and films

With evidence demonstrating the benefit of brief educational interventions, recent studies have begun to explore the impact of these when delivered via computer programmes and online applications. Initially internet-based interventions involved self-assessment of current alcohol consumption and information about

Table 7.1 Effectiveness of educational interventions for alcohol use disorders

Treatment	Form of treatment	Psychiatric disorder	Level of evidence for efficacy	Comments
Educational interventions	Bibliotherapy	Alcohol use disorders	Ia	Shown to have a small beneficial effect that can be enhanced by additional professional psychotherapeutic work. Works best in mild to moderate alcohol misuse
Educational interventions	Miscellaneous educational intervention including Internet, formal classes, films	Alcohol use disorders	IIa	Has different impact in different populations but in general is thought to be of some help but often needs some enhancements with other more formalized treatments. Films do not appear to be effective

the consequences of excessive drinking. But programmes have now been developed which are more interactive and include personalized motivational strategies and interventions based on cognitive behavioural therapy and other psychological treatments. Web-based interventions have been shown to bring about medium term reductions in alcohol consumption among problem drinkers and increase educational performance in students that are sustained over 12 months (Riper et al., 2008; Kypri et al., 2008).

While showing people educational videos about alcohol can also help people reduce their consumption, their impact may be no greater than providing written information about alcohol (Miller & Wilbourne, 2002; Eaden et al., 2006).

Summary

There is a strong evidence base to recommend educational intervention for all patients including at risk, problem, and dependent drinkers. It can be considered mildly to moderately effective and appears most effective with people who have mild to moderate problems with alcohol. Education can be enhanced significantly by combining it with motivational techniques, skills training, and psychotherapy since education as a stand-alone intervention is generally less effective than when combined with other strategies. The importance of educational interventions is reflected in official guidelines (UK Alcohol Forum, 2001; Scottish Intercollegiate Guideline Network, 2003; WHO, 2004) that endorse these approaches as part of first-line treatment. Self-help manuals linked to brief advice are generally recommended as second-line treatment in official guidelines (Scottish Intercollegiate Guideline Network, 2003). The impact of other forms of educational information is less certain. Interventions discussed in this chapter are summarized in Table 7.1.

8

Complex interventions for alcohol use disorders

Based on "Complex interventions for alcohol use disorders" by Valerie J. Slaymaker,
Kirk J. Brower and Mike Crawford in Effective Treatments in Psychiatry, Cambridge
University Press, 2008

Introduction

Complex interventions for alcohol use disorders utilize multiple therapeutic components and strategies based on a common underlying philosophy of treatment and target various facets of the disorder in a complementary and frequently simultaneous fashion. Most treatment for moderately to severely alcohol-dependent patients is complex because (a) aetiology, development, and course of alcohol use disorders are heterogeneous and influenced by multiple factors, (b) no single treatment strategy or technique is effective across all alcohol-dependent patients,

and (c) the active ingredients of most, if not all, psychosocial therapies for alcohol dependence are unknown.

Four complex interventions are reviewed: Alcoholics Anonymous (AA), the Minnesota Model of Treatment, therapeutic communities (TCs), and combined pharmacotherapy and psychotherapy. With the exception of AA, complex interventions are generally delivered within specialized addiction treatment settings.

Alcoholics Anonymous

Founded in 1935, Alcoholics Anonymous (AA) is an extensive global mutual-help organization with over 100 000 groups in 150 countries. Similar groups exist for those addicted to specific substances (Narcotics Anonymous, Cocaine Anonymous, Marijuana Anonymous).

AA aims to help members maintain total abstinence from alcohol and drugs by living in accordance with the Twelve Steps: recognizing problem drinking and alcoholism, developing hope for recovery, conducting a thorough self-inventory of personal shortcomings, implementing a behavioural plan to address the consequences of alcoholism, making restitution for harmful actions, engaging in regular behaviour intended to maintain recovery, developing spirituality and serenity, and helping other alcoholics. Regular attendance at meetings is strongly encouraged; newcomers are advised to attend 90 meetings in 90 days when possible. The programme's philosophy encourages modification of maladaptive cognitions (referred to as "stinkin' thinkin'"), behavioural changes (avoidance of drinking events, drinking friends, or relatives), and development of adaptive coping skills (call sponsor for needed support). Since this multifaceted approach combines elements of cognitive and behavioural change, social support (fellowship), and spiritual growth, AA is a complex intervention.

Frequently misunderstood as a religious organization, AA's spiritual principles are broad and consistent with many religious orientations. Members are encouraged to define a "Higher Power" for themselves and to find their own way of relating to that Higher Power since when alcoholics rely primarily on their individual selves for recovery, they are thought to be in danger of relapsing. They need a power greater than themselves for recovery. The programme's spiritual connotations cause difficulty for some.

AA is one of the most common sources of help for alcoholism in the US (Weisner et al., 1995). Worldwide membership is estimated at over 2 000 000. It is free, available to anyone who desires to stop drinking, omnipresent, and compatible with professional interventions.

The American Society of Addiction Medicine (ASAM, 2001), Department of Veterans Affairs, National Institute on Alcohol Abuse and Alcoholism (NIAA, 2000b), American Psychiatric Association (APA, 2006a), and addiction researcher groups (Humphreys et al., 2004) recommend self-help group participation adjunctive to professional treatment. The Substance Abuse and Mental Health Services Administration's (SAMHSA) Centre for Substance Abuse Treatment's practice guidelines recommend AA and related groups for alcohol and drug addicted people including adolescents, adults, older adults, pregnant women, and those with co-occurring mental health disorders (US Department of Health and Human Services, 1999).

Given AA's wide availability and accessibility, controlled, prospective studies with random assignment to AA versus no-AA are difficult as researchers are unable to establish control groups for comparison studies (Humphreys, 2003). Further, AA has a policy against engaging in or supporting research. Most studies have had to rely primarily on correlational and predictive analyses to explore the relationship between AA attendance or affiliation and drinking and psychosocial outcomes.

Reviews of AA effectiveness and efficacy consistently conclude that AA membership and participation is related to improved drinking and psychosocial outcomes (Tonigan et al., 2002; Humphreys, 2003; Emrick & Tonigan, 2004). These effects do not appear to be explained by participants' increased motivation (McKellar et al., 2003). Length of participation impacts outcome directly; higher first-year involvement levels predict better 2-year follow-up outcomes (McKellar et al., 2003) and better use and psychosocial outcomes at 8-year follow-up (Moos & Moos, 2004). AA involvement appears to work by increasing self-efficacy or the confidence to resist drinking, which in turn positively impacts abstinence (Morgenstern et al., 1997), a finding supported by Project MATCH

(Connors et al., 2001). AA participation predicted self-efficacy levels which in turn predicted percentage of days abstinent at 1 year and 3 years (Owen et al., 2003). AA seems to work via the development of social support networks that encourage sobriety (Humphreys et al., 1999; Owen et al., 2003). Participation appears to reduce utilization of additional treatment services. Those in programmes emphasizing AA attendance were more likely to be abstinent at 1-year follow-up with significantly lower health care costs compared to those in cognitive behavioural programmes (Humphreys & Moos, 2001).

Data suggests that AA is effective for many alcohol-dependent persons. Given the strength of the evidence, the ubiquity of meeting times and places, the importance of social support for recovery, its cost-free nature, and compatibility with professional treatment, AA is an important treatment option to be considered for all alcohol-dependent patients. Family members should be encouraged to attend Al-Anon, a twelve-step mutual-help group for people close to the patient.

The Minnesota Model of Care

The Minnesota Model can be traced to a Minnesota state psychiatric hospital in the early 1950s where Nelson Bradley, a physician, and Dan

Anderson, a psychologist, began to revolutionize addiction treatment. Local AA members urged the pair to examine two new and innovative programmes in Minnesota, Pioneer House and Hazelden, leading to programmes firmly rooted in AA's twelve-step philosophy. They developed a comprehensive alcoholism treatment philosophy conceptualizing alcoholism as a biological, psychological, social, and spiritual disease that was a primary, progressive, and chronic illness. They brought groups of professionals (physicians, psychologists, nurses, social workers, spiritual care providers) into multidisciplinary teams. They separated alcoholics from the mentally ill, unlocked doors, and brought recovering alcoholics in to interact with patients. Recovering people were also given paid positions as counsellors and fully participated on the professional treatment team.

Anderson (1981) later took a leadership position at Hazelden where the Minnesota Model continued to evolve. Addiction was a chronic biopsychosocial and spiritual disease often complicated by other medical and psychiatric disorders. Treatment, provided in residential, outpatient, extended care and halfway house settings, was delivered by professional teams addressing cognitive, behavioural, spiritual, emotional, and medical functioning with ongoing abstinence from alcohol and drugs as the goal. The Twelve Steps are fully integrated into the core treatment process and care plan. Cognitive behavioural strategies identify and restructure the "stinkin' thinkin'" associated with substance use. The model emphasizes treating all patients with dignity and respect. Confrontation is not used. Motivational enhancement approaches facilitate problem recognition and subsequent treatment engagement.

Treatment centres utilizing this philosophy of care are known interchangeably as Minnesota Model, Hazelden Model, twelve-step-based, or twelve-step facilitation (TSF; Nowinski et al., 1992) programmes. Despite integration of the Twelve Steps, this professionally delivered treatment is unique and distinct from the mutual and self-help of AA and is one of the most commonly used treatment approaches in the United States (Institute of Medicine, 1990). It has experienced worldwide dissemination.

Numerous studies, including early evaluations, quasi-experimental designs, and randomized trials, have demonstrated the efficacy of the Minnesota Model in improving substance use and psychosocial functioning (Ouimette et al., 1997; Humphreys & Moos, 2001). The earliest randomized trial conducted in the late 1980s in Finland found more patients treated in this model attended AA meetings compared to those in traditional hospital-based programmes. Significantly more patients treated in the Model were abstinent during 8–12 month follow-up (Keso & Salaspuro, 1990).

Project MATCH, the first large-scale, randomized, multisite study, examined whether over 1700 patients could be "matched" to one of three treatment approaches: TSF, cognitive behavioural therapy (CBT), and motivational enhancement therapy (MET). TSF was as effective in promoting abstinence and reducing drinking at 1 year as CBT and MET. At 3-year follow-up, a significantly higher abstinence rate was found for TSF participants compared to the other two conditions (Project MATCH Research Group, 1998).

Therapeutic communities

"Therapeutic communities (TCs)", first applied in the UK in the early 1950s, were developed independently by recovering individuals with substance use disorders as a mutual self-help alternative to traditional medical and psychiatric care (De Leon, 2004). TCs are highly structured hierarchical settings. Community members progress through stages characterized by length of time in treatment, motivation and commitment, TC status, and specific goal achievements. Individuals in TCs are community members or residents, not patients or clients. The TC is self-operating. Cooking, cleaning, and repairs within its expertise are performed by residents. Status is assigned according to length and progress in treatment. Community rules and expected conduct are clearly defined. Contingency management is utilized. Adherence to rules and treatment expectations are rewarded with increases in privileges and community status; rule violations by loss of privileges and status that can be regained with appropriate behaviour and progress. Early in treatment, motivation may be mostly external; later in treatment, members hopefully conform because they actively seek community affiliation. In the final treatment stages members are ideally motivated by their commitment to enhance the community and provide leadership. TCs are widely used in the USA.

TCs for substance use disorders can be broadly categorized into "traditional" and "modified" TCs. Traditional TCs emerged in the 1960s and refer to abstinence-based residential treatment programmes of 15–24 months in duration (De Leon, 2004). The evidence for effectiveness of traditional TCs comes primarily from naturalistic treatment outcome studies (DeLeon, 2004); time in treatment is positively correlated with good outcomes. Traditional TCs serve primarily male heroin-dependent individuals without serious Axis I psychiatric disorders.

In the 1980s with the emerging US crack cocaine epidemic, TCs were modified to make them more widely available by reducing costs and accommodating special populations. TC concepts and treatment methods were introduced into shorter stay residential programmes (3–12 months) and non-residential outpatient programmes (partial hospital, other abstinence-based outpatient care, methadone maintenance). Modified TC outcomes demonstrate effectiveness, especially for patients with lower problem severity.

Combined pharmacotherapy and psychotherapy

Combining pharmacotherapy and psychotherapy for alcohol use disorders has the potential for achieving greater efficacy than either alone. Psychotherapy here includes all forms of therapy whether dynamic, twelve-step-based, or cognitive behavioural, among others. Theoretically, the two types of treatment could operate synergistically through different mechanisms. For example, naltrexone might reduce both urges to drink and drinking's reinforcing effects, while CBT might increase skills and confidence in managing high-risk drinking situations. Behavioural therapies can enhance medication compliance

and reinforce other recovery activities. Knowledge about which particular psychotherapy (CBT, MET, TSF) should be combined with which medication is limited. Relapse prevention medications are viewed as adjunctive to psychosocial treatment in the USA, and simple medication monitoring by itself is not considered sufficient treatment.

A note on the COMBINE study (also see p 49)

The primary analyses of the COMBINE study (Anton et al., 2006) investigated the main and interactive effects of three interventions: naltrexone (NTX), acamprosate (ACAM), and cognitive behavioural interventions (CBI). Primary analyses were based on randomization of subjects to eight treatment conditions based on combinations of NTX, ACAM, or placebo, and CBI versus no CBI. All treatment groups received medical management (MM). The two primary outcomes were percentage of days abstinent and time to relapse to first heavy drinking day during the 16-week trial.

To summarize the findings:

- A main effect for NTX in delaying time to relapse when compared to placebo.
- ACAM no better than placebo; ACAM and CBI combination no more effective than placebo plus CBI.

Table 8.1 Effectiveness of complex interventions for alcohol use disorders

Treatment	Form of treatment	Psychiatric disorder	Level of evidence for efficacy	Comments
Complex intervention	Alcoholics Anonymous	Alcohol dependence	Ib	AA attendance is difficult to study in clinical trials. Evidence suggests modest but consistent improvements in days of sobriety. Length of participation as well as concurrent professional treatment also leads to improved outcomes
Complex intervention	The Minnesota Model including twelve-step facilitation (TSF)	Alcohol dependence	Ia	Substantial evidence supports that these programmes significantly improve sobriety and social functioning. A number of studies show that in many the gains are maintained
Complex intervention	Therapeutic community	Alcohol dependence	III	Despite the complexity of the treatment and the low rate of retention until completion of the programme, there is some evidence that in certain populations, it is an effective treatment
Complex intervention	Combined pharmacotherapy and psychotherapy	Alcohol dependence	Ib	The COMBINE study and other open-label studies suggest that the combination of psychotherapy and medication can be useful. Most evidence supports NTX as the pharmacological agent with weaker support for ACAM and little for disulfiram. At present, no particular psychotherapy has any real advantage over any other in combination with medications

- NTX effective with no advantage in combining it with either ACAM or CBI.
- A significant interaction found for NTX and CBI: any combination that included either NTX or CBI performed better than placebo without CBI.
- A significant interaction occurred with NTX plus supportive therapy group having the longest initial abstinence duration.
- MM combined with placebo increased percentage of abstinent days significantly more than CBI alone.
- Results for CBI alone are negative (Anton et al., 2006).

These complicated results suggest that interactions between medication and psychotherapy vary according to both the particular outcome variable selected and the duration of the outcome period assessed. Nonetheless, alcohol dependence may be managed successfully in non-specialized settings, as long as frequent interactions between the patient and a medication-knowledgeable licensed health care professional occur over a sustained period of several months and some medication is utilized. Interventions discussed in this chapter are summarized in Table 8.1.

9

Complementary and alternative medicine for alcohol misuse

Based on "Complementary and alternative medicine for alcohol misuse" by Elizabeth A. R. Robinson, Stephen Strobbe and Kirk J. Brower in Effective Treatments in Psychiatry, Cambridge University Press, 2008

Introduction

This chapter focuses on acupuncture, biofeedback, and meditation. Although there are many other types of Complementary and alternative medicine (CAM) modalities, we will not review the other therapies, as the scientific literature on these therapies with regard to alcohol misuse is sparse.

Acupuncture

Acupuncture, based on traditional Chinese medicine, is defined as "stimulation, primarily by the use of solid needles, of traditionally and clinically defined points on or beneath the skin, in an organized fashion for therapeutic and/or preventative purposes" (Hanet al., 2004, p. 743). In traditional Chinese medicine, acupuncture is thought to promote health through stimulation of specific anatomical points that, in turn, facilitates the natural flow of *qi* or vital energy. The experience of properly administered acupuncture has been described as a subjective state of well-being and represents recruitment of natural, internal resources directed towards healing. Benefits are thought to be additive and cumulative. Western medicine has conceptualized acupuncture in terms of its effect on endogenous endorphins (Pomeranz, 1989). The most commonly used and researched acupuncture protocol in alcoholism treatment is a 5-point technique, often referred to as the "NADA protocol", or "acudetox".

Acupuncture studies have been criticized for a number of methodological limitations. Difficulties in designing double-blind, placebo-controlled treatment conditions occur because populations across studies differ as to (a) inpatient or outpatient status, (b) number and types of substances being used, (c) stage of disorder, and (d) symptoms being treated. Technique variations such as (a) type of acupuncture needles, either with or without electrical stimulation, (b) standardized acupuncture doses in terms of both quantity and frequency, and (c) different outcomes add to the problem.

In reviewing a number of controlled studies, Kazanjian and Rothon (2002) concluded that, "The trials that scored highly in methodological quality did not conclusively demonstrate the effectiveness of acupuncture for the management of alcohol and drug dependence" (p. ix). Two other randomized controlled trials published after Kazanjian and Rothon's review (Bullock et al., 2002; Trumpler at al., 2003) also did not support use of acupuncture in alcohol treatment. Thus based on RCTs, there is currently insufficient evidence to recommend routine use of acupuncture in the treatment of alcohol use disorders or alcohol withdrawal. Nonetheless, acupuncture may still have utility in the treatment of select populations but the inability to conduct true double-blind placebo-controlled trials remains a source of frustration and limitation.

Mind–body therapies: biofeedback and meditation

Mind–body therapies span a wide range of approaches, including biofeedback and meditation. They are intended to enhance the mind's capacity to affect bodily function and symptoms. Prayer is the most common CAM intervention that individuals use outside of professional treatment; about 36% of the US population has used prayer and *only* prayer to address a health problem. There is even less conclusive research on the efficacy of prayer than for acupuncture, biofeedback, and meditation.

Biofeedback

Biofeedback is a technique used to induce relaxation by training individuals to voluntarily control selected physiological parameters (e.g. blood pressure, muscle tone, or brainwaves). By monitoring and providing real-time information or feedback about those measured parameters during treatment sessions, individuals can learn to control them. At least three different techniques of feedback have been studied in alcohol-dependent patients: brainwave biofeedback utilizing electroencephalography (EEG) to train patients to increase the quantity of their alpha (8–11 Hz) and/or theta (4–7 Hz) frequency waveforms, electromyography (EMG) biofeedback that trains patients to relax selected muscle groups, and a third type that monitors physiological signs such as heart rate, blood pressure, and finger temperature. Biofeedback is not usually used in the US addiction treatment setting.

The methodological quality of biofeedback studies does not permit conclusions about efficacy. Therefore, its use to promote abstinence or prevent relapse to heavy drinking cannot be recommended.

Meditation

Over 30 years of published research indicate that meditation may help with a variety of presenting psychiatric problems, including depression, anxiety, stress disorders, and possibly substance misuse. A primary rationale for using meditation training in alcoholism treatment is the evidence that stress plays a role in substance use disorders (Brady & Sonne, 1999), and psychophysiological evidence that meditation may alter stress reactions (e.g. Carlson et al., 2004).

Reviews of effectiveness of meditation are unclear as the meditation technique is often not clearly defined and is often confused with relaxation training, which can be a noticeable benefit or side effect of meditating. The assumption that meditation and relaxation are synonymous is incorrect, but the prevalence of this assumption complicates reviews of meditation's use in alcohol treatment. Some researchers have tried to tease out the effects of meditation alone by testing interventions that combine meditation with other components.

A useful definition of meditation: "... meditation refers to a family of self-regulation practices that focus on training attention and awareness in order to bring mental processes under greater voluntary control and thereby foster general mental well-being and development and/or specific capacities such as calm, clarity, and concentration" (Walsh & Shapiro, 2006, pp. 228–229). Meditation practices differ in the focus of attention one cultivates, the extent internal experience is altered or manipulated versus merely observed, and the goal. Attention can be concentrated, e.g. focused on a specific object, or one can cultivate moment-to-moment awareness, attending to and observing whatever internal experience is dominant (e.g. physical sensations, thoughts, or emotions). Transcendental meditation (TM) and Benson's Relaxation Response (Benson & Klipper, 2000) approach are examples of concentration approaches that use sounds or phrases (mantras) as the focus of attention, whereas mindfulness approaches emphasize awareness of the present moment.

Transcendental meditation

Transcendental meditation (TM) was introduced to the West in the 1970s from India. TM is taught in a standard seven-step course which includes group and individual instruction. Unlike other forms of meditation training, the training itself is secret and is not manualized. Claims made for TM's positive effects are passionate and enthusiastic, but they beg for corroboration by independent researchers and more rigorous designs and measures (Alexander et al., 1994).

Since the early 1970s, many studies have investigated the impact of TM on drinking behaviours, although only one study has recruited a sample of individuals with alcohol problems, used no-treatment and "treatment as usual" control groups, and random assignment (Taub et al., 1994). When the TM and biofeedback group data were combined and compared to the combined "treatment as usual" and the "no treatment" groups, differences were statistically significant favouring the TM and biofeedback groups.

Secular mantra-based techniques

Benson, a physician, impressed by the results and his experience with transcendental meditation, developed a secularized version of TM called "The Relaxation Response". This technique instructs users to silently say the word "one" in time with one's breath. Two 20-minute practice sessions a day are recommended.

One study of this approach with alcohol problems was a well-designed randomized controlled trial of four conditions among 41 heavy-drinking college students (Marlatt et al., 1984). Significant decreases in alcohol consumption occurred in all three active conditions from baseline to post-treatment, but unfortunately these gains were not maintained at follow-up. Another study (Murphy et al., 1986) investigated the impact on alcohol consumption of meditation, exercise (i.e. running), and a no-treatment control among 43 heavy social drinkers randomly assigned to three conditions. Pre–post alcohol consumption dropped significantly for both active treatment conditions (meditation and exercise).

Mindfulness

Mindfulness meditation fosters development of moment-to-moment awareness, with a range of meditations that each utilize an aspect of the present moment as a base for attention. In brief, mindfulness is the non-judgemental observation of our current experience of internal and external stimuli, as they arise and pass away. Jon Kabat-Zinn (1990) developed a secularized version, Mindfulness-Based Stress Reduction

(MBSR), that he and others have used with some success for chronic pain patients, anxiety disorders, and psoriasis (Grossman et al., 2004). Rigorous RCTs by Segal and colleagues (2002), replicated by Ma & Teasdale (2004), have established the usefulness of Mindfulness-Based Cognitive Therapy (MBCT) of depression (see Chapter 21). Subsequent work shows that mindfulness-based interventions are useful with a range of presenting problems. Mindfulness is a key component of Linehan's well-established Dialectical Behaviour Therapy for individuals with borderline personality disorder, many of whom have substance use problems (Linehan et al., 1999).

Zgierska in a recent thorough review (2009) describes 8 RCTs of mindfulness-based interventions carried out with individuals with substance use disorders. Subjects in several of these studies were predominantly individuals with alcohol use disorders. These feasibility pilot studies all used random assignment to either control (or TAU), or alternative treatment strategies to investigate the impact of mindfulness interventions. Zgierska and colleagues (2008) found significant pre–post changes in a small intensive outpatient sample in alcohol use, stress, craving, and depressive symptoms. Bowen and colleagues (2006) also found significant pre–post and group differences in an incarcerated population taught mindfulness meditation.

Vieten et al. (2010) describes pre–post improvements in negative affect, emotional reactivity, perceived stress, positive affect, and psychological well-being with a mindfulness-based intervention. Brewer and colleagues (2009) found that a mindfulness-based intervention was more effective than cognitive behavioural therapy in reducing reactions to stress provocation in an RCT with substance use disorders. In addition, several NIH-funded rigorous studies are underway that should provide more definitive information on the usefulness of mindfulness approaches with substance disorders.

Empirical evidence remains insufficient and not of rigorous quality at this time to assert definitively that teaching alcoholics meditation techniques will support their sobriety. Nevertheless, there is reason to suspect from these preliminary studies, theory, neurophysiological effects (e.g. Ostafin, 2008), and the efficacy of similar approaches with comorbid disorders, that mindfulness approaches may be shown with further research to have an impact on alcohol treatment and recovery.

Conclusion

There is little conclusive empirical work to date to support the use of CAM techniques in either alcohol dependence or withdrawal, largely

Table 9.1 Effectiveness of complementary and alternative medicine for alcohol misuse

Treatment	Form of treatment	Psychiatric disorder	Level of evidence for efficacy	Comments
Alternative medicine	Acupuncture	Alcohol use disorders	III	Because of the nature of acupuncture, difficult to do placebo-controlled trials. Evidence is contradictory and plagued by methodological issues
Alternative medicine	Biofeedback	Alcohol use disorders	III	Methodological issues prevent us from making any recommendations
Meditation	Transcendental meditation (TM)	Alcohol use disorders	Ib	One study revealed increases in days abstinent and greater total abstinence in TM group and in biofeedback group as well
Meditation	Secular-based meditation	Alcohol use disorders	IIb	While there appeared to be some benefit for meditation, other active control groups also showed improvement. Improvement was not maintained after meditation ended

because adequate studies have not been carried out. However, preliminary results are promising and warrant replication with larger samples and more rigorous designs. At the very least, CAM techniques, especially biofeedback and meditation, can help patients feel more in control over their bodies, minds, and behaviour and may well temper cravings, anxiety, and other physiological states involved in both alcohol use and recovery from alcohol dependence. Interventions discussed in this chapter are summarized in Table 9.1.

Drug misuse

Drug misuse

10

Empirically validated psychological therapies for drug dependence

Based on "Empirically validated psychological therapies for drug dependence" by Tara M. Neavins, Caroline J. Easton, Janet Brotchie and Kathleen M. Carroll in Effective Treatments in Psychiatry, Cambridge University Press, 2008

Introduction

Substantial gains have been made in the development of effective psychological therapies for adult drug abuse and dependence. There are effective pharmacotherapies for some classes of drug dependence (e.g. opioids) with positive outcomes in patient motivation, medication compliance, self-efficacy, and overall reduced treatment cost that improve dramatically with the addition of psychological therapies. For other classes of drugs (e.g. cocaine) where pharmacological interventions do not yet exist, psychological approaches are the state-of-the-art treatments. Many psychological approaches have been

evaluated in rigorous controlled clinical trials. Available treatment manuals and training materials facilitate use of these approaches by a variety of clinicians within and across a multidisciplinary approach.

Three issues deserve mention: (1) 'Talk' therapies remain the most common form of drug dependence treatment in the USA excluding detoxification or methadone maintenance. (2) Psychological treatments found effective in clinical trials often are not incorporated into mainstream clinical practice while many widely utilized treatments lack empirical evidence or randomized trial data. (3) For the majority of illicit drugs

79

(e.g. cocaine, amphetamines, meth-amphetamines, sedative/hypnotic/anxiolytics, cannabis, phencyclidine (PCP), hallucinogens, club drugs (MDMA) and inhalants) no generally effective pharmacotherapies exist. Behavioural approaches remain the only available treatment for most types of drug dependence.

In the UK, the focus has been on two approaches to treatment of prob-lematic drug use: (1) UK statutory treatment providers concentrate on providing pharmacological interven-tions to primary heroin-using clients. Clients who use other substances receive minimal interventions with non-opioid-using clients rarely becoming the focus of treatment, even for non-opioid use in opioid users. While the UK needs to imple-ment more evidence-based psycho-logical interventions, there are few evidence-based psychological inter-ventions provided within the drug treatment system. (2) The primary goal of psychological interventions has been harm reduction, focusing on changing risk-related behaviours rather than changing drug use per se.

Goals of psychological therapies in treating drug dependence

Psychological therapies differ from pharmacotherapy in their time to effect, durability of action, and target symptoms. Psychological therapies tend to require more time to achieve effectiveness but often have longer-lasting effects after completion. Most cognitive behavioural and behaviour-al therapies can be used across vari-ous treatment settings (e.g. inpatient, outpatient, residential) and modal-ities (e.g. group, individual, and fam-ily). Psychological therapies often rely on teaching coping skills or employ-ing motivational approaches and are applicable across types of substance abuse (Rounsaville & Carroll, 1997).

Cessation of drug use

Treatments rooted in motivational psychology, including motivational interviewing (Miller & Rollnick, 1991) and Motivation Enhancement Therapy (Miller et al., 1992), use strat-egies to bolster the patient's own motivational resources. Patients may first need to see reasons for chang-ing their behaviour before they can benefit from treatment. Motivational therapies are client-centred, un-derstand the ambivalence that many individuals face, and explore the pros and cons of continued substance use in attempting to increase moti-vation for treatment and abstinence. Motivational strategies provide client feedback that serves to increase moti-vation to change (Rounsaville & Carroll, 1997; Carroll, 2000).

Teaching coping skills and relapse prevention

Social learning theory posits that substance use may represent a means of coping with difficult situations, positive and negative emotional states, and invitations by peers to engage in use. By the time use has become dependence, it may be the individual's single, overgeneralized pattern of coping with a variety of situations and states. Patients need to understand high-risk situations that increase temptation to use and to learn more effective means of coping with those circumstances. Relapse prevention (Marlatt & Gordon, 1985), a means of increasing self-control and learning to cope with cravings, has been found particularly effective with cocaine-dependent individuals (Carroll et al., 1991; National Institute on Drug Abuse, 2004). Many cognitive behavioural therapies focus primarily on skills training to prevent relapses (Marlatt & Gordon, 1985; Carroll, 1998). Other behavioural therapies address high-risk situations (Childress et al., 1993).

Changing reinforcement contingencies

When abstinence is achieved, addicts may not know how to structure time previously consumed with obtaining and using drugs. Behavioural therapies and voucher-based contingency management (Budney & Higgins, 1998) assist with identifying and creating fulfilling and reinforcing alternatives to drug use (Carroll et al., 2001).

Fostering management of painful affects

Substance abusers have a compromised ability to identify and explicate their affect states. An important component of cognitive behavioural (CBT) and behavioural therapies (BT) is helping addicts create ways of coping with strong negative affects and teaching them to recognize sources of disturbing emotions (Rounsaville & Carroll, 1997).

Improving interpersonal functioning and enhancing social support

A network of social support is protective in preventing relapse (Marlatt & Gordon, 1985). Many cognitive behavioural and behavioural therapies emphasize teaching how to create and maintain a social network without substance users (Carroll, 2000). Supportive non-using peer networks such as Alcoholics Anonymous help clients terminate treatment successfully because they have not become dependent on one therapist or agency.

Fostering compliance with pharmacotherapy

Psychological treatments may be vital adjuncts to pharmacotherapies by increasing levels of compliance. The majority of techniques to improve compliance are psychosocial. Research consistently demonstrates the benefit of adding CBT and BT treatments to pharmacological treatments for substance use (Carroll, 1997).

Psychological therapies and opioid dependence

Behavioural therapies in the context of methadone maintenance

Methadone maintenance (MM) treatment revolutionized opioid addiction treatment with outcomes far surpassing those produced by non-pharmacological treatments (Rounsaville & Carroll, 1997; Carroll, 2000). MM allowed addicts to remain in treatment to reduce illicit opioid use, to decrease risk of HIV infection and other medical complications by decreasing intravenous drug use, and to create opportunities to address psychosocial issues (Sorenson & Copeland, 2000). But it is not uncommon for MM clients to sell take-home methadone or use other substances, especially alcohol, benzodiazepines, and cocaine, while on methadone.

Newer medication (e.g. buprenorphine and buprenorphine/naloxone) show promise, as they appear less apt to be diverted, have lower abuse potential, produce fewer side effects, and may also help alleviate pain (Johnson et al., 2003).

McLellan et al. (1993) randomly assigned 92 opiate-dependent individuals to: (1) MM alone, (2) MM with standard services, including regular counselling, or (3) enhanced MM, including regular counselling plus on-site medical, employment, and family therapy services. Those in the MM alone condition fared most poorly with improved outcomes associated with higher levels of behavioural treatment.

Contingency management approaches and opioid dependence

The effectiveness of decreasing opioid use via contingency management (CM) as an adjunct to MM treatment has wide empirical support (Rounsaville & Carroll, 1997; Carroll, 2000). Patients who meet specified target behaviours, e.g. drug-free urine specimens, attaining certain treatment goals, or attending treatment sessions, receive a reinforcer (reward). An example is methadone take-home privileges being conditional upon demonstration of decreased drug use or drug-free urines. Positive contingencies such as a voucher-based CM system appear more beneficial than negative contingencies (Silverman et al., 1996). While few studies have evaluated the efficacy of formal psychotherapy in enhancing MM outcomes, psychotherapy appears to assist addicts achieve and maintain better outcomes.

Behavioural couples therapy and opioid dependence

Empirical support for behavioural couples therapy in opioid dependence is increasing. Studies comparing individual to behavioural couples therapy reveal that those in couples therapy self-report significantly fewer drug-using days, fewer drug-related consequences, and greater lengths of abstinence, a difference maintained during 12-month follow-up (O'Farrell & Fals-Stewart, 2000).

Psychological therapies and cocaine dependence

In contrast to opioid dependence treatment, where behavioural therapies appear most effective when combined with pharmacotherapies (such as MM), the literature reveals strong evidence for effectiveness in cocaine dependence with purely behavioural treatments because no pharmacotherapy is currently available.

Investigations support comparatively brief, purely behavioural approaches as both sufficient and effective for the majority of patients. These include:

- Voucher-based CM is where abstinence is positively reinforced, drug use results in loss of reinforcement, and competing reinforcers to drug use are developed. Patients may receive redeemable points that increase in value with each successive clean urine or decrease when urines are not clean (Higgins et al., 2000).

- Low-cost CM, a "low-cost" alternative to traditional, fixed financial reimbursement, provides clients with prizes at variable intervals. Individuals in CM had significantly longer episodes of sustained abstinence from cocaine and opioids than in the standard condition. Gains were maintained over 6 months (Petry et al., 2004). CM produced quicker results than CBT though CBT produced similar post-treatment 6-month success. Combining CM and CBT did not lead to better outcomes than either condition alone (Rawson et al., 2002).

- CBT emphasizes: (1) exploring the positive and negative outcomes of use, (2) creating a functional analysis of substance use by understanding use in relation to its antecedents and consequences, (3) developing strategies for coping with high-risk situations including craving (4).

- preparing for emergencies and coping with relapse, and (5) identifying and confronting thoughts about substance use (Carroll, 1998). CBT appears more effective with individuals with more severe cocaine problems or comorbid disorders. It is significantly more effective than less intensive approaches, is equivalent to or more effective than manualized disease model approaches, and appears durable with reduced use even 1–2 years after treatment (McKay et al., 1999).

Disease model approaches to cocaine dependence and other substances of abuse

The NIDA Collaborative Cocaine Treatment Study (CCTS), a multisite randomized trial of psychotherapeutic treatments for cocaine dependence (Crits-Christoph et al., 1999), demonstrated effectiveness of a manualized treatment approach known as Individual Drug Counselling (IDC; Carroll, 2000). This study compared Cognitive Therapy plus Group Drug Counselling, Supportive-Expressive Therapy (short-term psychodynamic-oriented therapy), IDC focusing on abstinence from drugs and areas of impaired functioning, and Group Drug Counselling alone. Outcomes

were quite good with all groups significantly reducing their cocaine use. The best cocaine outcomes were for subjects who received IDC (Carroll et al., 2000), offering compelling support for the efficacy of manual-guided disease model approaches (Carroll, 2000).

Psychological therapies and amphetamine and methamphetamine dependence

Despite the prevalence of amphetamine and methamphetamine dependence, no empirically validated pharmacological and only one empirically validated behavioural treatment of methamphetamine dependence currently exists. Baker et al. (2001), in an RCT of brief psychological treatments for regular amphetamine users, found that CBT participants reported more than two times less daily amphetamine use than participants using the self-help booklet (control condition). Results remained good at 6-month follow-up.

The Matrix Model, a manualized, intensive, 16-session treatment that broadens CBT by supplementing it with family education, drug education, and Alcoholics or Narcotics Anonymous meetings, offers promise for methamphetamine abuse and dependence (Rawson et al., 2004).

Table 10.1 Effectiveness of empirically validated psychological therapies for drug dependence

Treatment	Form of treatment	Psychiatric disorder/ target audience	Level of evidence for efficacy	Comments
Behavioural therapy	Contingency management	Opioid dependence	Ia	Multiple studies including community-based programmes support the effectiveness in reducing opiate usage
Behavioural therapy	Voucher-based contingency management	Cocaine dependence	Ia	High acceptance, retention, and rates of abstinence
Psychological therapy/ psychotherapy	Motivational enhancement plus vouchers	Cannabis dependence	IIa	Both types of psychological therapy more effective than drug counselling alone
Psychological therapy/ psychotherapy	Supportive-expressive or cognitive	Opioid dependence Cocaine dependence	Ib	Both types of psychological therapy more effective than drug counselling alone
Psychological therapy/ psychotherapy	Cognitive-behavioural therapy	Cocaine dependence	Ia	Very effective in severe cocaine abuse and in people with comorbidities, and effects appear to be durable
Psychological therapy/ psychotherapy	Cognitive-behavioural therapy	Amphetamine dependence	IIb	CBT groups reported two times less daily amphetamine usage

Table 10.1 (cont.)

Treatment	Form of treatment	Psychiatric disorder/ target audience	Level of evidence for efficacy	Comments
Psychological therapy/ psychotherapy	Cognitive-behavioural therapy	Cannabis dependence	1b	CBT groups reported two times less daily amphetamine usage
Psychological therapy/ psychotherapy	Individual drug counselling (a manualized treatment)	Cocaine dependence	1b	As effective as CBT and Supportive–Expressive therapy with best outcomes for Individual Drug Counselling and cocaine
Psychological therapy/ psychotherapy	Behavioural couples therapy	Opioid and cocaine dependence	1b	Shown to be more effective than individual counselling

Empirical support for effectiveness remains to be determined. Low-cost CM of amphetamine and methamphetamine dependence appears to keep people in treatment longer, produce more substance-free urines, and lead to longer abstinence periods (Petry et al., 2005).

Psychological therapies and cannabis dependence

Treatment of cannabis dependence is understudied. No effective pharmacotherapies exist. Motivational approaches combined with vouchers appear most effective (Budney et al., 2000), though there is evidence for effectiveness of purely motivational approaches.

Drug dependence amongst young adults (ages 18–25) has begun to receive greater attention recently. The majority of clinical trials address marijuana use. Motivational enhancement therapy and CM led to significantly less cannabis usage and

fewer legal problems. Adding CBT to these approaches supported production of drug-free urines (Carroll et al., 2006).

Summary and conclusions

While a variety of effective psychological treatments for drug dependence disorders have been identified, this knowledge has not been well integrated into general clinical practice (Carroll, 2000). Frequently cited barriers include a lack of an organized system for disseminating effective treatments to the clinical community and failure of researchers to design their studies with critical clinical questions in mind and consideration for cost-effectiveness. Encouraging signs are emerging. Several rigorous trials evaluating psychological treatments have taken seriously the need to report cost-effectiveness data and cost savings (Carroll, 2000). Interventions discussed in this chapter are summarized in Table 10.1.

11

Treatment of stimulant dependence

Based on "Treatment of stimulant dependence" by Mehmet Sofuoglu, Kostas Agath and Thomas R. Kosten in Effective Treatments in Psychiatry, Cambridge University Press, 2008

Introduction

Cocaine and amphetamine addictions are major worldwide public health concerns. The estimated annual prevalence of cocaine abusers in people over 15 years old is 0.3% globally, 0.4% in Europe, 1.7% in the Americas; for amphetamine abusers it is 0.6% globally, 0.7% in Europe, 0.7% in the Americas. Of all treatment cases of substance misuse, not including alcohol, cocaine abuse represents 29% in the USA and 5% in the European Union. Over the last decade, cocaine consumption in the USA has decreased while consumption of both cocaine and amphetamine-type stimulants in Europe has increased.

Methamphetamine abuse is an international public health problem, with two-thirds of the world's 33 million amphetamine abusers living in Asia (United Nations Office for Drug Control and Crime Prevention, 2000; Ahmad, 2003).

In the USA there are an estimated 2 million dependent cocaine and amphetamine users (SAMHSA, 2008). In the UK cocaine misuse is higher than the use of amphetamines. Of the treatment service users in the UK, 6% report cocaine and 4% report amphetamine as a primary drug (National Treatment Agency, 2002), although misuse with multiple substances is frequent, with 50% of heroin users reporting using stimulants in the last 3 months, and about a third of stimulant users being problem drinkers. Crack cocaine misuse is twice as frequent as cocaine powder misuse (Greater London Alcohol and Drug Alliance, 2004).

The risks associated with stimulant use are substantial and include increased risk of HIV, hepatitis C and B infection, increased crime and violence, as well as medical, financial, and psychosocial problems.

Smoking free base cocaine (crack) is preferred though intranasal and intravenous routes are also common. Effects of snorted cocaine generally occur within 15–20 minutes; peak effects from intravenous or smoked cocaine occur within 3–5 minutes. Amphetamines, taken orally or intravenously, produce actions similar to cocaine. A smoked version of methamphetamine (Ice, Crank) is also available. Methamphetamine can produce euphoria lasting 12 to 24 hours.

Clinical aspects of stimulant use

As in DSM-IV, stimulant dependence is characterized by compulsive use of stimulants at the expense of important activities and responsibilities. Stimulant use is continued in spite of the physical or psychological problems caused by drug use. The individual has a chronic desire for or makes unsuccessful attempts to decrease or quit stimulant use. Dependence may have physiological components characterized by tolerance or withdrawal. Stimulant abuse, on the other hand, is a maladaptive drug use with associated social and medical consequences but without the typical compulsive drug use pattern of drug dependence (American Psychiatric Association, 1994).

Stimulant intoxication is characterized by euphoria, hyperalertness, grandiosity, anxiety, restlessness, stereotypical behaviour, psychomotor agitation, and impaired judgement with physical signs and symptoms including tachycardia, bradycardia, dilated pupils, elevated or lowered blood pressure, perspiration or chills, nausea or vomiting, weight loss, chest pain, cardiac arrhythmia, confusion, seizures, dyskinesia, or dystonias. Treatment of stimulant intoxication includes close monitoring in a safe environment until symptoms subside. Usually benzodiazepines are sufficient to alleviate the symptoms of intoxication. Antipsychotics should be reserved for cases when psychosis is present (Kosten, 2002).

Stimulant-induced psychotic disorder is seen in high-dose, chronic stimulant users, often during binge episodes or during withdrawal (Satel & Edell, 1991), and can include delusions, hallucinations, paranoid thinking, and stereotyped compulsive behaviour. Amphetamines are more likely to induce paranoia than cocaine. Treatment of stimulant intoxication paranoia involves close clinical monitoring and short-term treatment with antipsychotics.

Following heavy use, stimulants can produce a state of mental confusion and excitement, known as stimulant delirium (Ruttenber et al., 1997), disturbances in consciousness and disorientation and perceptual disturbances such as visual and auditory hallucinations. Delirium indicates stimulant overdose; patients need intensive monitoring for medical complications including seizures, cardiac arrhythmias, and vascular and pulmonary complications (Shanti & Lucas, 2003). Benzodiazepines are preferred over antipsychotics for control of agitation because antipsychotics may decrease seizure threshold and worsen the hyperthermia associated with stimulant overdose. Acutely, benzodiazepines can help minimize the need for physical restraints.

Stimulant withdrawal is characterized by: depressed mood; fatigue; vivid, unpleasant dreams; insomnia or hypersomnia; increased appetite; and psychomotor retardation or agitation following cessation of stimulant use (American Psychiatric Association, 1994). Greater amounts and sustained duration of use are associated with more severe withdrawal symptoms and seem to be associated with poor treatment outcome (Kampman et al., 2001a; Sofuoglu et al., 2003). Clinically, stimulant withdrawal is generally self-limited and does not require specific treatment.

Treatment for stimulant use disorder

Treatment for the stimulant user is still not well established. The growing knowledge base about the neurobiological actions of stimulants has not translated into effective pharmacotherapies.

Most clinical trials for the pharmacological and behavioural treatments for stimulant dependence have focused on cocaine; those treatments are now being tested for the treatment of amphetamine use. Nonetheless, research on stimulant misuse treatment is characterized by heterogeneity of study populations and large variations in dropout rates (Sofuoglu & Kosten, 2006; Hill & Sofuoglu, 2007). The most frequently used outcome measures are cocaine urine testing and treatment retention. Secondary outcome measures are craving, depressive symptoms, and various other self-reported measures.

Pharmacotherapy of cocaine dependence or misuse

Antidepressants

The rationale to use antidepressants as a treatment for stimulant addiction is the proposed downregulation of synaptic monoamine receptors. The downregulation is opposite to the upregulation of monoamine receptors caused by chronic stimulant use. A number of antidepressants including imipramine, desipramine, bupropion, and SSRIs have been studied as a treatment for cocaine dependence. A recent review concluded that there was no evidence supporting the clinical use of antidepressants in the treatment of cocaine dependence (de Lima et al., 2002) irrespective of treatment setting, co-existing opioid dependence, or comorbid depression. Two small studies attribute some effect to fluoxetine; some other studies attribute some effect to desipramine.

Because of high dropout rates, the idea of adding psychotherapy to medication treatment was suggested. A randomized clinical trial of desipramine and contingency management (CM) found that neither treatment alone significantly reduced cocaine abuse in buprenorphine-maintained cocaine abusers, but the combination of treatments showed efficacy in increasing cocaine-free urines (Kosten et al., 2003).

Dopamine agonists (amantadine, bromocriptine)

Reviews and meta-analyses conclude that dopamine agonists are not superior to placebo in reducing cocaine abuse or in improving retention, irrespective of treatment setting, comorbid opioid dependence, or alcohol abuse (Soares et al., 2002).

Disulfiram

A number of randomized controlled trials found disulfiram, at 250 mg/day, to be effective for the treatment of cocaine dependence, and the beneficial effects do not seem to be mediated through a decrease in alcohol use. Disulfiram has shown efficacy in cocaine users alone or users with concurrent alcohol abuse or dependence (Carroll et al., 1998), with increased retention and decreased cocaine use; and in methadone or buprenorphine-maintained opioid and cocaine-dependent subjects (Petrakis et al., 2000; George et al., 2000; Carroll et al., 2004).

Antiepileptics

Tiagabine, an antiseizure medication, at 24 mg/day (in twice daily dosing) was more effective than placebo in reducing cocaine use. Tiagabine may be a promising medication for cocaine dependence pharmacotherapy

(González et al., 2003). Topiramate, an antiseizure medication, at 200 mg/day, decreased cocaine use behaviour in a randomized controlled study.

Baclofen

Baclofen at 60 mg/day reduced cocaine use more than placebo, and was more effective in the subgroup of patients with greater cocaine use at baseline.

Adrenergic blockers

Cocaine activates the adrenergic system, which mediates the physiological responses to cocaine including an increase in heart rate, blood pressure, and arousal. In an RCT, propranolol, a non-selective beta-adrenergic blocker, led to better retention and greater drug-free urines than placebo in cocaine-dependent subjects (Kampman et al., 2001b); at 100 mg/day, propranolol was more effective than placebo only in those with severe cocaine withdrawal symptoms at baseline. Adrenergic blockers may be effective in attenuating some of the physiological effects of cocaine, especially in the subgroup with high cocaine withdrawal severity.

Other pharmacological data

Dexamphetamine was found to be better than placebo in increasing retention, though the results were not always consistent and positive. Naltrexone, when used in conjunction with relapse prevention, was associated with decreased cocaine use. Buspirone helped with the symptoms of withdrawal (but not treatment retention) from day 5 onwards in a 4-week study.

Pharmacotherapy of amphetamine dependence or misuse

A recent meta-analysis of studies with fluoxetine, imipramine, desipramine, and amlodipine concluded that none was effective in the treatment of amphetamine misuse and dependence (Srisurapanont et al., 2002); fluoxetine decreased craving at the start of the treatment.

Psychosocial treatments

Summarizing the role of psychosocial treatment in stimulant misuse is difficult given the large number of treatments and diversity of treatment populations, settings, and protocols. Some of these are summarized in Chapter 10. A recent meta-analysis grouped psychosocial treatments into three groups: supportive (counselling, relaxation, acupuncture, etc.), re-educative (CBT, drug counselling,

12-step approach, cue exposure, contingency management, community reinforcement approach, etc.), and re-constructive (dynamic therapy, family therapy, interpersonal psychotherapy, supportive-expressive therapy, etc.) and showed that (a) re-educative therapies marginally but significantly reduce cocaine use especially during the first 6 months of the intervention, and (b) re-constructive therapies increase treatment retention up to 1 year (Fridell, 2003).

Other approaches

In cocaine-dependent individuals, adding a *twelve-step-based drug counselling programme* was better than CBT or supportive–expressive therapy alone. The *community reinforcement approach* (CRA), a multimodal treatment comprising a mixture of relapse prevention, skills training, 12-step approach, and other interventions, was effective in cocaine dependence but not in methadone maintenance. The use of vouchers improved its effectiveness. There is no consensus on the efficacy of *acupuncture* in cocaine dependence.

Psychiatric comorbidity

In treatment-seeking cocaine users, major depression, bipolar disorder, post-traumatic stress disorder (PTSD) and phobias, ADHD, and antisocial personality are common comorbid psychiatric disorders that may increase the risk for drug use. Treatment adherence can also be more difficult in this comorbid group. Thus, a treatment plan needs to address both the stimulant addiction and the comorbid disorder. Guidelines for the pharmacotherapy of stimulant addiction and psychiatric comorbidity have not been developed.

Concomitant addictions

Opioid addiction

Cocaine use is especially common in individuals who are addicted to other drugs of abuse. In opioid users in methadone maintenance, cocaine use ranges from 30% to 80% (Grella et al., 1997). In opioid- and cocaine-dependent patients, treatment with methadone or buprenorphine alone does not reduce cocaine use. In opioid-dependent cocaine users, a combination of buprenorphine and desipramine reduced both opioid and cocaine use (Oliveto et al., 1999), and the anticonvulsant tiagabine, in combination with methadone, reduced cocaine and opioid use.

Alcohol addiction

Thirty percent of treatment-seeking cocaine users report alcoholism.

Table 11.1 Effectiveness of treatments for stimulant dependence

Treatment	Form of treatment	Psychiatric disorder/target audience	Level of evidence for efficacy	Comments
Pharmacotherapy	Antidepressant	Cocaine dependence	Ib	Score is lower here because most studies that have shown improvement have been difficult to replicate. Some evidence in small study for fluoxetine and imipramine but the evidence is very weak
Pharmacotherapy	Disulfiram	Cocaine dependence	Ia	Better retention in programme and better impact on decreasing cocaine usage
Pharmacotherapy	Dopamine agonists Amantadine, bromocriptine	Cocaine dependence	Ib	Amantadine may be better at retaining people in a treatment programme, especially in the short term, while bromocriptine may be better at reducing craving
Pharmacotherapy	Tiagabine Topiramate	Cocaine dependence	Ib	Appears to reduce cocaine usage and cocaine use behaviour
Pharmacotherapy	Baclofen	Cocaine dependence	Ib	Better than placebo
Pharmacotherapy	Adrenergic blockers	Cocaine dependence	Ib	Better than placebo (and may have some efficacy in cocaine + alcohol abuse)

	Treatment	Condition	Evidence	Description
Pharmacotherapy	Antidepressant (tricyclics, bupropion)	Cocaine dependence plus depression	IIa	Reduction of depressive symptoms and cocaine craving
Psychosocial treatment	Cognitive behavioural therapy	Cocaine dependence	Ia	Has been shown to be effective especially for reducing cocaine usage for the first 6 months, and better than a 12-step programme in achieving that goal. It may also be better than a 12-step approach in patients with comorbid depression
Psychosocial treatment	Contingency management	Cocaine dependence	Ib	Has been shown to be effective in initiating abstinence and to prevent relapse. It may be more effective than CBT in the initiation of abstinence phase of treatment
Psychosocial treatment	Individual 12-step counselling	Cocaine dependence	III	Probably has some impact when joined with group 12-step approach
Psychosocial treatment	Community reinforcement approach	Cocaine dependence	III	Effective in cocaine dependence but not in methadone maintenance. May be more effective when combined with CM
Combined treatment		Cocaine dependence	IIa	Only the combination showed significant improvement

Table 11.1 (cont.)

Treatment	Form of treatment	Psychiatric disorder/target audience	Level of evidence for efficacy	Comments
	Psychotherapy (contingency management) and pharmacotherapy (desipramine)			
Combined treatment	CBT and desipramine	Cocaine dependence and depression	III	Improved treatment retention and abstinence
Alternative treatment	Acupuncture	Cocaine dependence	IIa	Results are inconsistent. Probably good in a multimodal treatment but not as a stand-alone treatment

Concomitant alcohol use is a poor prognostic factor in stimulant users. Disulfiram at 250 mg/day has been shown to decrease both alcohol and cocaine use in these dual abusers (Carroll et al., 1998).

Summary and conclusion

Before treatment initiation, stimulant users require a comprehensive psychiatric, medical, and laboratory examination. Psychiatric comorbidity is common in stimulant users and needs to be addressed together with stimulant addiction. Stimulant users commonly use other drugs of abuse which can result in serious overdose and death. To date, no effective drugs are available for stimulant dependence, although progress has been made in the development of pharmacotherapies. Behavioural treatments aimed at maintaining drug abstinence and preventing relapse have shown favourable results and are essential components to assist adherence to pharmacotherapy. Interventions discussed in this chapter are summarized in Table 11.1.

Acknowledgement

Supported by the National Institute on Drug Abuse grants P50-DA12762 K05-DA0454 (TRK), R01-DA 14537, and K12 00167 (MS).

12

Treatment of opioid dependence

Based on "Treatment of opioid dependence" by Leslie L. Buckley, Nicholas Seivewright, Mark Parry, Abhijeetha Salvaji and Richard Schottenfeld in Effective Treatments in Psychiatry, Cambridge University Press, 2008

Introduction

Opioid dependence is characterized by relapse, increased mortality, significant medical morbidity, psychiatric sequelae, and impaired social function. Costs to families and society are secondary to impaired social and occupational functioning and increased criminal behaviour or violence. Opioid abuse and dependence can involve drugs obtained on the street or using opioid pain medications for non-medical purposes. Illicit drug use is generally more common in males, but the majority of new initiators of non-medically prescribed painkillers are females.

Clinical features

Opioids relieve pain and induce euphoria through agonist effects in activating CNS μ-receptors that result in opioid intoxication. Morphine, heroin, and methadone are full agonists; others (buprenorphine) are partial agonists. Compounds with high affinity but no efficacy for the receptor (naltrexone) are antagonists. Opioids vary in duration of action: heroin and morphine have a relatively short duration; maintenance medications, methadone, buprenorphine, naltrexone, have longer half-lives that allow increased stability and daily (or less frequent) dosing.

Disorders related to opioids are divided into substance-induced disorders (intoxication, withdrawal, and other manifestations of acute intake or withdrawal) and substance use disorders. Opioid use results in initial euphoria or "rush" with warm flushing of the skin and heaviness in the extremities; nausea is common especially among first-timers. Acute euphoria may be followed by a longer less intense period of tranquillity, euphoria, apathy, or dysphoria. Tolerance (little or no euphoria) develops with repeated chronic use.

Opioid withdrawal syndrome includes dysphoric or anxious mood; nausea, vomiting, diarrhoea or stomach cramps; muscle aches; lacrimation, rhinorrhea, pupillary dilation, piloerection; mild tachycardia and hypertension; sweating, yawning, fever, chills, and insomnia accompanied by strong opioid cravings. Withdrawal from shorter-acting opioids (heroin) begins 6–8 hours after the last dose, peaks within 2–3 days, and usually subsides within 5–10 days. Insomnia, restlessness, and dysphoria may persist for months. Longer-acting opioids can delay withdrawal onset for several days.

Opioid overdose is a medical emergency. The opioid antagonist, naloxone, should be administered to treat overdose.

The psychological and physical effects of opioids depend upon the opioid used, rapidity of onset and intensity of the opioid's effect, route of administration, and the individual's use history. As tolerance develops, continued use is maintained not for positive effects but to avoid extremely aversive withdrawal. After a withdrawal period, opioid tolerance is decreased, and there is significant overdose risk in resuming high doses used before withdrawal.

Evidence-based treatments for opioid dependence

Various strategies are used to treat those with opioid dependency. Pharmacological interventions include medically assisted withdrawal (MAW), medications to minimize withdrawal symptoms, antagonists to block acute opioid effects, and opioid agonist maintenance treatment with long-acting opioid agonists or partial agonists to prevent withdrawal and, at higher doses, decrease craving. Psychotherapeutic treatments, twelve-step approaches and psychosocial interventions are important comprehensive treatment components.

It is important to define successful treatment and prioritize short- and long-term treatment goals since opioid dependence is chronic, with alternating abstinence and frequent relapse. Ultra-rapid successful withdrawal, if followed by relapse a week later, may have greater risk (drug overdose) than benefit. Interventions should prioritize decreased mortality risk and prevention of transmission of chronic infectious diseases and other medical complications. Other goals include sustained remission from opioids, improved psychosocial functioning including employment, and decreased criminal behaviour.

Medically assisted withdrawal

Through medically assisted withdrawal (MAW), the opioid-dependent patient is provided with pharmacological relief of withdrawal symptoms often through substitution of a longer-acting opioid agonist (methadone) or partial agonist (buprenorphine) followed by gradual tapering, or through pharmacological treatment to reduce autonomic withdrawal symptoms (clonidine, lofexidine). Other pharmacological treatments reduce nausea, gastrointestinal symptoms, muscle pains, and sleep disturbance during withdrawal. Antagonist-precipitated withdrawal symptoms treated by clonidine and others may shorten withdrawal and facilitate initiation of antagonist maintenance treatment. The process is complete after discontinuation of all opioids without withdrawal symptoms in the absence of medications used to treat withdrawal symptoms. Successful completion of withdrawal is confirmed by lack of precipitated withdrawal in response to intramuscular naloxone and oral naltrexone. The time from opioid discontinuation to symptom-free toleration of oral naltrexone depends on whether long- or short-acting opioids are being discontinued. In healthy adults untreated withdrawal is not life-threatening but is extremely unpleasant and can lead to relapse.

Complications of MAW include suicide secondary to withdrawal-induced anxiety and dysphoria, spontaneous abortion, medical complications, and post-withdrawal overdose after relapse. Patients need information about risks and benefits of MAW and alternative treatments. MAW should be accompanied by support and counselling on relapse prevention and ongoing drug abuse treatment (drug counselling, family therapy, and naltrexone maintenance treatment).

Methadone in MAW

Methadone, a long-acting, full μ-opioid receptor, used in progressively decreasing doses, reduces symptoms of withdrawal during MAW.

Buprenorphine in MAW

Buprenorphine, a unique opioid, a partial agonist with very high affinity at the μ-opioid receptor, can reduce or prevent symptoms of withdrawal. Because it displaces full μ-receptor agonists, it can also cause withdrawal symptoms in patients with high physical dependence (maintained at daily doses > 40–50 mg of methadone). To minimize precipitated withdrawal, buprenorphine should not be administered to patients receiving > 40 mg methadone daily and should only be given when withdrawal symptoms are present. Slow dissociation from the μ-receptor allows self-tapering and milder (though sometimes more prolonged) withdrawal.

Pharmacological treatments for withdrawal symptoms

Clonidine and lofexidine

These α_2-adrenergic agonists treat symptoms of opioid withdrawal by alleviating autonomic symptoms of withdrawal. Clonidine, used for hypertension, is often combined with medications to reduce muscle pains and cramps, diarrhoea, anxiety, insomnia, and nausea. Blood pressure and heart rate should be monitored; caution should be taken for orthostatic hypotension. Lofexidine, not approved in the USA but with RCTs supporting effectiveness, has no effect on blood pressure and less sedative effect than clonidine (Carnwath and Hardman, 1998).

Antagonists in MAW

Naltrexone

Naltrexone, with high affinity for blocking the μ-opioid receptor (where it is inactive and dissociates slowly from it), can precipitate severe prolonged withdrawal symptoms. There is little evidence that naltrexone in MAW results in superior abstinence rates or retention in treatment (O'Connor & Kosten, 1998). Three-day pretreatment with buprenorphine prior to naltrexone-precipitated withdrawal can decrease withdrawal symptom severity. Limited evidence supports ultra-rapid MAW using naltrexone under general anaesthesia or conscious sedation.

Opioid antagonist treatment (of dependence)

Opioid antagonists treat opioid dependence by reversing an opioid overdose or and preventing relapse by blocking opioid effects at opioid receptors.

Naloxone

Naloxone, a short-acting rapidly metabolized opioid antagonist reverses opioid overdose effects in emergencies. Naloxone, which is not well-absorbed sublingually or orally, is combined with buprenorphine in a combination tablet (Suboxone) to prevent injection misuse of buprenorphine. Naloxone (0.8 mg IM) can confirm physiological opioid dependence in individuals seeking maintenance treatment or MAW and verify withdrawal completion prior to initiating naltrexone.

Naltrexone maintenance treatment

Naltrexone, a long-acting opioid antagonist, blocks opioid effects by competitively occupying but not activating opioid receptors. Side effects include nausea, headache, dizziness, nervousness, and fatigue. Naltrexone abstinence-based treatment is initiated only on complete withdrawal from opioids. Its helps to reduce extremely high MAW relapse (Kirchmayer et al., 2002). Combining naltrexone treatment with psychotherapy improves outcomes (Carroll et al., 2001).

The most frequent indication for naltrexone maintenance is in milder dependence with social support where detoxification is easy and motivation to remain opioid-free is high. Outside of academic research centres formal naltrexone treatment programmes are rare.

Opioid agonist maintenance treatment

Results and meta-analyses of clinical trials consistently support the effectiveness of opioid agonist maintenance treatment for reducing illicit opioid use, mortality, medical morbidity (including HIV), criminal activity associated with dependence, and improving psychosocial functioning (Farre et al., 2002; Mattick et al., 2002a; 2002b). The patient is stabilized on long-acting, orally available, medically prescribed opioid agonists or partial agonists that prevent withdrawal symptoms and, with sufficient doses allowing for cross-tolerance, reduces craving and blocks or reduces the acute rewarding effects of illicit opioid use. It facilitates behavioural monitoring for illicit use, psychosocial/behavioural treatments, and lifestyle change necessary for longer-term abstinence and recovery. Drug counselling during opioid agonist maintenance treatment enhances outcome.

Methadone, the first US medication for maintenance treatment, remains the most commonly used agonist in the USA, UK, and Europe. Buprenorphine and LAAM (L-α-acetylmethadol) are currently FDA-approved for maintenance treatment in the USA, though LAAM, a methadone derivative, is no longer marketed in the USA or approved for use in the EU. Buprenorphine, more recently approved, is generally comparable in outcome to methadone (Ling et al., 1996; Johnson et al., 2000; West et al., 2000).

Methadone maintenance treatment (MMT)

Methadone, a full μ-opioid receptor agonist used since the mid-1960s, is repeatedly documented as an effective opioid dependence treatment. Its average half-life of approximately 24 hours allows for once-daily dosing. Numerous medications (e.g. antiretrovirals, antidepressants, anticonvulsants, and antibiotics) interact with methadone metabolism, decreasing methadone levels and inducing withdrawal symptoms or increasing methadone levels, potentially putting patients at risk of side effects or death. MMT, initiated at low dose (up to 30 mg daily) sufficient to prevent or ameliorate withdrawal symptoms, is gradually increased over several weeks to a dose sufficient to reduce craving and illicit opioid use. Higher doses (60–100 mg) are associated with better treatment retention rates and decreased illicit drug use (Johnson et al., 2000; Faggiano et al., 2003). In MMT, there is a risk of death from overdose related to excessive initial doses or too rapid and excessive dose increases, especially during the first 1–2 weeks of treatment.

Because of potential lethality and high risk of abuse (methadone has street value), MMT in the USA is controlled and delivered in specialized clinics which provide counselling and may offer medical, social work, legal, or vocational services.

Buprenorphine maintenance treatment

Buprenorphine, a partial μ-receptor agonist, has mixed properties that confer greater safety in overdose, less interaction with other euphoriant drugs, and quicker transfer to naltrexone after detoxification. The partial agonist profile makes detoxification more attractive and less problematic than with methadone (Kosten, 2003).

RCTs performed in the USA (Johnson et al., 1995) and in Europe (Petitjean et al., 2001; Kakko et al., 2003) and meta-analyses of comparisons with methadone (West et al., 2000) find broadly equivalent overall results with reduced illicit drug use, injecting, and associated problems. The clinician should wait until there are withdrawal signs before initiating treatment because buprenorphine may precipitate withdrawal symptoms through displacing opioid-occupied opioid receptors. Buprenorphine is generally well tolerated with a dose-dependent ceiling effect resulting in decreased risk of adverse events such as respiratory depression. Higher daily doses (12–16 mg) are more effective than lower doses (4–8 mg) (Ling et al., 1996; Schottenfeld et al., 1997). Buprenorphine is mainly prescribed in tablet form; there is significant abuse risk by injection.

Buprenorphine, an alternative to methadone, may be preferable where slow reduction or detoxification is desired especially in individuals with moderate degrees of dependence. Severely dependent individuals may require a more potent opioid, usually methadone.

Diamorphine

Diamorphine is essentially heroin. In the UK where it can be prescribed in the 'British system' of drug treatment, it is used in a small minority of treatment-resistant patients.

Office-based care

Until recently, US MMT has been delivered through specially licensed

treatment programmes ensuring procedures that decrease the likelihood
of diversion for illicit use. Recent
evaluations support the feasibility of
office-based medical maintenance
with efficacy comparable to specialized programmes (King et al., 2002).

Psychosocial treatment in agonist maintenance

Management of opioid dependence
involves pharmacological treatments
to a greater extent than in some other
forms of drug misuse where psychosocial interventions may be the only strategies. Counselling here is adjunctive
(O'Malley et al., 1972), but prescribing
in isolation can be dangerous. Combined pharmacological and psychological treatment appears to optimize
outcomes.

Cognitive behavioural therapy (CBT)
and supportive–expressive therapy
(SE) appeared superior to standard
drug counselling (DC) in methadone
patients, especially in patients with
psychiatric comorbidity (Woody et al.,
1983). Motivational interviewing
achieves reduced opioid-related problems, better treatment compliance,
and improved retention than MMT
alone (Saunders et al., 1995). Network
therapy, recruiting family members
and friends to assist in treatment
compliance, increases negative urine
screens (Galanter et al., 2004).
Twelve-step programmes, Narcotics

or Methadone Anonymous, also provide assistance.

More intense treatments such as
day programmes (Ravndal, 2001)
have not proven more effective than
less intensive weekly counselling. The
UK NTORS study of long-term non-
pharmacological modalities (Gossop
et al., 2001) found that all treatments
markedly reduced opioid and benzodiazepine use and injecting. MMT
and residential rehabilitation were
remarkably similar at 1-year and
4–5-year follow-up. An RCT involving
three different levels of psychosocial
support in MMT – minimal treatment, MMT with standard drug counselling, and MMT with standard drug
counselling plus additional vocation,
legal and medical services – found
significant outcome improvement
with each additional intervention
(McLellan et al., 1993).

Treatment in pregnancy

The use of illicit opioids during pregnancy is associated with risks to the
mother and foetus and upon delivery,
to the neonate, who may experience
withdrawal symptoms. Comprehensive
MMT, including coordinated medical
and psychosocial services, reduces epi-
sodic withdrawal and improves the
health status and well-being of the
woman and foetus. Buprenorphine
appears to be safe in pregnancy
(Lacroix et al., 2004) but is not yet

Table 12.1 Effectiveness of treatments for opioid dependence

Treatment	Form of treatment	Psychiatric disorder/target audience	Level of evidence for efficacy	Comments
Psychopharmacology	Alpha$_2$ adrenergic agonists	Medically assisted opiate withdrawal	Ib	Clonidine and lofexidine can both help relieve some of the more unpleasant autonomic side effects. Lofexidine has less hypotension and sedation than clonidine. They do not relieve symptoms of insomnia, restlessness, nausea, lacrimination, rhinorrhea, or nausea
Psychopharmacology	Naltrexone	Opioid antagonist (maintenance) treatment	IIb	Little effect as measured by retention rates in people with little motivation to cease use. Those with high motivation (executive, professionals, probationers) have much higher retention and success rates. Improvement in retention can occur when accompanied by psychosocial interventions
Psychopharmacology	Methadone	Opioid agonist (maintenance) treatment	Ia	Effective in reducing drug usage, decreasing morbidity and mortality from the drug usage, decreases criminal activity, and increases social functioning

Table 12.1 (cont.)

Treatment	Form of treatment	Psychiatric disorder/target audience	Level of evidence for efficacy	Comments
Psychopharmacology	Buprenorphine	Opioid agonist (maintenance) treatment	Ia	Effective as methadone in reducing drug usage, decreasing morbidity and mortality from the drug usage, decreases criminal activity, and increases social functioning. It may be easier to dose than methadone and may have a greater early retention rate
Psychopharmacology	Diamorphine	Opioid agonist (maintenance) treatment	Ia	Not available in USA. Major problem is that it perpetuates the idea of injecting something rather than changing the person to an oral form of maintenance
Psychosocial and maintenance	Standard treatment versus standard treatment plus CBT versus standard treatment plus supportive–expressive therapy	Opioid dependence maintenance treatment	IIb	Psychosocial treatments by themselves are ineffective, but with psychopharmacological treatment, the addition of other psychosocial interventions to standard treatment enhances outcome. Supportive–expressive and CBT did equally well

Psychosocial and maintenance	Motivational interviewing plus methadone maintenance	Opioid dependence maintenance treatment	Ib	Motivational intervention revealed reduced opioid-related problems, better compliance with treatment, and improved retention
Psychosocial and maintenance	Enhanced services plus methadone maintenance	Opioid dependence maintenance treatment	Ib	Comparing methadone alone, methadone plus standard drug counselling, and methadone plus standard drug counselling plus enhanced services (vocational, medical, legal), the methadone maintenance alone did most poorly with the enhanced services doing the best
Psychosocial and maintenance	Contingency management or community reinforcement plus methadone maintenance	Opioid dependence maintenance treatment	IIa	Some evidence for effectiveness, but evidence not as strong as it is for alcohol or cocaine dependence

approved for use in pregnancy in the USA. Neonatal withdrawal is less marked than after MMT.

Conclusion

Methadone maintenance remains the most thoroughly studied and documented effective treatment. Buprenorphine studies are encouraging, and office-based care reveals potential for enhanced safety and increased access to agonist maintenance. Opioid antagonists are effective for selected groups, while combined antagonist maintenance and psychotherapeutic approaches show promise. MAW provides less uncomfortable withdrawal and an opportunity to encourage ongoing treatment involvement and decreased relapse. Interventions discussed in this chapter are summarized in Table 12.1.

13

Treatment of sedative–hypnotic dependence

Based on "Treatment of sedative–hypnotic dependence" by Karim Dar and Manoj Kumar in Effective Treatments in Psychiatry, Cambridge University Press, 2008

Introduction

The sedative–hypnotic drugs discussed here all facilitate GABA transmission (as does alcohol). In lower doses they reduce anxiety and in larger ones induce drowsiness and sleep. The common drugs are benzodiazepines, Z-drugs (zopiclone, zolpidem, and zaleplon), and barbiturates. There are more similarities than differences between them. Barbiturates were popular between 1910 and 1960, benzodiazepines from the 1960s through the 1990s (though still very commonly used), and Z-drugs in the last 20 years. The change in preferred drug group has largely been a consequence of

concerns over dependence and, to a lesser extent, adverse effects, that are perceived to be less with each succeeding class.

Dependence on these drugs is not always easy to identify. Some people show classical addiction (dependence) syndromes (prominent drug-seeking behaviour, marked tolerance to the drug's effects, and dramatic withdrawal syndromes including epileptic seizures) that tend to be manifest when patients take doses well above those recommended therapeutically. 'Low-dose dependence' refers to withdrawal problems after stopping medication in those who have been taking these drugs consistently in therapeutic dosages (Hawley et al., 1994). The distinction between anxiety symptoms and those of withdrawal syndromes is difficult as these overlap. However, there are differences. In withdrawal syndromes there are varying degrees of hyperexcitability of voluntary musculature and hyperacuity of sensation leading to muscle twitching, aches and pains, hypersensitivity to light, smell and sounds, a metallic taste in one's mouth, and, rarely, convulsions (Tyrer et al., 1990).

Benzodiazepine dependence

Pharmacological treatments

There are several approaches to the treatment of benzodiazepine dependence:

- Gradual tapering doses of the drug creating dependence.
- Substitution of short-acting benzodiazepines with a longer-acting benzodiazepine, which is then reduced over a period of weeks.
- Substitution by other drugs with less dependence followed by gradual reduction.
- Direct treatment of withdrawal symptoms.

Gradual reduction of benzodiazepines

Gradual reduction of benzodiazepines, the most commonly used detoxification method for benzodiazepine dependence, with or without cognitive behavioural therapy, has been shown to increase successful withdrawal rates in several studies (Murphy & Tyrer, 1991; Oude-Voshaar et al., 2003). A recent systematic review found that only gradual reduction (tapering) was an unequivocally effective strategy (Oude-Voshaar et al., 2006b). Discontinuation schedules vary widely from a 7-day schedule to discontinuation over many years. Short-term withdrawal over 7 days or less has been reported to be successful in some studies (Rickels et al., 1990). Blinded tapering of dose with gradual substitution of placebo plus psychological support over 8–9 weeks was successful (Curran et al., 2003). Although there is little evidence for choosing inpatient over outpatient treatment for most patients, inpatients are more likely to complete the detoxification regimen and dosage reductions may be more rapid. Gradual reduction/withdrawal strategies can be employed equally successfully in sedative–hypnotic tolerant patients with phenobarbital as well as with benzodiazepines (Perry et al., 1981). There is no clear optimal rate or duration of reduction.

Gradual discontinuation programmes succeed in two-thirds of patients and can be combined with additional pharmacological or psychological treatment (Oude-Voshaar et al., 2006a), although a systematic review shows no strong support for any specific adjunctive therapies (Oude-Voshaar et al., 2006b). Most studies have methodological problems: small numbers of subjects, lack of randomization, and blinding. There is limited data on long-term outcome of benzodiazepine withdrawal, but some degree of relapse is common (Zitman & Couvée, 2001). Discontinuation may be particularly difficult in patients with personality disorder, comorbid mental or physical illness, or multiple drug use. Inpatient detoxification is useful for complex dependence. Patients need support through and after the withdrawal period. A recent Cochrane Review (Denis et al., 2006a) concluded that "all included studies agreed that gradual taper was preferable to abrupt discontinuation". A meta-analysis (Parr et al., 2008) reported that "gradual dose reduction (OR = 5.96; CI = 2.08–17.11) provided superior cessation rates at post-treatment to routine care".

Substitution and tapering with barbiturates

Another method for treating benzodiazepine dependence is substitution with phenobarbitone and then instituting a gradual stepwise reduction in dose (Smith & Wesson, 1985). This method is rarely used in the UK or Europe though not uncommon in the USA. There are no RCTs examining efficacy and outcomes. This method is not recommended currently for routine treatment and should be restricted to inpatient settings with those on high benzodiazepine doses.

Substitution and tapering with carbamazepine

Though initially thought to be of value, carbamazepine is seldom if ever used to treat benzodiazepine dependence in Europe. A randomized, placebo-controlled trial found no significant differences from placebo in withdrawal symptom severity or in 12-week post-withdrawal outcomes (Schweizer et al., 1991). Patients taking more than 20 mg diazepam-equivalent appeared to derive benefit. Carbamazepine can offer some anticonvulsant cover for those with an epilepsy history. Recent UK guidelines suggest that carbamazepine may be used instead of benzodiazepines to control withdrawal symptoms from high doses of benzodiazepines (Lingford-Hughes, 2004), but probably should be reserved for carefully selected people with dependence on very high doses of benzodiazepines and an epilepsy history.

Additional pharmacological treatment

Parr et al.'s (2008) review comparing gradual dose reduction (GDR) alone versus GDR plus substitutive pharmacotherapy found that only 3 of 17 studies using substitutive pharmacotherapy demonstrated greater cessation rates at post-treatment; and no studies showed superiority from substitutive pharmacotherapy at follow-up. They concluded that at present "current evidence is insufficient to support the prescription of adjunctive pharmacotherapy".

Maintenance treatments

Maintenance prescribing of benzodiazepines occurs mostly in specialist methadone maintenance clinics in the UK. Preliminary open studies suggest that maintenance prescribing reduced other benzodiazepine use; no controlled trials are published to support this treatment and current expert opinion (Department of Health, 2003a; Lingford-Hughes, 2004) does not support this, and it is best avoided due to overdose risks, injecting, and diversion. For those who take benzodiazepines by mouth in therapeutic dosage, it has been suggested that continuation of the drug is a perfectly acceptable alternative to frequent attempts to promote withdrawal and there are data to support this (Liebrenz et al., 2010).

Z-drugs dependence

Annual prescriptions for the Z-drugs, zaleplon, zolpidem and zopiclone, a class of drugs heavily promoted in US direct-to-consumer advertising, are rising (Department of Health,

2003a). Prescribers may believe that changing to a Z-drug can avoid problems associated with regular hypnotic use though little data support this.

Dependence on Z-drugs is a recognized risk for some patients. Its incidence may be increasing (National Institute for Clinical Excellence, 2004). The misuse is characterized by significant dose escalation and withdrawal symptoms. Patients with a history of drug or alcohol misuse or other psychiatric disorder are most vulnerable though others are as well (Hajak et al., 2003). There is little data on the frequency of withdrawal symptoms associated with these drugs especially compared to the benzodiazepines.

Since there are as yet no published studies on treating Z-drug dependence, prevention is probably the best form of treatment. Normal criteria for benzodiazepine prescriptions should be applied when prescribing non-benzodiazepine sedatives and hypnotics, as they act upon the same receptor, the benzodiazepine–GABA–chloride complex. The same caution as with benzodiazepines should be taken when considering the prescription of Z-drugs to at-risk populations, those with drug abuse/dependence or psychiatric illness histories (Hajak et al., 2003). Z-drugs should be used cautiously for short-term treatment of insomnia because of this potential risk of dependence. It is assumed that gradual withdrawal would be as useful as with the benzodiazepines.

Barbiturate dependence

Currently use and abuse of barbiturates is seen infrequently. There have been no RCTs in the last decade evaluating treatment for barbiturate dependence. Published literature from the early 1970s has serious methodological problems. Smith and Wesson (1971) developed a protocol that used phenobarbital substitution, stabilization, and tapering to treat barbiturate dependence, a technique still considered to be the "gold standard". More recently Robinson et al. (1981) successfully used repeated oral loading doses of phenobarbital, titrating doses against symptoms, for barbiturate withdrawal. Substitution of barbiturates with diazepam has been successful (Perry et al., 1981). The major clinical concern with barbiturate withdrawal is to prevent grand mal seizures and toxic confusional states. Though evidence is very limited, a gradual withdrawal, preferably on an inpatient basis, with substitution and tapering with a long-acting barbiturate such as phenobarbitone, appears the safest option.

Psychological treatments

Certain psychological interventions, particularly CBT strategies focusing on anxiety management, have been thought useful in benzodiazepine dependence and withdrawal treatment (Tyrer et al., 1985; Sanchez-Craig et al., 1987), but there are no studies examining psychological interventions for barbiturate or Z-drug dependence.

Two RCTs involving participants who met the criteria for panic disorder utilizing the CBT approach in combination with slow tapering of benzodiazepines demonstrated efficacy (13/17; 76% successfully discontinued) over similar tapering regimens with supportive medical management (4/16; 25% discontinued) (Otto et al., 1993) (77% of the CBT patients remained benzodiazepine free at 3-month follow-up).

In a 3-month RCT in a general practice setting, 180 people attempting to discontinue long-term benzodiazepine use were assigned to taper plus CBT or taper alone plus usual care. Tapering alone led to a significantly higher proportion of successful discontinuations (62% vs. 21%); adding CBT did not increase the success rate (58% vs. 62%) and was thought to be of limited value (Oude-Voshaar et al., 2003). Other studies also failed to find that CBT added efficacy (Sanchez-Craig et al., 1987; Spiegel et al., 1994). But a randomized comparison study (a combination of group CBT and benzodiazepine tapering versus gradual tapering only over an 8-week period) involving participants aged over 65 years found more success for complete withdrawal in the combined treatment (77% versus 38%), this favourable outcome persisting at 12 months (70% versus 24%) (Baillargeon et al., 2003).

Thus there is no reliable evidence for psychological treatment as a stand-alone treatment method. Most studies have significant methodological shortcomings. The recent BAP guidelines (Lingford-Hughes, 2004) and a systematic review (Oude-Voshaar et al., 2006b) conclude that additional psychological therapies do not appear to increase the effectiveness of graded discontinuation from benzodiazepines but should be considered on their own merits. A more recent systematic review (Parr et al., 2008) which included seven studies with 454 participants compared psychological interventions and GDR with GDR alone. Psychological treatment plus GDR were superior to both routine care (OR = 3.38; CI = 1.86–6.12) and GDR alone (OR = 1.82; CI = 1.25–2.67). The authors concluded that "psychological interventions may provide a small but significant additional benefit over GDR alone at post-cessation and at follow-up".

In the Parr et al. (2008) meta-analysis common elements found in psychological interventions were relaxation training, CBT for insomnia, and in the case of multicomponent programmes, self-monitoring of consumption and symptoms, goal setting, management of withdrawal and coping with anxiety. These interventions therefore include aspects both to assist participants to deal with withdrawal symptoms and to address symptoms that triggered the person's prescription of benzodiazepines initially. It would therefore be critical to consider incorporating these elements in treatment regimens.

Minimal interventions

Minimal interventions include advisory letters, provision of other information, single consultation with a GP, and short courses of relaxation. Books written for patients are also available (Tyrer, 1986). An RCT found that a letter from the GP suggesting a reduction in benzodiazepine use reduced dosages by 50% with about 20% of patients stopping altogether (Heather et al., 2004). In another recent trial with 284 patients on long-term benzodiazepines, 39% of those receiving either of two brief

Table 13.1 Effectiveness of treatments for sedative–hypnotic dependence

Treatment	Form of treatment	Psychiatric disorder/target audience	Level of evidence for efficacy	Comments
Gradual withdrawal (with or without switching to a longer-acting benzodiazepine)	Gradual reduction with longer-acting benzodiazepines. NB. In practice diazepam is often used for this purpose as in chronic doses its major long-acting metabolite (nordiazepam) is the active ingredient and the range of doses (10 mg, 5 mg, & 2 mg) for this drug is a practical advantage	Benzodiazepine dependence	Ia	Support for gradual dose reduction exists. Little support for additional adjunctive pharmacotherapy during gradual dose reduction
Phenobarbitone substitution	Gradual reduction after phenobarbitone substitution	Benzodiazepine dependence	III	Limited to occasional use with inpatients on high doses of benzodiazepines
Carbamazepine substitution	Carbamazepine	Benzodiazepine dependence	IIb	Despite some shortcomings, this is a frequently recommended form of treatment, though little is known about its long-term impact

Table 13.1 (cont.)

Treatment	Form of treatment	Psychiatric disorder/target audience	Level of evidence for efficacy	Comments
Psychological treatment	CBT and other forms of behavioural therapy	Benzodiazepine dependence	III	Little evidence for the effectiveness of this treatment as a stand-alone intervention but may be somewhat helpful as an adjunct to other pharmacological treatments
Antidepressant substitution	Tricyclic antidepressant substitution/SSRI	Benzodiazepine dependence	III	Minimal evidence of efficacy and acceptability
Brief psychological interventions and bibliotherapy	Non-specialized interventions using small resources	All tranquillizer dependence	II	Is probably more valuable than formal CBT and similar approaches and appears to have a small but significant benefit

interventions (a short consultation or a letter from their GP advising gradual reduction in benzodiazepine intake) achieved at least a 25% reduction in their benzodiazepine use, though 24% of a control group randomized to "usual GP care" also reduced benzodiazepine use by at least 25%. A minimal intervention in the form of brief advice from the GP supplemented by a self-help booklet compared with a control group who received "routine" care resulted in 18% of the intervention group versus 5% in the control group reducing usage. At 6-months follow-up, 43% in the intervention group versus 20% in the control group reported reduced benzodiazepine usage. More subjects (20% versus 7%) in the intervention group stopped benzodiazepines completely (Bashir et al., 1994).

Though these studies excluded several categories of patients, such as psychiatric illness, poly-substance misusers, etc., the cumulative findings demonstrate that in selected patients, an appreciable success rate of close to 20% with fairly simple interventions can be achieved even after many years of benzodiazepine use. Furthermore, they are cost-effective. Parr et al. (2008) carried out a meta-analysis of three studies (n=532) and reported that brief interventions to cease benzodiazepine use were more effective than routine care or not raising the issue at all (OR = 4.37; CI = 2.28–8.40).

Alternative treatments

There is a general lack of research in the literature on the role and efficacy of alternative treatments in addictive disorders.

Summary and conclusion

Treatment of tranquillizer dependence is not especially satisfactory. Only gradual withdrawal, often using a different benzodiazepine over a variable time scale, shows satisfactory efficacy. Other forms of pharmacological substitution have limited value. Interventions discussed in this chapter are summarized in Table 13.1.

14

Treatment of cannabis dependence

Based on "Treatment of cannabis dependence" by Brent A. Moore,
Henrietta Bowden-Jones, Alan J. Budney and Ryan Vandrey in Effective Treatments
in Psychiatry, Cambridge University Press, 2008

Introduction

Cannabis use remains the most prevalent form of illicit drug use in English speaking countries and the European Union. Population rates of cannabis use have been found to be highest in New Zealand (20%) and Australia (17%), lower in the USA (11%) and Canada (7%), and range from 2% (Finland) to 11% (UK) across the European Union, with rates higher among young adult populations (SAMHSA, 2002; European Monitoring Centres for Drugs and Drug Addiction, 2003). The World Health Organization estimates that 2.45% of the world uses cannabis regularly or, to put it in perspective, 141 million people. Cannabis is second only to alcohol as a factor in fatal road accidents (10% in the UK) because cannabis impairs psychomotor performance. In the UK, reclassification of cannabis into a class C drug has worried some that the change would have people believe that it is less harmful than previously thought. This possible misconception is unfortunate because research has shown that an increased perception of the risks of cannabis is strongly correlated with decreased rates of use over time (Johnston et al., 2002).

Almost all users smoke either marijuana cigarettes ('joints') or use pipes to smoke marijuana or hashish. Problems associated with regular cannabis use include: impairment in memory (including difficulty in recalling previously learnt items), concentration, motivation, health, interpersonal relationships, and employment. In addition, there is lower participation in conventional adult roles, more history of psychiatric symptoms and hospitalizations, and greater participation in deviant activities (Budney et al., 2003). Physical health problems include respiratory complications and pulmonary damage secondary to chronic smoking.

There has been little empirical research into treatment for cannabis dependency. There are so few randomized controls that no meta-analyses are found in the Cochrane database, although the database now includes a systematic review of the few trials conducted (Denis et al., 2006b).

Cannabis withdrawal

Compared to the dramatic medical and physiological symptoms associated with severe opioid, sedative, or alcohol withdrawal, cannabis withdrawal was considered most likely to have little clinical significance. Research on tobacco identified a reliable and clinically meaningful withdrawal syndrome less dramatic than with other drugs of abuse and the discovery of the endogenous

cannabinoid system indicated that a neurobiological basis for cannabis dependence existed. A valid and reliable cannabinoid withdrawal syndrome characterized by symptoms of anger or aggression, decreased appetite or weight loss, irritability, nervousness, restlessness, sleep difficulty, and less common symptoms of chills, depressed mood, stomach pain, shakiness, and sweating has been documented (Haney et al., 1999; Budney et al., 2004). These appear similar to nicotine withdrawal (Vandrey et al., 2005). Cannabinoid withdrawal has been directly linked to the CB1 receptor in the endogenous cannabinoid system and is pharmacologically specific to the active component in cannabis, tetrahydrocannabidol (THC). Oral THC can alleviate cannabis withdrawal symptoms (Budney et al., 2007).

Reduction in DA activity in brain reward systems appears to be associated with similar characteristics of withdrawal for cannabis as it is with other drugs of abuse such as cocaine, opiates, amphetamines, nicotine, and alcohol. Reduction of this DA activity is a possible explanation of the chronic and persistent dysphoric symptoms of protracted withdrawal (George et al., 1998). Attempts to escape from the dysphoric moods and irritability may be associated with relapse.

Cannabis dependence

Strong evidence from epidemiology, basic neurobiology, animal research, and human laboratory and clinical studies indicates that cannabis can and does lead to a dependence syndrome similar to that with other drugs of abuse (Budney & Moore, 2002). In the USA, approximately 12 million individuals have at some point in their lives met diagnostic criteria for cannabis dependence (SAMSHA, 2002). Dependence rates increase substantially with more frequent use from approximately 20% for individuals who report using cannabis at least five times in the past year to more than 70% for almost daily users (Coffey et al., 2002). The percentage of people reporting chronic use and rates of initiation of use among youth and young adults have increased over the last decade accompanied by a decreased perception of the risk of regular cannabis use by youth over this same time period (Johnston et al., 2002).

Cannabis-dependent individuals seeking treatment generally have long histories of regular use (average more than 10 years), use cannabis daily, and have a range of use-related psychosocial problems (Budney et al., 1998). Most commonly reported problems are: feeling bad/guilty about their use, procrastination, low productivity, low self-confidence, interpersonal/family problems, memory problems, and financial difficulties. Cannabis-dependent individuals report repeated unsuccessful attempts to stop using and perceive that they are unable to quit. Approximately 50 to 70% of cannabis-dependent users also use tobacco (Moore & Budney, 2001), creating additional risk of respiratory and other health problems (See Chapter 15). Tobacco use is associated with increased psychosocial problems and poorer treatment response among cannabis-dependent people (Moore & Budney, 2001).

When compared with cocaine-dependent outpatients, cannabis-dependent people have similar types of problems, but cannabis abusers generally reveal a less severe dependence syndrome. Cocaine-dependent people endorse greater polydrug abuse and more employment difficulties. Otherwise, few between-group differences are observed (including demographics) (Budney et al., 1998). Though cannabis-dependent people rarely show the same crises that other drug-dependent people display, they do reveal psychosocial impairment that warrants clinical attention.

The number of individuals who seek treatment for cannabis abuse at registered treatment agencies has doubled since the early nineties (SAMSHA, 2002). Approximately

15% present with cannabis as the primary abused drug, a proportion similar to heroin (18%) and cocaine (13%). Australia and Europe have also seen similar increases in individuals seeking cannabis abuse treatment with the rate in Australia second only to alcohol (Australian Institute of Health and Welfare, 2003; European Monitoring Centres for Drugs and Drug Addiction, 2003).

Behavioural interventions (see Chapter 10)

Behavioural interventions have demonstrated efficacy with cannabis abusing populations (Denis et al., 2006b). The first randomized controlled trial revealed no significant differences between the treatments, a 10-week group therapy, social support or cognitive behavioural therapy (CBT), and relapse prevention. A second study with increased numbers of CBT sessions found no differences between active treatments, but treatments were more efficacious than a waiting list (Stephens et al., 2000). McCambridge and Strang (2004) found that a single session of motivational interviewing (MI) decreased cannabis use frequency by 66% vs. 27% for controls. At 3 months, 16% of the intervention group but only 5% of controls had discontinued cannabis use. "Intention to stop" was a strong predictor of ultimate success.

Those receiving MI were 3.5 times more likely to make the decision to stop. Additional studies comparing brief interventions to longer treatments indicate that more treatment (1 session vs. 6 sessions of CBT) led to decreased cannabis use (Copeland et al., 2001).

Results from a large multisite trial comparing two sessions of Motivation Enhancement Therapy (MET) (p. 80) with a nine-session CBT+MET and a delayed treatment condition found that the longer treatment was associated with reduced use and less negative consequences (Babor et al., 2004). Recently, a larger trial compared 14 weeks of CBT alone, CBT with Contingency Management (CM) in the form of abstinence-based vouchers (pp. 82–83), or abstinence-based voucher CM alone found that abstinence-based vouchers led to greater levels of continuous documented abstinence. CBT did not increase abstinence during treatment but led to greater maintenance of abstinence following treatment compared to voucher-based CM alone (Budney et al., 2006). Similar types of interventions have demonstrated efficacy in alcohol, cocaine, and opiate dependence. We can therefore conclude that MET and CBT are effective in the treatment of cannabis dependence. While longer treatments (12- and 14-week CBT or CM combined with CBT) have been shown to be more effective than brief treatments, the optimal duration to maximize cost-effectiveness has not been determined.

Studies of contingency management (CM) alone or paired with CBT or MET indicate that all can be effective (Budney et al., 2006; Carroll et al., 2006; Kadden et al., 2007). Abstinence-based vouchers led to greater documented continuous abstinence during treatment. When combined with CBT or MET, CM led to greater maintenance of abstinence following treatment.

Unfortunately, relapse rates associated with cannabis dependence treatment also appear similar to other drugs of abuse (Moore & Budney, 2003), indicating that cannabis dependence is not easily treated with the currently available psychosocial treatments alone. There is substantial need for additional treatments.

Psychopharmacological interventions

Cannabis withdrawal may contribute to cannabis dependence and relapse. Decreasing cannabis withdrawal severity may aid cessation. Several studies have examined pharmacological interventions for this role (see Vandrey & Haney, 2009).

Nefazadone, a serotonin reuptake inhibitor and $5HT_2$ receptor antagonist, decreased ratings of anxiety and muscle pain, but all other ratings of withdrawal symptoms (irritable, miserable, trouble sleeping) remained high. The dopamine reuptake blocker, bupropion, was found to increase irritability, depression, restlessness, and trouble sleeping perhaps due to bupropion's stimulant properties. Divalproex (sodium valproate) was found to decrease cannabis craving, but ratings of anxiety, irritability, and tiredness increased (Haney et al., 2004). While oral THC was effective in reducing craving and suppressed ratings of anxiety, feeling miserable, trouble sleeping, and chills, participants failed to distinguish active drug from placebo (Haney et al., 2004; Budney et al., 2007). Nonetheless these studies with tetrahydrocannabidol (THC) show some promise. Other promising medications may include partial agonists as well as cannabinoid antagonists.

Alternative and other treatments

There is no evidence that acupuncture or hypnosis works in helping people cease use of cannabis. While psychodynamic psychotherapy and family therapy have been used to treat cannabis dependence, there is little data available as to their effectiveness.

Table 14.1 Effectiveness of treatments for cannabis dependence

Treatment	Form of treatment	Psychiatric disorder/target audience	Level of evidence for efficacy	Comments
Psychotherapy	Cognitive behavioural therapy	Cannabis dependence	Ia	With or without motivational interviewing, treatment group improved to a greater degree than no treatment group. Longer treatment may lead to greater effectiveness
Psychotherapy	Contingency management (alone or with CBT or MET)	Cannabis dependence	Ia	Voucher-based incentives led to greater levels of continuous abstinence
Psychotherapy	Motivation enhancement therapy/motivational interviewing	Cannabis dependence	Ia	Found to be more effective than waiting list controls. The longer the exposure to this treatment, the better the results
Psychopharmacology	Tetrahydrocannabidol	Cannabis dependence	IIa	THC effective in reducing craving and in lowering withdrawal symptoms
Psychopharmacology	Divalproex	Cannabis dependence	IIb	Evidence is conflicting. Can decrease craving but anxiety, irritability, and fatigue increased

Summary and conclusions

Cannabis dependence is a substantial worldwide problem. While demand for treatment services has continued to rise in the past decade, the total number of individuals seeking treatment for cannabis dependence is only a small proportion of the estimated number of dependent individuals. Research suggests that psychosocial interventions such as CBT, MET, relapse prevention, and CM are effective in treating cannabis dependence and should be considered as first-line treatments. However, rates of abstinence initiation and relapse appear similar to other drugs of abuse. Where there are differences, CBT and CBT with CM have been most effective. Drug treatment may help improve the treatment of cannabis dependence but good data are lacking. This should therefore be considered a second-line adjunct to behavioural treatments. Interventions discussed in this chapter are summarized in Table 14.1.

15

Treatment of nicotine dependence

Based on "Treatment of nicotine dependence" by Andrea H. Weinberger, Pamela Walters, Taryn M. Allen, Melissa M. Dudas, Kristi A. Sacco and Tony P. George in Effective Treatments in Psychiatry, Cambridge University Press, 2008

Introduction

Cigarette smoking, the most common form of tobacco use with over 1.1 billion users worldwide, is the single largest preventable cause of substantial morbidity and mortality in developed countries. Approximately 23% of the general population in the USA and 29% in the UK smoke cigarettes (Giovino, 2002). Cigarette smoking prevalence in the USA has decreased from 45% (1960s) to 23% (2002). About 430 000 people in the USA die annually from smoking-attributable medical illnesses (chronic respiratory diseases, substantially higher risk of cancers and cardiovascular disease, two times the chance of fatal ischaemic heart disease and four times for fatal aortic aneurysm) (Giovino, 2002). Smoking may cause 450 million deaths worldwide in the next 50 years. A 50% reduction in smoking could prevent 20–30 million premature deaths in the next 25 years. Quitting smoking can substantially improve one's health.

Remaining smokers generally have lower education attainment, lower socio-economic status, less interest in behavioural treatments for cessation, and more medical, substance abuse and psychiatric comorbidities, greater difficulty in quitting smoking, and have often failed to quit despite many different interventions. Meanwhile controlled trials with nicotine replacement therapies (NRTs) over the past 15 years reveal declining quit rates. Women, now smoking at higher rates, may experience more intense nicotine withdrawal and depressed mood when attempting to quit and may be less NRT responsive. A large proportion of smokers who failed quit attempts do not respond to conventional pharmacotherapies.

Clinical features of nicotine dependence

Most cigarette smokers smoke daily and have physiological dependence on nicotine (Rigotti et al., 2002) that involves daily smoking for several weeks, toleration of nicotine's aversive effects, and experience nicotine withdrawal symptoms (dysphoria, anxiety, irritability, middle of the night insomnia, increased appetite, and craving for cigarettes) upon cessation (American Psychiatric Association, 2006b). Positive effects of cigarette smoking (taste, satisfaction) appear mediated by non-nicotine components of tobacco. Secondary positive effects of nicotine and tobacco include mood modulation, stress reduction, and weight control. Conditioned cues can elicit urges to smoke even after prolonged abstinence.

National guidelines

Clinical guidelines include: The US Public Health Service's "Treating Tobacco Use and Dependence" (Fiore et al., 2000); American Psychiatric Association Practice Guidelines for the Treatment of Nicotine Dependence (APA, 2006); Royal College of Physicians' guidelines (1998, updated in 2000) (West & Shiffman, 2001). The UK's NHS guidelines suggest the following strategies: nicotine replacement therapies (NRTs) or bupropion prescribed only as part of an abstinent contingent treatment programme where the smoker commits to stop smoking; smokers offered advice and encouragement; an initial NRT or bupropion prescription sufficient to last only 2 weeks after the target quit date or 3–4 weeks of bupropion; second prescriptions given only after reassessment demonstrates the person's continuing attempts to quit or the NHS does not support further attempts for 6 months. Smokers under the age of 18 years, pregnant or breastfeeding, or who have unstable cardiovascular disorders should consult a health care worker before beginning either treatment. In the UK, bupropion is not recommended for people under 18 or pregnant or breastfeeding women.

Evidence-based treatments for nicotine dependence

Stepped-care approaches

The majority of smokers quit on their own or with minimal treatment. Most existing algorithms/guidelines rely on a stepped-care approach: minimal interventions early on, more intensive ones for those unable to stop with minimal interventions (Hughes, 1994; Rigotti, 2002). In treating smoking cessation, the following should be considered: assessment of motivation and intention to quit, availability of support and counselling (though scant data support positive impact on success rates), previous attempts and methods used to stop, smoker's preferences as to quit method and possible side effects of that method, and any contraindications of that method for that smoker.

Medication treatments

Pharmacotherapies for nicotine dependence can be divided into NRT and non-nicotine medications. Non-medication somatic therapies include acupuncture and devices.

Nicotine replacement therapies (NRTs)

The goal of NRT is to relieve withdrawal and allow the patient to focus on habit and conditioning factors when attempting to quit. After acute withdrawal, the therapy is gradually reduced so withdrawal is minimal. NRTs rely on systemic venous absorption and do not produce the rapid high arterial nicotine levels achieved through inhalation of cigarette smoke. NRTs are much less addictive but should be discontinued if the person restarts smoking.

All commercially available forms of NRT are effective and increase quit rates by approximately 1.5–2 fold. A meta-analysis of six NRT products containing 97 RCTs involving 38 0000 smokers followed for 6 months after commencing treatment found an odds ratio of smoking cessation for any NRT versus placebo of 1.74 (95% CI 1.64–1.86); at 12 months, 1.69 (95% CI 1.57–1.82) (Silagy et al., 2002). A review of eight nicotine gum studies, three inhaler studies, and one microtab study (774 subjects) found strong evidence for oral nicotine therapies to reduce total withdrawal discomfort, irritability, and anxiety with some evidence for effect on depressed mood and craving (less for gum than for the others) (West & Shiffman, 2001).

Nicotine gum

Several placebo-controlled RCTs have established the safety and efficacy of nicotine gum. Gum contains 2 or 4 mg of nicotine which is released from a resin by chewing. The recommended dose is one piece of 2 mg gum/hour

(4 mg gum for highly nicotine-dependent smokers). Originally recommended for 3 months treatment duration, it appears that longer treatment may be more effective. Absorption peaks 30 minutes after chewing. Cigarettes achieve nicotine levels that are 5–10 times higher. Side effects are rare. About 5–20% continue gum for 9 or more months, but few for more than 2 years (Hughes, 1991). Abuse is minimal. Combinations of nicotine gum and patch may help more treatment-resistant heavy smokers.

Transdermal nicotine patch

The efficacy of the nicotine transdermal patch (NTP) is well documented (Fiore et al., 1994). Nicotine is readily absorbed across the skin. Patches are for 24 or 16 hours (waking) use and are applied daily, beginning with smoking cessation. Nicotine levels peak 6–10 hours after initial administration and remain fairly steady thereafter. After 4–6 weeks patients usually taper to a lower dose; after 2–4 more weeks the patch is removed. No taper is needed. Total treatment duration is 6–12 weeks. Nicotine levels from patches are typically half those in smoking. Abrupt cessation usually causes no significant withdrawal symptoms. Two nicotine patches are available over-the-counter. Patches have no significant adverse effects (Silagy et al., 1994).

Nicotine nasal spray

Two double-blind, placebo-controlled RCTs have established the safety and efficacy of nicotine nasal spray (Schneider et al., 1995; Blondal et al., 1997). Quit rates doubled after 3–6 months. The spray, administered to each nostril every 4–6 hours, contains nicotine in solution similar to other nasal sprays (Schneider et al., 1995). Nicotine levels rise more rapidly than nicotine gum, with peak levels occurring within 10 minutes. Smokers can use the spray ad lib up to 30 times/day for 12 weeks, including a taper. Nicotine nasal spray has modest reinforcing effects, so follow-up of nasal spray users is recommended.

Nicotine vapour inhalers (NVI)

Two 4–6-month double-blind, placebo-controlled RCTs demonstrate superiority of NVI over placebo inhalers (Schneider et al., 1996; Bolliger et al., 2000) with a 2–3-fold increase in quit rates (17–26%). NVI are cartridges (plugs) of nicotine placed inside hollow cigarette-like plastic rods and produce nicotine vapour when warm air passes through them. Absorption is primarily buccal. Nicotine levels increase more quickly than gum, less quickly than nasal spray. Smokers may puff the inhaler ad lib. Dosing is 6–16 cartridges daily. No serious medical side effects have been reported, though half report throat irritation or coughing. About 10% of smokers continue inhalers for extended periods, and follow-up of inhaler users is recommended.

Nicotine polacrilex lozenges

A 6-week double-blind, placebo-controlled RCT of 2 and 4 mg nicotine lozenges established their superiority to placebo (Shiffman et al., 2002). Nicotine is absorbed buccally (swallowing is very gastrointestinally irritating). High-dose lozenges may be more efficacious in more highly dependent smokers.

Non-NRT psychopharmacological treatment

Sustained release bupropion

Bupropion, an atypical antidepressant agent in a sustained release (SR) formulation (Zyban®), is efficacious and safe for treating nicotine dependence (Hurt et al., 1997) and is considered a first-line smoking cessation pharmacological treatment. How bupropion aids in smoking cessation is unclear but is likely to involve dopamine and norepinephrine reuptake blockade and antagonism of high-affinity nicotinic acetylcholine receptors. Bupropion therapy goals include: (1) smoking cessation, (2) reduction of nicotine craving and withdrawal symptoms, and (3) prevention of cessation-induced weight gain. In the UK bupropion is licensed only for smoking cessation. The target dose is 300 mg daily (150 mg bid), started 7 days prior to the target quit date (TQD) at 150 mg daily, increasing to 150 mg bid after 3–4 days. Unlike NRTs, there is no absolute requirement that smokers completely cease smoking by the TQD. The main contraindication for bupropion is past history of seizures of any aetiology. Bupropion treatment dose-dependently reduced weight gain associated with smoking cessation and significantly reduced nicotine withdrawal symptoms at 150 and 300 mg/day doses (Hurt et al., 1997).

A double-blind, placebo-controlled, randomized multicentre trial evaluated the combination of bupropion and NTP in four conditions: each active condition alone, in combination, or a placebo. Both bupropion + patch and bupropion alone were significantly better than placebo and patch alone. The combination was not better than bupropion alone though weight suppression after cessation was most robust with it. A higher than expected rate of treatment-emergent hypertension (4–5%) developed with the combination (Jorenby et al., 1999).

Varenciline tartarate

Varenicline tartarate (Chantix® in USA, Champix® in Europe), an $\alpha_4\beta_2$ nicotinic receptor partial agonist, is approved as a first-line smoking cessation agent in the USA and Europe. Results of two independent but identical phase III trials comparing varenicline (1 mg bid) to bupropion SR (150 mg bid) and placebo revealed quit rates significantly higher with varenicline (p < 0.0001). Both drugs had significantly higher quit rates than placebo (Jorenby et al., 2006).

Other non-nicotine pharmacotherapies

Non-nicotine pharmacotherapies tested for utility for treating nicotine dependence (but not FDA approved) include:

Nortriptyline – a tricyclic antidepressant shown in several double-blind, placebo-controlled trials to be superior to placebo (Prochazka et al., 1998) with efficacy comparable to bupropion.

Clonidine – a pre-synaptic alpha$_2$ agonist that in three meta-analytical reviews was found to double quit rates (Covey & Glassman, 1991; Law & Tang, 1995), helping reduce acute nicotine withdrawal symptoms. It may assist smokers with high anxiety levels during early cessation.

Mecamylamine – decreases positive subjective effects from cigarettes though there is little evidence to recommend it.

Psychosocial treatments

Behavioural therapy

Behavioural therapy (BT) assumes that learning supports development, maintenance, and cessation of smoking. BT's goals include: (1) providing skills to aid quitting; (2) teaching skills to avoid high-risk situations; and (3) supporting and extending effects of proven nicotine dependence pharmacotherapies. Over 100 controlled prospective studies verify BT's efficacy. Quit rates are twice that of control groups (Baille et al., 1994; Law and Tang, 1995). BTs, usually part of a multimodal package, are first-line treatments.

BTs use a stepped-care approach, minimal interventions first, and, failing these, more intense levels of BT combined with pharmacotherapies. Since nearly two-thirds of patients relapse in the first week after attempting smoking, most treatment is timed to occur before or just after cessation initiation.

Table 15.1 Effectiveness of treatments for nicotine dependence

Treatment	Form of treatment	Psychiatric disorder/target audience	Level of evidence for efficacy	Comments
Nicotine replacement therapy	Nicotine gum	Adult smokers	Ia	Gradually and successfully reduces craving and withdrawal (slow absorption)
Nicotine replacement therapy	Transdermal nicotine patch	Adult smokers	Ia	Gradually and successfully reduces craving and withdrawal (slow absorption)
Nicotine replacement therapy	Nasal spray	Adult smokers	Ia	Rapidly reduces craving and withdrawal (rapid absorption)
Nicotine replacement therapy	Nicotine inhaler	Adult smokers	Ia	Rapidly reduces craving and withdrawal (rapid absorption)
Nicotine replacement therapy	• Nicotine polacrilex lozenges	Adult smokers	Ib	Gradually and successfully reduces craving and withdrawal (slow absorption)
Psychopharmacology	Bupropion	Adult smokers	Ia	Significantly better than placebo at short-term smoking cessation and at 1-year follow-up. It is dose-dependent in its ability to reduce smoking, weight gain, and withdrawal symptoms at the 150 mg and 300 mg (SR) doses

Table 15.1 (cont.)

Treatment	Form of treatment	Psychiatric disorder/target audience	Level of evidence for efficacy	Comments
Psychopharmacology	Varenicline	Adult smokers	Ia	Superior to placebo and bupropion in the short term (3 months) and at 1-year follow-up. Reduces craving and withdrawal symptoms, but little effect on weight gain. These effects are dose-dependent, with best outcomes at the 2 mg/day divided dosing schedule
Psychopharmacology	Nortriptyline	Adult smokers	IIa	Listed as a second-line agent but is superior to placebo
Psychopharmacology	Clonidine	Adult smokers	IIa	Listed as a second-line agent but is superior to placebo. May be best for people with concomitant anxiety. There are negative reports re. effectiveness as well
Psychopharmacology	Mecamylamine	Adult smokers	IIa	Some evidence for efficacy but only in combination with nicotine patch
Psychopharmacology	Naltrexone	Adult smokers	IIa	Some evidence for efficacy but only in combination with nicotine patch
Psychopharmacology	MAOIs	Adult smokers	Ib	Small studies suggest that they may be helpful in the short term

Combined treatment	TNP and bupropion	Adult smokers	Combination not better than bupropion alone and possible side effect of hypertension in the combination. Bupropion alone better than TNP alone	Ib
Psychosocial treatment	Multimodal cognitive behavioural therapy	Adult smokers	Increases quit rates twofold over control groups. It deserves a Ib because the programmes and populations may differ greatly from study to study	Ib
Psychosocial treatment	Self-help and other brief interventions	Adult smokers	Appear to have a modest but slight increase in quit rates, though little evidence that they work by themselves or with people who are heavy smokers	IIb
Psychosocial treatment	Motivational interviewing	Adult smokers	Appear to have a modest but slight increase in quit rates, solid methodological studies have yet to be conducted	IIb

Cognitive behavioural interventions (skills training/ relapse prevention therapies)

Cognitive behavioural therapy (CBT), in combination with NRT or bupropion, is recommended if initial treatments fail. In CBT, patients anticipate "likely to smoke" situations and plan coping strategies for them. Cognitive coping includes identifying and challenging maladaptive thoughts, substituting more effective thought patterns to prevent a slip from becoming a relapse, and not viewing the slip catastrophically. Allen Carr's "Easy Way to Quit Smoking" method is CBT based (Carr, 2004).

Motivational interventions (MI)

Few studies have rigorously evaluated MI efficacy for smoking cessation. Preliminary positive findings suggest that MI may be helpful either alone or adjunctive to pharmacological and psychosocial interventions.

Self-help materials and other brief interventions

Major goals of self-help materials and procedures are to increase motivation to quit and impart cessation skills. Minimal behavioural interventions such as community support groups, call-back telephone counselling, and computer-generated self-help materials can augment smoking cessation rates in controlled settings, but do not seem to add power to other interventions (Lancaster & Stead, 1999). Training programmes for physicians in basic behavioural supportive cessation counselling may enhance cessation rates, especially in hospitalized medical inpatients. Pharmacists and other health care people may employ these brief interventions with some success. Community interventions, mass media campaigns and posters, etc., appear to influence, at best, lighter smokers with very limited impact on adolescents.

Alternative treatments

There is little hard data for the effectiveness of either acupuncture or hypnotherapy.

Interventions discussed in this chapter are summarized in Table 15.1.

16

Treatment of co-occurring psychiatric and substance use disorders

Based on "Treatment of co-occurring psychiatric and substance use disorders" by Douglas M. Ziedonis, Ed Day, Erin L. O'Hea, and Jonathan Krejci in Effective Treatments in Psychiatry, Cambridge University Press, 2008

Introduction

Co-occurring mental illness and addiction are common among individuals with mental health problems, and result in worse treatment outcomes, greater risk of suicide, heightened craving, withdrawal symptoms, cognitive impairment, wider fluctuations in mental status, poorer medication compliance, and increased hospitalizations and emergency room visits (SAMSHA, 2003). The goal of integrated treatment is to address both the mental health and substance abuse problems and associated symptoms

simultaneously (Ziedonis et al., 2005).

Assessment and diagnosis

The initial assessment involves establishing a timeline of the progression of substance use and mental illness to understand the relative age of onset, how the problem areas are interrelated, and the relationships of life events to exacerbations and remissions. It is important to clarify whether symptoms were present during extended drug-free periods and the impact of each disorder on the presentation, clinical course, and outcome of the other disorders. Structured screening instruments can help the assessment process. Corroborative information is also invaluable and can assist in providing details about periods of sobriety and treatment compliance. Assessing motivation in addressing both disorders is important for treatment planning. Often the levels of motivation vary for the different problems. Most individuals have multiple addictions and multiple psychiatric problems. Integrated treatment is best. However, treatment sometimes begins with the problem area the patient is internally motivated to address or externally required (Ziedonis et al., 2005).

Treatment models with emphasis on integrated care

Integrated treatment is expected in both mental health and substance abuse treatment settings; however there is a great range of services and skills at different agencies. While the literature supports integrated services be delivered simultaneously within the same programme, it is not always feasible and may need to be done at multiple sites during the same time period. The SAMHSA four quadrant model provides a way for agencies to identify the level of severity of both mental illness and addiction they are able to manage (SAMHSA, 2003; APA, 2006). The Dual Diagnosis Good Practice Guideline (UK) recommends patients with severe mental health and substance misuse problems receive "high quality, patient focused and integrated care ... delivered within mental health services" (Department of Health, 2002). Integrated treatment should include treatment matched to motivation and recovery, assertive outreach techniques, family and social support interventions, cultural sensitivity, and multiple psychotherapeutic modalities (SAMSHA, 2003; APA, 2006). These components improve treatment adherence and reduce dropout, relapse, and rehospitalization (SAMSHA, 2003; APA, 2006).

Clinical treatment interventions

Psychopharmacology

Whilst evidence-based pharmacological treatments have been well established for treating specific psychiatric disorders, we have less confidence in the evidence for treating co-occurring disorders.

Treatments used in co-occurring disorders include the same medications used to treat a specific addiction disorder (detoxification, protracted abstinence, or maintenance) and to treat the co-occurring specific mental disorder. Since there are often several drugs available for treating the specific psychiatric disorder, the specific medication choice(s) must consider abuse liability, overdose risk, interaction between medication and substances abused, and the body organs affected by the substances, especially issues of seizure risk, sedation, and liver toxicity (APA, 2006; Smelson et al., 2008). In outpatient care consider starting at a low dose and slowly increasing over time as needed. Some medications (methylphenidate, amphetamines, benzodiazepines, stimulants) used in some psychiatric disorders (anxiety disorders, ADHD) raise concerns because of abuse potential in comorbid substance use disorder.

Psychosocial treatments

Integrated psychosocial treatments
Psychosocial treatments remain the cornerstone of addiction treatment and are effective in treating co-occurring disorders. The common psychosocial addiction treatments are motivational enhancement therapy (MET), relapse prevention, and 12-step facilitation; the common mental health treatments are cognitive behavioural therapy (CBT) and social skills training (Ziedonis et al., 2005). Dual recovery therapy (DRT) integrates CBT approaches from both fields for specific subtypes. The time-limited care coordination (TLC) approach integrates DRT with assertive community treatment using a critical time intervention (Susser et al., 1997) and peer support (Yanos et al., 2001) and can improve treatment attendance and medication compliance (Smelson et al., 2010) and demonstrates the advantages of wrap-around services (SAMHSA, 2003).

Specific co-occurring mental illness subtypes

Major depression and dysthymia

Depression is very common in substance abusers, and many individuals with depression have an addiction (APA, 2006). No particular FDA-approved antidepressant is more efficacious, although adverse effects of hepatic and cardiac toxicity, seizure risk, and agitation should be considered. Sleep disturbances, primarily insomnia, are common (Mackenzie et al., 1999) and may be addressed non-pharmacologically (stress reduction techniques, sleep hygiene). Selective serotonin reuptake inhibitors (SSRIs) and other newer antidepressants such as bupropion and mirtazapine are commonly first-line treatments (APA, 2006). A meta-analysis concluded that antidepressant medications exert modest beneficial effects for depressive symptoms but concurrent substance abuse therapy is necessary (Nunes & Levin, 2004). Integrative psychotherapies are critical additions (APA, 2006).

Bipolar disorder

Substance use disorders co-occur more often with bipolar disorder (> 50%) than with other mental illnesses. Unfortunately for individuals with a co-occurring bipolar disorder and substance abuse, both disorders exacerbate each illness. Bipolar disorder is associated with impulsivity and poor compliance and substance abuse worsens bipolar illness course, increasing the severity and frequency of manic, depressive, and mixed episodes. There is limited data to suggest specific FDA-approved medication for bipolar disorder in this population; clear evidence supports integrating cognitive behavioural therapies (Westermeyer et al., 2003).

Anxiety disorders

Anxiety disorders can be diagnosed in around 25% of individuals with alcohol dependence and 43% in drug dependence and often precede the onset of addiction (Grant et al., 2004). Because of the addictive nature of some pharmacotherapies

(e.g. benzodiazepines) caution should be taken in prescribing medications to patients with comorbid anxiety and substance abuse (APA, 2006). There is a need to do more psychosocial treatment studies for this population, and Hesse (2009) has found limited evidence to date.

Panic disorder

Individuals with co-occurring panic and substance use disorders may respond well to combination SSRI and psychosocial therapy. Benzodiazepines are not recommended because of abuse and dependence risks. Panic-like symptoms may be experienced in various phases of substance use (intoxication, withdrawal) or may have preceded the substance abuse (McKeehan & Martin, 2002). Psychoeducation and CBT, with an emphasis on graded exposure or systematic desensitization, can help patients manage these symptoms (McKeehan & Martin, 2002).

Post-traumatic stress disorder (PTSD)

PTSD is very common among patients with substance use disorders (12–34%), particularly among women (30–59%). PTSD symptoms are common triggers for substance use. Integrated psychosocial treatments provide education about both disorders, teach coping skills to gain control over symptoms, and help patients understand the link between their PTSD and substance use (Rotunda et al., 2008). In terms of medication options, recommendations from guidelines for treating PTSD alone are usually followed (see Chapter 28) and are often used in conjunction with cognitive behavioural therapies (APA, 2006).

Adult attention deficit disorder (ADD)

A nationally representative household data study revealed that 15.2% of individuals in the community with ADD also have an addiction compared to 5.6% of individuals without ADD and 10–24% in clinical samples (Mariani & Levin, 2007). Treating co-occurring ADD and substance use is complicated because of considerable symptom overlap. Although psychostimulant medication (e.g. methylphenidate and amphetamine) are the most commonly used drugs to treat ADD without an addiction, clinicians are reluctant to prescribe stimulants to patients with an addiction because of abuse liability and lack of evidence for co-occurring disorders (APA, 2006). Selecting medications with lower abuse liability (atomoxetine or bupropion) provides a safer and more effective approach (Kollins, 2008). Research on the

effectiveness of psychosocial treatments in this population is understudied (Mariani & Levin, 2007).

Personality disorders

Personality disorders, most often antisocial, borderline, histrionic and narcissistic, occur in about half of individuals with substance use disorders although accurate diagnosing is difficult. Integrated treatment blends behavioural approaches for personality disorders with traditional substance abuse treatments. Linehan's dialectical behavioural therapy (DBT) has been modified to treat co-occurring borderline personality and substance use disorders. Research supports its effectiveness (Linehan et al., 1999). DBT appears to help treatment retention (Bornovalova & Daughters, 2007).

Schizophrenia

About 50–70% of individuals with schizophrenia have current alcohol or other drug abuse disorder and 60–85% are tobacco dependent (Ziedonis et al., 2005). Integrated treatment usually occurs in mental health settings and must address the positive and negative symptoms of schizophrenia, cognitive limitations, social support, suicidal ideation, and low motivation. There are specific therapy manuals for treatment of

Table 16.1 Effectiveness of treatments for co-occurring psychiatric and substance use disorders

Treatment	Form of treatment	Psychiatric disorder/target audience	Level of evidence for efficacy	Comments
Integrated treatment (psychosocial)	Multimodal treatment that addresses simultaneously substance abuse and psychiatric disorder. An integrated model uses recovery-oriented approaches, motivational interviewing, interpersonal psychotherapies, and behavioural skills training	Dual diagnosis patients	Ib	There are many different studies using different methodology and since no two studies are exactly alike, then Ia not given here. But the overall impression is that integrated treatment is more effective than serial or parallel treatment across a wide range of psychiatric diagnoses and various substances. The best integrated care is delivered by a single team that approaches "both" problems
Psychosocial treatment	Motivational interviewing	Dual diagnosis patients	IIb	Attendance in the programme appears to be the main benefit, but also some studies reveal that motivational interviewing

				can significantly reduce the comorbid substance misuse
Psychosocial treatment	Dialectical behaviour therapy	Comorbid personality disorder and substance misuse	IIb	Preliminary evidence supports this intervention with at least short-term improvement in use of substances and personality pathology
Pharmacotherapy	Anticonvulsants	Comorbid bipolar disorder and substance abuse	IIb	Various studies suggest that patients with dual diagnosis tolerate anticonvulsants, particularly valproate, better than lithium
Pharmacotherapy	Antidepressants	Comorbid depression in substance abuser	Ib–II	SSRIs are probably first line and TCAs second-line treatment here but the evidence is better for the effectiveness of TCAs especially with people on methadone maintenance
Pharmacotherapy	Atypical antipsychotics	Comorbid schizophrenia and substance abuse	IIb	Atypicals appear more effective than typicals. Some evidence that clozapine, olanzapine, and risperidone may be useful to reduce severity of both disorders with the largest evidence base for clozapine

co-occurring schizophrenia and addiction, including dual recovery therapy (Ziedonis & Stern, 2001), modified cognitive behavioural therapy with motivational enhancement (Bellack & DiClemente, 1999; Bellack et al., 2006), and the substance abuse management module (SAMM) (Shaner et al., 2003). These approaches all include elements of motivational enhancement therapy, relapse prevention, and social skills training. These approaches are supportive of patients being involved in 12-step recovery meetings (e.g. Alcoholics Anonymous; see Ziedonis et al., 2005 for full review).

For individuals with co-occurring schizophrenia and substance abuse problems, there is a need to manage the psychosis with antipsychotic treatment and the use of atypicals, although based on smaller studies, may have somewhat greater evidence (APA, 2006). However the atypical antipsychotics as a drug group do have serious side effects that must be monitored, including weight gain, hyperlipidaemia, elevated glucose, mood, and neurological symptoms (also see Chapter 17).

Nicotine dependence

Most individuals with any psychiatric disorder are addicted to tobacco, and 42% of all the cigarettes consumed in the United States are by these individuals (Lasser et al., 2000). Treatment planning should consider motivational level to quit and other factors (also see Chapter 15). There are seven FDA-approved medications for nicotine dependence, including five types of nicotine replacement therapies (gum, patch, lozenge, inhaler, and nasal spray) and two FDA-approved non-nicotine treatments (bupropion SR and varenicline). All these medications do have important side effects to consider when deciding with a patient what might be the best choice (APA, 2006), including serious neuropsychiatric side effects with varenicline and bupropion. Tobacco use among these patients should be considered when selecting a medication given that smoking substantially lowers blood levels of clozapine, olanzapine, and numerous traditional antipsychotics (haloperidol, chlorpromazine) by increasing P450 1A2 isoenzyme hepatic metabolism (Ziedonis et al., 2005). Combining psychosocial treatments with medications increases abstinence rates by 50% compared to the delivery of either intervention alone (Zhu et al., 2000). The APA guideline recommends the core psychosocial treatments of CBT and MET (APA, 2006).

Interventions discussed in this chapter are summarized in Table 16.1.

Schizophrenia

17

Pharmacological treatment for schizophrenia

Based on "Pharmacological treatments for schizophrenia" by Stephen R. Marder and Peter B. Jones in Effective Treatments in Psychiatry, Cambridge University Press, 2008

Introduction

This subject is one of the most debated in psychiatry. Fundamentally we have the problem of a very severe mental illness for which we have effective treatments in the short term – but at a price. All these treatments are pharmacological and non-curative; they suppress the symptoms of schizophrenia while they are being taken but as schizophrenia is a heterogeneous condition which usually has a long-term course, when the drugs are withdrawn there is a strong possibility of relapse. Added to this we have a great number of potential adverse effects that make the

treatments unpopular with patients. In this chapter we will also include schizo-affective disorder and related conditions as part of the schizophrenia diagnostic spectrum. In deciding on drug treatment it is desirable to look at each of the phases of a person's illness, the acute, stable and stabilization phases (Lehman et al., 2004).

Treatment in the acute phase

The acute phase of schizophrenia is characterized by psychotic symptoms such as hallucinations and delusions and often disturbed behaviour. There are often depressive and anxiety symptoms also. In this phase patients are most responsive to drug therapy and antipsychotic drug treatment is currently the most appropriate therapy. A large number of randomized trials and meta-analyses have shown that approximately 60% of patients treated with an antipsychotic drug will have a substantial remission in symptoms compared with fewer than 20% taking placebo. The positive symptoms of schizophrenia (hallucinations, delusions, and disturbed behaviour) tend to respond rather better than the negative symptoms (lack of social involvement, reduced drive and interest) but even these symptoms tend to improve when treatment is given in the acute phase.

Efficacy of typical and atypical antipsychotic drugs

When the atypical (sometimes called second generation) antipsychotic drugs were introduced in the early 1990s there was hope that these agents would be more effective than the typical (first generation) drugs as well as having less serious adverse effects. This hope was stimulated by the exciting finding that clozapine, allegedly one of the second generation drugs but actually older than many first generation ones, was more effective than other drugs for a broad range of symptom dimensions including positive, negative, and mood symptoms (Kane et al., 1988). Further support came from early studies of risperidone and olanzapine, all supported by the manufacturers of these drugs. However, a careful meta-analysis by Geddes et al. (2000) concluded that the advantages of the atypical agents were only apparent when patients received excessive doses of the comparison drug, which was almost always haloperidol, in the clinical trials. Subsequent meta-analyses have largely confirmed the Geddes findings (Leucht et al., 1999; 2009) but one by Davis et al. (2003) suggested that risperidone, olanzapine, and possibly amisulpride, were superior to haloperidol even allowing for dosage differences.

The cumulative evidence of the last 10 years has sadly confirmed that any differences in efficacy between the atypical and typical antipsychotic drugs are too small to recommend one group over another. On the other hand, there clearly are differences in response with individual patients that justify several drugs being available for prescription. Although the atypical antipsychotic drugs were introduced on a wave of euphoria that these compounds did not have the major adverse effect of movement disorders and later development of tardive dyskinesia, recent studies, notably the CATIE and

CUtLASS studies (Lieberman et al., 2005; Jones et al., 2006), have shown that there is no meaningful difference between the effects of typical and atypical antipsychotics and large meta-analyses have confirmed this (Geddes et al., 2000; Leucht et al., 2009). There is also very little difference between the adverse effects of these compounds when they were used in the CATIE study (Miller et al., 2008).

The only exception is clozapine, a drug which is older than all the other second generation antipsychotics (and therefore does not deserve this label), which has been shown to be clearly more effective in resistant cases of schizophrenia and generally is more effective than other antipsychotic drugs of all types (Lewis et al., 2006). This was confirmed in the second phase of the CATIE study (McEvoy et al., 2006) in which those patients who discontinue their treatment because of lack of efficacy were randomly assigned under double-blind conditions to risperidone, olanzapine, quetiapine, or clozapine. For the main outcome, discontinuation rates, only 56% of patients on clozapine discontinued compared with 71% on olanzapine, 86% on risperidone, and 93% on quetiapine.

This may seem a surprising conclusion in view of many favourable results about atypical drugs over the past 15 years. The reasons why Peter Jones concluded everyone was 'beguiled' (Washington Post, 2006) into thinking that atypical antipsychotics were superior reflect a combination of drug company-sponsored studies (which tend to inflate the effect size of their own drugs), comparison with haloperidol (the antipsychotic drug with one of the highest propensities for movement disorders), and dosage differences (with the older drugs being given in larger doses than the atypical drugs and therefore creating more adverse effects).

The other growing concern has been with the tendency of some atypical drugs to have the additional problems of appetite stimulation and weight gain. This has been associated with a higher incidence of subsequent obesity and type II diabetes, the combination commonly called the metabolic syndrome (Mackin et al., 2007). Because of these concerns treatment guidelines for schizophrenia now suggest regular monitoring of weight, glucose, lipids, and blood pressure during the course of treatment. Unfortunately, clozapine, despite its superior efficacy, also has a strong propensity to lead to weight gain and the metabolic syndrome. With olanzapine, which tends to be the atypical drug favoured by many patients, weight gain was the most pronounced adverse effect (Lieberman et al., 2005) and this adverse effect has been constantly replicated in studies since this time.

Pharmacological treatment in the stable phase

In the stable or maintenance phase antipsychotic drugs should usually be combined with psychosocial interventions. This has been encapsulated in the recovery model of schizophrenia which gives more responsibility to the patient to improve life satisfaction, sustaining hope and optimism and empowering people to gain greater personal control of their own treatment (Resnick et al., 2004).

There is incontrovertible evidence that those who stop antipsychotic drugs after recovery from the acute phase are significantly more likely to relapse, with one meta-analysis showing that 72% of patients relapsed in the year following change to placebo compared to only 23% who stay on atypical antipsychotic drugs (Davis et al., 1989). Even when patients have been stable for many years withdrawal of antipsychotic drugs is associated with a much greater risk of relapse (Hogarty et al., 1976). Very similar findings have been shown in meta-analyses of relapse with the atypical antipsychotic drugs (Leucht et al., 2003).

Because of these findings standard treatment guidelines (Lehman et al., 2004; National Collaborating Centre for Mental Health, 2010) suggest that those that have had multiple episodes of schizophrenia should remain on long-term maintenance treatment unless the adverse effects of the drugs concerned exceed the benefits. If a decision is made to reduce the antipsychotic drugs it should be done through gradual dose reduction and close monitoring.

Treatment-resistant schizophrenia

Approximately 40% of patients with schizophrenia treated with antipsychotic drugs will continue to experience positive symptoms that are resistant to medication. Treatment resistance was defined in 1988 by Kane et al. as

(1) persistent positive psychotic symptoms,

(2) moderately severe illness (Brief Psychiatric Rating Scale (BPRS) score greater than or equal to 45),

(3) persistence of illness shown by no stable period of good occupational social functioning and

(4) illness refractory to medication despite at least three periods of treatment or at least 6 weeks' duration with antipsychotic drugs.

It used to be thought that atypical antipsychotic drugs were more effective in this population (Marder et al., 2002) but the CATIE and CUtLASS studies suggest there is no advantage for atypical antipsychotic drugs in those that

Table 17.1 Effectiveness of drug treatment for schizophrenia and related psychoses

Treatment	Form of treatment	Psychiatric disorder	Level of evidence for efficacy	Comments
Typical antipsychotic drugs	Chlorpromazine (also see Appendix) sulpiride	Acute schizophrenia and related acute psychoses (including schizoaffective disorder)	Ia	
Clozapine	Tablets with routine monitoring of blood neutrophil levels	Refractory schizophrenia	Ia	Significantly greater improvement with clozapine than with typical antipsychotic drugs – greater for negative symptoms
Risperidone	Tablets (normal and quick absorption), liquid and depot injection	Acute and maintenance treatment of schizophrenia	Ia	Unequivocal evidence of efficacy with marginal evidence of increased benefit over typical antipsychotic drugs with no conclusive comparative studies yet with injectable form
Olanzapine	Tablets (normal and quick absorption), IM injection	Acute and maintenance treatment of schizophrenia	Ia	Unequivocal evidence of efficacy with some evidence of increased benefit over typical antipsychotic drugs offset by greater adverse effects (particularly metabolic ones)

Table 17.1 (cont.)

Treatment	Form of treatment	Psychiatric disorder	Level of evidence for efficacy	Comments
Amisulpride	Tablets	Acute and maintenance treatment of schizophrenia	Ia	Unequivocal evidence of efficacy with marginal evidence of increased benefit over typical antipsychotic drugs
Quetiapine	Tablets	Acute and maintenance treatment of schizophrenia		
All typical and atypical antipsychotic drugs	Tablets, injections and depot injections	Relapse prevention	Ia	All highly effective and significantly reduces relapse compared with placebo maintenance
Combined antipsychotic drugs (typical plus atypical or in same group)	Both tablets and injections	Treatment refractory schizophrenia	Ia	No clear benefit of polypharmacy
Antipsychotic drugs plus ECT	Any form	Treatment refractory schizophrenia	Ia	Slight benefit of combined therapy

are to some extent resistant. The exception is clozapine, whose effect sizes are larger than those of other antipsychotic drugs (McEvoy et al., 2006; Lewis et al., 2006). However, despite the better results for clozapine, fewer than half of those with treatment-resistant schizophrenia respond to the drug (Chakos et al., 2001).

A recent revision of the Texas Medication Algorithm Project (TMAP) (Miller et al., 2004) suggested the following procedure be followed if a patient showed no response to a trial of a typical antipsychotic drug. First it is reasonable to try an atypical antipsychotic drug. After two failures with different atypical drugs then it is time to change to clozapine. If adherence to medication is an issue then it is then reasonable to replace the oral drug with a depot injection of either a typical or atypical antipsychotic drug.

It might be thought that failure to respond to one antipsychotic drug might justify adding another to the drug regime, and in practice this form of polypharmacy is remarkably common, even though vigilant pharmacists are reducing its presence in inpatient care. Studies that have added the atypical antipsychotic drug, risperidone, to clozapine have shown no extra benefit (Josiassen et al., 2005; Yagcioglu et al., 2005; Honer et al., 2006). ECT may still have a place in the treatment of refractory patients either alone or in combination with antipsychotic drugs (Lehman et al., 2004). It remains an indication for the treatment of catatonic schizophrenia.

Conclusions

Patients with schizophrenia benefit greatly by taking antipsychotic medication at all phases of schizophrenia. The benefits of all antipsychotic drugs, both typical and atypical, are very similar and there is no advantage in terms of efficacy from either group of drugs. There are also strong arguments for suggesting that the division into first and second generation antipsychotic drugs is of little or no value (Tyrer & Kendall, 2009). All antipsychotic drugs have adverse effects that reduce adherence to therapy and, although these adverse effects differ to some extent between different agents, on balance the evils of one group, movement disorders and tardive dyskinesia with typical antipsychotics, are the same as weight gain, dyslipidaemia diabetes, and earlier mortality with the atypical ones, and in any case these adverse effects overlap. Because there are considerable differences between antipsychotic drugs in terms of adverse effects, the clinician should make the choice according to these criteria rather than those of efficacy. Interventions discussed in this chapter are summarized in Table 17.1.

18

Psychosocial and pharmacological treatments for schizophrenia

Based on "Psychosocial and pharmacological treatments for schizophrenia" by Peter B. Jones and Stephen R. Marder in Effective Treatments in Psychiatry, Cambridge University Press, 2008

Introduction

This chapter is so titled because psychosocial treatments for schizophrenia should be regarded as partners with antipsychotic drug treatment rather than independent, as they were in the past. Psychosocial interventions comprise more than the supportive psychotherapies that should accompany any treatment modality. They can be used to target residual positive symptoms, negative symptoms, and the sometimes puzzling phase where people fail to return to pre-morbid or predicted levels of functioning despite resolution of symptoms.

There is considerable convergence about the multidisciplinary management of many chronic illnesses. Education, informed decision making, reducing long-term risks, and focusing on increasing function and quality of life (preferably with input from the patient) are central to modern management of diseases such as diabetes mellitus, asthma, chronic inflammatory conditions – and schizophrenia.

Common principles of psychosocial interventions

The aims of these interventions include increased function, improved quality of life and recovery, as well as the reduction of specific symptoms and avoidance of relapse. Systematic reviews of psychosocial interventions (Pilling et al., 2002a; 2002b) confirm the value of this general approach, not only given to people with schizophrenia but also to families and carers.

In examining psychosocial interventions it should also be emphasized that analytical theories of aetiology based on a person's relationship with parents, family dynamics, and communication (Lidz et al., 1965; Wynne et al., 1958) have been shown to have no basis in fact (Hirsch & Leff, 1971). Instead we have good evidence that high levels of expressed emotion in families and groups, particularly when expressed in the form of hostility, criticism, and emotional overinvolvement, increase the risk of relapse in schizophrenia (Brown et al., 1972). When interventions were found that reduced expressed emotion (e.g. Vaughn & Leff, 1976) the chances of relapse were reduced.

Specific interventions

Psychoeducation

Knowledge and understanding generally lead to better decisions and improving these two aspects for a patient is one of the most basic of interventions. Education about illness can improve engagement with services, better adherence to drug treatment, early detection of signs of relapse, planning strategies for dealing with such signs, and ways to deal with or avoid circumstances that may have precipitated episodes of illness.

Schizophrenia may be more likely to develop in vulnerable individuals, particularly those with a family history of schizophrenia, those who use cannabis, have exposure to major life events, and are abused in childhood. It is possible, but remains to be established in research studies, that if these vulnerabilities are tackled early or avoided then the pathological consequences of schizophrenia will not occur. Information should also be shared about symptoms and it may be particularly useful in the first episode of schizophrenia to give this information in a sensitive and appropriate manner. There is good evidence that this type of information leads to a better outcome than standard care alone (Pekkala & Merinder, 2002).

Family interventions

Unfortunately in the later stages of schizophrenia there is often disengagement from family and the role of family interventions is then limited. At an earlier stage in illness there is now very good evidence that educating and working with families can become a highly valuable component of the management of schizophrenia. Families are the major support system available outside hospital and are not only an important resource of care but have a major influence on the course and outcome of the disorder.

Originally the main interventions were reduction of expressed emotion and the development of greater understanding for families. Wherever possible, family members and others connected with someone with schizophrenia should be involved in management. Such involvement benefits from an intervention that educates them about schizophrenia, its effects on the person with the illness and on the family, as well as providing an avenue of support.

Psychosocial family interventions

Psychosocial family interventions have several aims. They build a therapeutic alliance with carers so they are more likely to take on the work involved in improving relationships, including lowering the level of expressed emotion, the creation of a more positive family atmosphere, and the identification of specific problems and their solutions. Engagement with the family is best done early in the first episode and certainly during the acute phase of schizophrenia.

A second component of intervention is a relatively structured component that educates the family about the illness, often referred to as psychoeducation, something which is important for the sufferer themselves and is considered separately in that context. This intervention is usually begun and maintained by a member of the community mental health team although relatives of other people with schizophrenia could provide additional support and information. Learning from other families with similar experiences can be useful and provides much needed support to relatives. These two aspects usually need to be supplemented with individual interventions specifically designed for each family to assess their own circumstances. Sometimes there may be formal family therapy from a systems therapist, sometimes ongoing problem solving and support, or reformulation when new problems arise or circumstances change.

There is considerable empirical evidence to support this style of family intervention; a Cochrane Review of 14 randomized trials indicated that patients' mental state improved with family therapy (Pharoah et al., 2003). In particular dropout rates are low, indicating that these interventions are acceptable to patients and families. However, no clear effects were defined in the domain of social functioning but there were positive trends regarding employment and independent living. There is also a reduction of about 20% in the total cost of care.

Cognitive therapy

Cognitive therapy was originally developed for the treatment of depression but has been extended in the last 20 years to the treatment of schizophrenia (Kingdon & Turkington, 1995). Although there is evidence that cognitive therapy for psychosis has some benefit it is not clear to what extent this is related to the direct treatment of psychotic symptoms. A Cochrane Review (Jones et al., 2004) and 19 randomized controlled trials suggest that CBT does not reduce long-term relapse and re-admission compared with standard care but it did decrease the risk of staying in hospital and improved mental state over the medium term, but not after 1 year. Patients were not especially well engaged with treatment and comparison with supportive psychotherapy showed no important differences. More recently, studies have suggested that much of the improvement in the patient with schizophrenia is related to the treatment of depression and anxiety, which, as already noted,

are prevalent in the acute phase of schizophrenia (Garety et al., 2008). If CBT is only effective in treating the ancillary symptoms of schizophrenia it does not mean that it is ineffective in schizophrenia but does qualify the enthusiasm and indications for the treatment.

Compliance therapy

Patients with schizophrenia often stop taking their antipsychotic drugs, and compliance therapy, encouraged by the benefits of motivational interviewing in patients with substance misuse, aims to improve the collaboration between the patient and psychiatrist and their medication consumption. Unfortunately, despite initial positive findings a more recent large-scale multinational study (Gray et al., 2006) found no difference in quality of life after 1 year. However, a recent trial of a related form of adherence therapy (Staring et al., 2010) yielded positive results and it is clear that any gains in this area of care would yield great benefits to patients and service planners.

Cognitive remediation

This is a set of practical interventions at the interface between clinical neuropsychology, behaviourism, occupational therapy, and education, a fusion similar to the approaches used in the early stages of dementia. The therapy aims to identify the cognitive impairments and functional sequelae, and thence to help people find strategies to improve function in spite of them; it has met with some success (Wykes & Huddy, 2009). The area is likely to become increasingly fused with other therapeutic approaches.

Recovery movement

The recovery movement is relevant to the psychosocial treatment of schizophrenia. It developed in the consumer movement in the 1980s, was influenced by the 12-step programme of Alcoholics Anonymous, and arose mainly as a reaction to the standard treatments available for schizophrenia at the time. As these are mainly pharmacological, are associated with many adverse effects, and specifically linked to diagnosis, it is not surprising that early advocates of the recovery movement were antipathetic to all these, and were basically anti-biological in their orientation (Resnick et al., 2004). It has been embraced to a varying extent by rehabilitation services, governments, and psychiatrists, as its core principles of hope, empowerment, life satisfaction, and knowledge are desired by all patients in their own declaration of independence to rival that of Thomas Jefferson, and

have been put in similar ringing tones, with patients starting on "a journey of healing and transformation enabling them to live a meaningful life in a community of his or her choice while striving to achieve his or her full potential" (Wikipedia, 2010).

This approach is more of a philosophy than a treatment movement. However, some of the principles embraced by advocates of recovery can be especially relevant in the treatment of schizophrenia. These principles encourage clinicians to ask patients about their personal goals and to recommend non-pharmacological interventions that can help them reach those goals. In addition, recovery principles recognize that patients with schizophrenia are capable of improving their lives even if symptoms of their illness are only partially responsive to their medications. If patients feel that the only way they can stay "well" is to take drugs that they do not like on a long-term basis then any alternative vision that is more positive is going to be embraced. It also has some basis, as some patients – the exact proportion can only be a guess – do get better without, or in spite of, the standard treatments that we provide in psychiatric practice. However, there is no longer an understanding that recovery is an alternative to a biological approach, but an ambitious vision within which drug treatments play a part.

Table 18.1 Effectiveness of psychosocial interventions in schizophrenia

Treatment	Form of treatment	Psychiatric disorder	Level of evidence for efficacy	Comments
Psychoeducation	Individual	Schizophrenia – all forms	Ia	Reduced relapse and admission compared with standard intervention
Psychoeducation	Family	Schizophrenia – all forms	Ia	Reduction of symptoms in patients and reduced burden and expressed emotion in families
Cognitive therapy	Individual	Schizophrenia – all forms	Ia	Modest gains only, with improved mental state over first few months but not after 1 year
Cognitive therapy	Individual	Schizophrenia – negative symptoms	Ib	Some evidence of greater gain with negative symptoms
Compliance therapy	Individual	Schizophrenia	Ia	Non-specific gains, possibly achieved as much by education as by specific compliance therapy
Medication management	Individual or group	Schizophrenia – acute	III	Insufficient evidence of gain
Cognitive remediation	Individual and group	Schizophrenia – acute to chronic	Ib	Some evidence of improved cognitive function and self-esteem
Social skills training	Group	Schizophrenia – all types	Ib	Some inconclusive evidence of specific gains in social functioning
Vocational rehabilitation	Individual or group	Schizophrenia – all types	Ia	Improvement in functioning and possibly insight. Definite evidence of gain

It nonetheless has been criticized for its loose use of language and its political connotations, which have led to it being taken on by governments and health systems, and this has aroused added concern. As Oyebode (2004) comments "legitimization by governments both authenticates and authorizes a change in use of language or, as some might say, a misuse of language. What is certain is that the involvement of governments in this endorsement of a peculiar departure in ordinary language use demonstrates that we are here dealing with the politics of health care and not the clinical aspects".

It has proved difficult to join up the principles of evidence-based psychiatry with the recovery movement, despite valiant attempts (Andresen et al., 2003; Resnick et al., 2004; 2005), and as the "journeys" that a patient takes in this movement are individual ones they are impossible to standardize. Some of the principles of recovery are integral to nidotherapy (Tyrer et al., 2003b; see Chapter 36), but go far beyond the manipulation of the environment. There sorely needs to be some kind of rapprochement that allows this movement to be taken on board by professionals interested in evidence-based psychiatry so that it does not just become the province of enthusiasts who are wishing to move it forward at breakneck pace (Roberts & Wolfson, 2004; Bora et al., 2010).

Conclusions

Psychosocial treatments for schizophrenia are effective as ancillary to drug treatment (Table 18.1) and are likely to expand further unless we are able to synthesize new drugs that are effective antipsychotics with few adverse events. The growth of the recovery movement has led to greater optimism and we await the evidence of its long-term effects.

Mood disorders

Blood disorders

19

Psychopharmacology of mood disorders

Based on "Psychopharmacology of mood disorders" by William H. Coryell and John Geddes in Effective Treatments in Psychiatry, Cambridge University Press, 2008

Introduction

Depression is currently the fourth leading cause of disease burden (Üstün et al., 2004) and as drug treatment is the most widely used form of treatment this subject is highly relevant to prescribing practice. Deciding when to prescribe a drug is at least as important as what to prescribe, in what dose, and for how long. This chapter therefore examines the considerations that need to be addressed before prescription begins as well as the process by which a drug treatment is chosen.

Requirements before prescription of an antidepressant drug

Although diagnosis is not the subject of this book it is nonetheless extremely important for the clinician to be aware of the following before deciding to prescribe a drug for depression:

(1) Does the patient satisfy the criteria for a depressive episode or illness? If they do not (or have only a mild episode) then other forms of treatment should be considered (National Institute for Health and Clinical Excellence,

2009d). In addition, if they have comorbid illness but do not have one of the other disorders described in other chapters that also shows response to antidepressants, then both patient and clinician are likely to be disappointed with the response;

(2) Has the illness episode lasted for several months? Although the diagnostic requirements for depression in both ICD and DSM classifications allow for the diagnosis to be made earlier there is good evidence that drug/placebo differences are less if the episode is a shorter one, as many of these will respond spontaneously in the same way as adjustment disorder (see Chapter 28);

(3) Is the depression secondary to another disorder such as alcohol dependence or another condition for which antidepressants are not indicated specifically? If so, that underlying disorder needs to be treated too, possibly before the antidepressant is given.

First-line treatment

Because there are very many antidepressant drugs with similar efficacy the choice of compound at the first point at which prescription is recommended is far from easy. It is likely to depend on knowledge of the patient's symptoms, previous experience in response to drugs, and how much the adverse event profile of the drug is likely to be perceived by the patient. Thus a drug such as trimipramine, which is highly sedative and has many anticholinergic effects, may be very suitable for a very agitated man who has major problems with sleeping, whereas it would be quite unsuitable for a patient who normally sleeps well and needs to concentrate hard during the working day. Weight gain is also common with tricyclic antidepressants, monoamine oxidase inhibitors, and mirtazepine and this is regarded as an adverse effect by many people, but for those who have lost weight as a consequence of depression this adverse effect can be a boon. Similarly, men with problems of premature ejaculation may benefit from treatment with SSRIs (Atmaca et al., 2002) even though delay in ejaculation may be considered a major problem by many others.

Costs may also come into the equation when prescribing an antidepressant. There is a 60-fold difference between the cheapest and most expensive antidepressants and yet the efficacy differences are tiny by comparison. There are conflicting reports about the influence of age and gender in predicting response to antidepressants. Nevertheless, a consensus is developing suggesting that younger people respond better to SSRIs and older ones to tricyclic antidepressants (Parker, 2002; Joyce et al., 2003; Parker et al., 2003), and that women tend to respond better to SSRIs than men (Kornstein et al., 2000; Grigoriadis et al., 2003; Joyce et al., 2003). If other conditions present with the depression the choice of antidepressant may also be influenced, as in obsessive compulsive disorder (see Chapter 27) SSRIs are more effective than tricyclic antidepressants. Dosage may also be an important factor. If the patient is likely to be unreliable about taking the antidepressant then a single dose a day schedule may be preferable to multiple dosing; a drug such as fluoxetine is an example of such a drug. Toxicity in overdose is also important as depressed patients can attempt suicide by overdose; a wide range of drugs is safe in overdose, including the tricyclic drug, lofepramine, as only a small part of it is metabolized to the active compound desipramine, and an overdose is not metabolized.

When all these considerations have been made SSRIs and mirtazepine can be considered as first-line treatments, with a recent meta-analysis of all studies suggesting sertraline may have the most favourable profile (Cipriani et al., 2009). Genetic differences may also be relevant in determining response (Uher et al., 2010) but more data are needed.

Second-line treatment

A large US study, the Sequenced Treatment Alternatives to Relieve Depression (STAR*D) trial, found that first-line treatment with a commonly used SSRI, citalopram, was followed by a remission rate of only 28% (Trivedi et al., 2006). This makes second-line treatment doubly important. When to consider a change is not easy, as antidepressants can take between 1 and 8 weeks to show benefit, but most people who have not improved at 2 weeks fail to recover by 8 weeks (Nierenberg et al., 1995). There are three options when the first drug appears to fail.

Option 1: addition of another drug

This has not been investigated widely in randomized controlled trials. Four studies have been carried out with patients who failed to respond to an SSRI at first prescription; two showed that the addition of another antidepressant (mirtazepine or mianserin) (Ferreri et al., 2001; Carpenter et al., 2002) aided response, and two others showed no value (Fava et al., 2002; Licht & Quitzau, 2002). In the STAR*D trial patients who failed to respond to citalopram were randomized to continued citalopram plus bupropion or buspirone. No difference in efficacy was found but there was a lower withdrawal rate in those randomized to bupropion (Trivedi et al., 2006).

Option 2: substitution of a new drug

In the STAR*D trial an option after initial non-response to citalopram was randomization to bupropion (sustained release), sertraline, or extended-release venlafaxine (Rush et al., 2006a); no difference was found between these three options.

Option 3: augmentation with a drug of a different type

In contrast to the other two options there have been many trials of augmentation with lithium, pindolol, and tri-iodothyronine. All these drugs have benefits in this situation. A meta-analysis with lithium suggested it was 3.7 times more likely to achieve a response than placebo (Bauer & Dopfmer, 1999) with benefit occurring with daily dosage greater than 600 mg and duration of treatment at least 12 days. The meta-analysis mainly included trials of tricyclic antidepressants but similar results have been found with SSRIs (Katona et al., 1995; Baumann et al.,

1996). Pindolol is a beta-blocking drug that blocks 5-HT$_{1A}$ autoreceptors and so prevents negative feedback following synaptic reuptake inhibition. It is successful, but only by hastening response, not in improving it (Ballesteros & Callado, 2004). However, PET scans suggest that the dosage used in these studies was too low and 7.5 mg daily is needed for the drug to occupy the receptors adequately, and at this level it is more effective (Sokolski et al., 2004). A meta-analysis of tri-iodothyronine also showed acceleration of antidepressant response although it was more likely to do so in women than men (Altshuler et al., 2001). As there is some evidence that poor responders are more likely to have thyroid function tests that incline towards hypothyroidism it might be appropriate to test thyroid function in resistant patients.

Olanzapine has also been shown in two trials to have some value in improving response to fluoxetine (Shelton et al., 2005).

Maintenance treatment

A meta-analysis of 4410 patients (31 trials) showed that patients who had responded to an antidepressant and were then randomized to placebo or continued drug experienced a 41% relapse rate with placebo and 18% with the antidepressants (Geddes et al., 2003). This evidence is strongest for patients being withdrawn from antidepressants within the first 2 years but still becomes manifest with withdrawal up to 5 years. The size of this discontinuation effect (twice as many patients relapse on placebo than do those who stay on antidepressants) is greater than the initial response rate from trials carried out in recent years (Walsh et al., 2002) and suggests that as soon as patients do respond the issue of withdrawal should be discussed and planned, including the option of long-term therapy. Indeed, it could be argued that this discussion should take place before treatment is started in less severely ill patients.

Bipolar affective disorder

Acute treatment: mania

Both typical and atypical antipsychotic drugs, lithium, carbamazepine and valproate are effective in the treatment of acute mania (Goodwin et al., 1969; Yatham, 2003). Because of the risk of relapse it is normally recommended that a mood stabilizer such as lithium or valproate should be given early in the course of this treatment if not already implemented. All the major atypical antipsychotics have been shown to be of value in acute mania (Yatham, 2003) and have the advantage that in most cases they are less likely to lead to depressive symptoms than does treatment with typical antipsychotic drugs. This is one of the few fundamental points of difference between these two groups. There is no good evidence supporting the use of any particular mood stabilizer in the acute phase.

Acute treatment: depression

As with acute mania, the longer-term implications of treatment of acute bipolar depression are important to be aware of at the beginning of therapy. This disorder can fluctuate wildly and there is now great concern about the dangers of precipitating a manic episode or inducing a rapid cycling disorder by giving antidepressants in bipolar depression. Despite this concern, the evidence does not really support this hypothesis; switch rates are as great for placebo as antidepressants (Gijsman et al., 2003).

The options are to do nothing in the first instance as so many episodes resolve spontaneously. Antidepressants may be prescribed but long-term studies do not suggest that they possess long-term benefit so it is wise to keep treatment episodes short. Atypical antipsychotic drugs may be effective antidepressants in this condition, and quetiapine is recommended for this purpose in NICE guidelines (National Collaborating Centre for Mental Health, 2005) following favourable reports of its efficacy. Olanzapine may also have similar benefit (Tohen et al., 2003). Lamotrigine also has presumptive evidence of efficacy, but this is based on a cumulative meta-analysis rather than clear evidence from single trials (Geddes et al., 2009).

Maintenance therapy

The four main mood stabilizers, lithium, valproate, carbamazepine and lamotrigine, have all been studied as prophylactic drugs for the maintenance therapy of bipolar disorder. Lithium has by far the best evidence as a prophylactic with a 40% lower chance of relapse when patients are allocated to lithium compared with placebo. Valproate has only shown weak effectiveness, carbamazepine has not been properly tested, and lamotrigine shows some benefit but has only been properly tested in rapid cycling patients. An important international trial (BALANCE) has just been completed and the results are of great interest (Geddes et al., 2010). Three hundred and thirty patients with bipolar disorder were randomized to valproate (in the form of Depakote), lithium, or the combination of lithium and valproate after recovering from the episode and followed up for 2 years. All outcomes, including the primary one of time to relapse recorded by the initiation of new treatment for a new mood episode, showed that the combination of lithium and valproate was the most effective (hazard ratio of 0.59, p = 0.0023 compared to valproate alone) with lithium alone superior to valproate alone (hazard ratio 0.71, p = 0.047), but no significant differences between the combination and lithium alone. The findings are unusual in confirming a combined treatment as more effective than single ones and as the trial was a large pragmatic one in 41 sites, it reflected real world practice so that the patients could be regarded as representative of ordinary clinical practice. It allows a much clearer evidence table to be constructed for the prophylaxis of bipolar disorder (see Table 19.2), in which lithium treatment, alone or in combination, would normally be considered to be the initial choice for prophylaxis unless there are major reasons for thinking otherwise (e.g. a young woman with only one previous episode who might be thinking of childbearing). In this situation it might be desirable to avoid mood stabilizers altogether in view of their hazards (Paton, 2008).

Table 19.1 Effectiveness of drug treatment of acute and resistant depression and maintenance treatment

Treatment	Form of treatment	Psychiatric disorder	Level of evidence to test efficacy	Comments
Tricyclic antidepressants	Mixed noradrenaline and 5-HT reuptake inhibitors	Depressive episode	Ia	Although the choice of first-line treatment will depend on many factors (see text) a recent combined meta-analysis of many other trials of SSRIs suggested that sertraline has the largest effect size and might be preferred (Geddes et al., 2009)
Buproprion		Depressive episode	Ia	
Selective serotonin reuptake inhibitors (SSRIs)	Selective 5-HT reuptake inhibition	Depressive episode	Ia	
Selective serotonin-noradrenaline reuptake inhibitor (SNRI)	Selective inhibition of both noradrenaline and 5-HT	Depressive episode	Ia	
Monoamine oxidase inhibitors (MAOIs)	Irreversible and reversible inhibitors of monoamine oxidase	Resistant depression	II	Better results with irreversible inhibitors (e.g. phenelzine) but these drugs have more adverse effects

Table 19.1 (cont.)

Treatment	Form of treatment	Psychiatric disorder	Level of evidence to test efficacy	Comments
SSRI augmentation	Mianserin and mirtazepine	Resistant depression	II	Some conflicting trial evidence
Tricyclic antidepressant/SSRI augmentation	Lithium	Resistant depression	Ia	Effective if lithium given ≥600 mg daily for at least 12 days
Tricyclic antidepressant/SSRI augmentation	Tri-iodothyronine	Resistant depression	Ia	Greater evidence of efficacy in women
SSRI augmentation	Pindolol	Resistant depression	Ia	Hastens response in low dosage (2.5 mg/day), may be more effective at 7.5 mg/day
SSRI augmentation	Olanzapine	Resistant depression	Ia	May speed up response
Maintenance therapy	Tricyclic antidepressants, SSRIs, MAOIs, SNRIs	Maintenance treatment after recovery	Ia	Early discontinuation likely to lead to relapse with all medication groups

Table 19.2 Drug treatment of bipolar disorder and its prophylaxis

Treatment	Form of treatment	Psychiatric disorder	Level of evidence to test efficacy	Comments
Typical antipsychotic drugs	Chlorpromazine, trifluoperazine, perphenazine, haloperidol	Acute manic episode	Ia	Although all these drugs are effective in the treatment of acute mania the antipsychotic drugs are normally essential as they are more rapid in action than the mood stabilizers
Atypical antipsychotic drugs	Olanzapine, risperidone, quetiapine, ziprasidone, aripiprazole	Acute manic episode	Ia	
Mood stabilizers	Lithium, valproate, carbamazepine, lamotrigine	Acute manic episode	Ia	
Atypical antipsychotic drugs	Quetiapine, olanzapine	Bipolar depression	Ia	Quetiapine currently recommended for this condition; olanzapine may be equivalent in efficacy

Table 19.2 (cont.)

Treatment	Form of treatment	Psychiatric disorder	Level of evidence to test efficacy	Comments
Mood stabilizers	Lamotrigine	Bipolar depression	Ib	Some evidence of efficacy in rapid cyclers
Prophylaxis of depressive and manic episodes	Valproate	Prophylaxis	Ib	Limited evidence of efficacy
Prophylaxis of depressive and manic episodes	Lithium	Prophylaxis	Ia	Strong evidence of efficacy in preventing both manic and depressive episodes, but BALANCE trial suggests best preventive combination is lithium and valproate combined

Summary

The drug treatment of mood disorders now has an impressive evidence base (Tables 19.1 and 19.2) in which the value of good randomized trials is illustrated by the relative confidence with which we can now make recommendations for treatment.

20

Brain stimulation and neurosurgical procedures for the treatment of mood disorders

Based on "Efficacy of brain stimulation and neurosurgical procedures for treatment of mood disorders" by Kunal K. Patra and Edward Coffey in Effective Treatments in Psychiatry, Cambridge University Press, 2008

Introduction

Until recently, this chapter could only have described electroconvulsive therapy (ECT), but with the growth of a new range of treatments competition is developing. This is helping to put the place of brain stimulation in a much wider context, particularly as many of the new treatments can be given without the necessity of an anaesthetic or other medication. However, none of the new treatments can yet be regarded as established ones that can be used in ordinary clinical practice as their evidence base is only now being developed.

Electroconvulsive therapy (ECT) in depression

ECT had been used for over 35 years before it could be said to have a proper evidence base. The first randomized trial of sham and real ECT was carried out by Lambourn and Gill (1978), and was the only study to show a negative finding. Dr Lambourn was one of my (PT) junior doctors at the time and carried out the study diligently, but the sample was small and unilateral ECT was the active treatment. All other sham versus real trials of ECT since have shown benefit for the active treatment (see Table 20.1 for summary) and meta-analyses and treatment guidelines all concur with this conclusion (Davis et al., 1993; Kho et al., 2003; NICE, 2009d). Despite this it is important to note that sham ECT showed some apparent benefit during these studies. I well remember one of my own patients who had failed to respond to ordinary ECT in the past, being included in the trial by Gregory et al. (1985), and making an apparently full recovery.

ECT can therefore be regarded as more effective than its placebo equivalent, and the important questions concern the most desirable way it should be given and how it compares with other antidepressants and other therapies. The first is a reasonable consensus; bilateral ECT is more effective than unilateral ECT (Gregory et al., 1985), but unilateral ECT leads to less memory disturbance, and that the way (i.e. electrode placement, duration of shock, voltage) in which ECT is given has little influence on outcome. A recent study compared bifrontal, bitemporal, and unilateral ECT and found unilateral treatment to be less effective than the other two, and bitemporal ECT to act much more quickly than bifrontal treatment (Kellner et al., 2010). The evidence for ECT in comparison with antidepressant drugs is a little less certain. On balance ECT appears to be more effective than antidepressive drugs but the benefits refer mainly to its increased speed of response rather than its overall long-term gain (Greenblatt et al., 1964; Medical Research Council, 1985; Folkerts et al., 1997) (Table 20.1).

Maintenance ECT in depression

There are no controlled studies on the effectiveness of maintenance ECT over a long period, largely because of the ethical concerns this would engender, and it is not recommended in official guidelines such as NICE. However, the Royal College of Psychiatrists (2005) demurred and in a report felt there was sufficient evidence from clinical experience and from case studies to support continuation ECT in some cases refractory to other treatment.

Electroconvulsive therapy (ECT) in other disorders

ECT has been used for the treatment of manic episodes and catatonia for

Table 20.1 Effectiveness of ECT

Author	Form of treatment, subjects, and psychiatric disorder	Method	Findings
Lambourn et al., 1978	Sham vs. real ECT: 32 right-handed in-and outpatients with depressive psychosis	Equal allocation: 6 right temporal (unilateral) treatments; concomitant benzodiazepines	No differences in Hamilton depression scores after 6 treatments
Freeman et al., 1978	Sham vs. real ECT: 40 inpatients with depressive illness	Equal allocation: 6 bilateral treatments (first two ECTs sham in sham group); concomitant antidepressants	After first two ECTs the real ECT group had significantly lower depression scores and had fewer treatments overall
Johnstone et al., 1980	Sham vs. real ECT: 70 inpatients with "endogenous depression"	Equal allocation: 8 bilateral treatments; concomitant benzodiazepines	Significantly greater improvement in ECT group
West, 1981	Sham vs. real ECT: 40 inpatients with depressive illness	Equal allocation: 6 bilateral treatments; concomitant amitriptyline	Ditto
Brandon et al., 1984	Sham vs. real ECT: 95 inpatients with depression	Equal allocation: 8 bilateral treatments; concomitant benzodiazepines	Better improvement at 2 and 4 weeks; no difference at 12 and 28 weeks
Gregory et al., 1985	Sham vs. bilateral and unilateral ECT: 69 inpatients with depression, concomitant benzodiazepines	Equal allocation: 6 bilateral and unilateral treatments; concomitant benzodiazepines	Better improvement in both ECT groups after 2, 4, and 6 treatments
Kellner et al., 2010	Bifrontal and bitemporal vs. unilateral ECT: 230 patients with bipolar and unipolar depression	Equal allocation with 10 treatments each	55% with right unilateral, 61% with bifrontal, and 64% with bitemporal ECT (differences not significant but faster response with bitemporal treatment)

Greenblatt et al., 1964	ECT vs. imipramine, isocarboxazid, phenelzine, and placebo: 281 inpatients with depression	9 ECT given, presumed bilateral	Order of improvement: ECT (76%), phenelzine (50%), imipramine (49%), placebo (46%), isocarboxazid (28%)
Medical Research Council, 1965	ECT vs. imipramine, phenelzine, and placebo: 250 outpatients and inpatients with depression	4–8 bilateral ECT given	ECT significantly superior to other treatments, imipramine second in efficacy
Gangadhar et al., 1982	ECT vs. imipramine and placebo – 2 separate trials of 16 patients resistant to tricyclic antidepressants	6 bilateral ECT given	ECT superior, but only after 2 weeks' treatment, not subsequently
Dinan et al., 1989	ECT vs. lithium and tricyclic antidepressants: 32 patients resistant to tricyclic antidepressants	6 bilateral ECT given	No difference in outcome between groups after 3 weeks
Folkerts et al., 1997	ECT vs. paroxetine: 39 right-handed inpatients with depression	6–9 unilateral ECTs	ECT significantly superior to paroxetine at 4 weeks

many years and appears in most recommended treatment guidelines despite relatively slim evidence for its value.

As the treatment is usually given in an emergency it is difficult to perform trials in these conditions but three studies have been carried out into the management of acute mania with ECT. The first of these was a trial of ECT against lithium carbonate in 34 inpatients with bipolar disorder. Improvement in clinical symptoms was greater between weeks 6 and 8 with ECT but after 8 weeks outcome was similar in both the short and long term (Small et al., 1988). In a second study combined lithium/ haloperidol therapy was compared with ECT in 27 patients in a manic phase of bipolar disorder. Only five patients were in the lithium/haloperidol group and none improved, whereas 13 (59%) achieved full remission in the ECT group (Mukherjee et al., 1994). In the last study 30 patients received sham or real ECT with both groups receiving chlorpromazine in a dose of 600 mg daily. Those receiving real ECT improved more quickly and completely than those in the sham group.

These findings suggest that ECT is an appropriate treatment for mania but should normally be considered as a second-line treatment.

Several studies find that augmentation of antipsychotics with ECT enhances efficacy in the treatment of delusions, hallucinations, and thought disorder in patients with acute psychotic episodes in schizophrenia (Chanpattana et al., 1999). Generally, ECT is not as effective for negative symptoms of schizophrenia such as blunted emotional expression and amotivation.

Transcranial magnetic stimulation

Transcranial magnetic stimulation (TMS) involves the passage of a pulsed magnetic field generated by an electrical coil through the scalp and into the brain. This depolarizes neurons in the brain and, although used mainly for brain stimulation in neurology, there are suggestions that the procedure may have treatment benefits for psychiatry also (George et al., 1999; 2003). The condition most commonly treated is depression and sufficient trials have now been carried out to allow meta-analyses to be carried out on the data. The results are not consistent and there is currently insufficient evidence to support the use of this treatment in depression (Martin et al., 2003; 2004). More recent trials have produced inconsistent results, with some showing good results in resistant depression (Anderson et al., 2007) and others showing little benefit. TMS does not seem to be as effective as ECT and ECT seems to be substantially more effective for the short-term treatment of depression (Eranti et al., 2007).

Vagal nerve stimulation (VNS)

Since early work showing that vagus nerve stimulation could prevent motor and autonomic components of epilepsy there has been interest in this technique in the treatment of depression. There are also reports of increased dopaminergic, serotonergic, and noradrenergic neurotransmission following stimulation of the vagus and this supports its possible value in treatment. After an early open study showing improvement in depressive symptoms (Sackeim et al., 2001) a randomized trial showed no significant difference in outcome with 235 resistant depressive patients already on antidepressant therapy with sham and real vagus nerve stimulation in the two treatment arms (Rush et al., 2005). There are some suggestions that the beneficial effects of treatment take longer to become apparent after VNS (George et al., 2005) but this has not been tested in *a priori* studies. At present it is therefore impossible to conclude that VNS has any benefit for the treatment of depression from the evidence available (Table 20.2).

Neurosurgical procedures

Ablative procedures

Psychosurgery is now rarely considered in psychiatric treatment but for a small minority of very handicapped patients with obsessive compulsive disorder (see Chapter 27) and major depression it is still a valid treatment option. Modern treatment is by stereotactic methods, and includes cingulotomy, subcaudate tractotomy, limbic leucotomy, and anterior capsulotomy (Cosgrove, 2000; Sienaert, 2011). The evidence available does not allow any clear conclusions to be drawn about its value.

Deep brain stimulation

This radical approach involves the stereotactic implantation of a small stimulus electrode into the specific parts of the brain using magnetic resonance imaging as a guide. It is mainly a treatment initiated for intractable movement disorders found in neurological clinics but it has been used both in obsessive compulsive disorder and likely drug-induced movement disorders, including tardive dyskinesia. There are preliminary suggestions that stimulation of the subgenual cingulate area is more likely to produce antidepressant effects (Mayberg et al., 2005). This evidence is not strong enough to lead to any specific recommendations.

Conclusions

Although ECT is becoming less used in many countries it remains a highly

Table 20.2 Summary of brain stimulation procedures in mood disorders

Treatment	Form of treatment	Psychiatric disorder	Level of evidence to test efficacy	Comments
Bilateral ECT	Suprathreshold dosage	Severe depressive episode	Ia	Unequivocal efficacy with only one negative study (see Table 20.1 and text)
Unilateral ECT	Suprathreshold dosage	Severe depression in elderly	Ia	Less effective than bilateral ECT but much less memory disturbance
Bilateral ECT	Suprathreshold dosage	Mania	III	Lacks trial evidence but many positive reports
Bilateral ECT	Not known	Maintenance treatment of depression	IV	No evidence of efficacy despite being repeatedly used
Repetitive transcranial magnetic stimulation (rTMS)	Up to three times weekly	Severe depression	Ib	May be effective but trials equivocal – may depend on form of treatment
Vagal nerve stimulation	Pulse generator treatment	Treatment-resistant depression	III	Open studies only to date

effective treatment with few adverse effects when given under optimal conditions. Electroconvulsive therapy is still the most efficacious treatment for major depression, particularly when symptoms are severe (Ebmeier et al., 2006). The results of the STAR*D trial were salutary with the cumulative remission rate from clinical depression being 67% after four sequential acute treatment schedules (Rush et al., 2006b). It is also, almost certainly, likely to be effective in acute mania and should be kept in reserve for this condition as a second-line treatment. Unilateral ECT is associated with less memory disturbance than bilateral ECT so it can be given to the right hemisphere in right-handed patients, but in those who are left-handed it is more difficult to be certain which is the dominant hemisphere, and the treatment has to be given to the non-dominant hemisphere if memory disturbance is to be reduced. In the present state

of knowledge – and this is unlikely to change dramatically in the next few years – unilateral ECT should be reserved for elderly patients or those with pre-existing memory disturbance. Bifrontal ECT has its advocates and allegedly has fewer effects on memory (Letemendia et al., 1993) but has not been shown to have any advantages in trials to date.

Transcranial magnetic stimulation probably has some benefit in the treatment of depression but for which type of problem and how it should be administered remain to be elucidated. Until then it should remain an experimental treatment. As it has the great advantage that it can be administered without an anaesthetic it would be an asset to care if its value could be clarified. Vagal nerve stimulation and deep brain stimulation still require a great deal more efficacy studies before they can be considered as clinical treatments in psychiatry.

21

Psychotherapy for depression: current empirical status and future directions

Based on "Psychotherapy for depression: current empirical status and future directions" by Scott Temple and John Geddes in Effective Treatments in Psychiatry, Cambridge University Press, 2008

Introduction

Psychological treatments for depression have made great advances in the last 30 years. As the enthusiasm for drug treatments has waned to some extent, the relative advantages of psychological approaches, particularly with regard to their very few adverse effects, has raised their profile enormously. In keeping with the evidence that depression is the leading cause of mental distress it is good to note that it also has the strongest evidence base for psychological treatment than any other mental disorder. As well as extremely robust evidence for established therapies there is also a growing literature on new approaches that should help to expand treatments successfully to include primary care, where most people with depression are seen, and all of these are discussed in this section.

Cognitive behavioural therapy (CBT)

Cognitive behavioural therapy has revolutionized many areas of treatment in psychiatry but it is important to remember that its founder,

Aaron T. Beck, introduced it for the treatment of depression. In analyzing the dreams of depressed patients in psychoanalytical training he was asked to find evidence of anger and repression. Instead he found depressive thoughts and themes and subsequently hypothesized that pathological depression was maintained and reinforced by depressive cognitive biases. These distorted thoughts and beliefs needed to be reversed if the mood was to improve (Beck, 2006). The refinement of this treatment, so that it is now given by thousands of practitioners from across the world from many different backgrounds, has led to many randomized trials that show it to be at least as good for the treatment of mild and moderate depression as antidepressant drugs (National Collaborating Centre for Mental Health, 2009a) and preferable to drug treatment as it has no significant adverse effects. There is also good evidence that CBT combined with antidepressant drugs is superior to drugs alone in more severe depression and, because it does not lose its efficacy to the same extent as antidepressants after treatment finishes, it may also have a prophylactic effect on the recurrence of major depressive episodes (Evans et al., 1992; Jarrett et al., 1999).

Interpersonal psychotherapy

Interpersonal psychotherapy (IPT) was developed in the context of depression being associated with loss, isolation, unresolved grief, role transition, and social withdrawal. These have long been noted in depressive disorder, but Gerald Klerman, who developed the treatment, argued that these were associated with interpersonal deficits that needed to be corrected (Klerman et al., 1984). A series of randomized controlled trials has shown interpersonal therapy to be undoubtedly effective (Dimascio et al., 1979; Weissman et al., 1979; Elkin et al., 1989; Gibbons et al., 2002), and of these the evidence derived from the large multicentre trial, the Treatment of Depression Collaborative Research Programme (TDCRP), has had the most impact and helped to establish IPT worldwide.

There has been considerable controversy over the relative advantages of CBT and IPT in the treatment of depression. The TDCRP compared the outcome of 250 patients randomized to four treatment arms (tricyclic antidepressant, placebo, IPT, and CBT) and was somewhat underpowered to test all four of these satisfactorily. The results showed both psychotherapies to be essentially similar in efficacy and better than placebo after 12 weeks but by the 16th week were no better than placebo. The tricyclic antidepressant, imipramine, was more rapid in its treatment effects and was superior to the psychotherapies after 12 weeks. The controversy arose mainly over subsidiary analyses that suggested a better response to IPT than CBT in severe depression, but as this was also associated with large treatment/site interactions it suggested that differences in the treatment and performance of the therapists was at least as important as the nature of the treatments themselves.

Further studies since the TDCRP have generally supported the initial suspicions that IPT and CBT are roughly similar in their efficacy and that both have the prophylactic ability to reduce relapse of depression (Kovacs et al., 1981; Simons et al., 1986; Frank et al., 1990; Evans et al., 1992). Further studies of CBT in comparison with SSRIs in the form of paroxetine also reinforce the earlier findings; treatment effects of the psychotherapy lag behind the drug but efficacy is at least as good if experienced therapists are used (DeRubeis et al., 2005; Hollon et al., 2005). The positive effects of CBT in the hands of experienced therapists are maintained over several years (Kingdon et al., 1996). There is increasing evidence that CBT might be marginally more effective than IPT in severe depression (Luty et al., 2007), and in patients who also have comorbid personality disorder (Joyce et al., 2007).

Mindfulness-based cognitive behavioural therapy

This treatment, based on a combination of cognitive therapy linked to mindfulness meditation – a treatment that is particularly focused on preventing depressive ruminations – has been introduced mainly as a prophylactic method of preventing further episodes of depression in those who have recovered from a major depressive episode. It is usually administered in groups over a period of eight sessions. In the initial randomized controlled trial of 145 patients who had recovered from a major depressive episode the follow-up evidence showed that mindfulness-based cognitive behavioural therapy (MCBT) was effective in reducing relapse, but only in patients with three or more previous episodes of depression (Teasdale et al., 2000). As this finding was found in a *post hoc* analysis more data were needed to put the place of this treatment in perspective and a follow-on study confirmed these findings (Ma & Teasdale, 2004). Exactly why the high frequency depression sufferers should show benefit only is far from clear; one obvious explanation is that they are much more likely to ruminate about depression. More studies are needed from other investigators.

Behaviour therapy and activation

This might be thought to be similar to the behavioural components of cognitive behavioural therapy but there are important differences. Jacobson et al. (2001) developed a more direct programme of behavioural activation that attempts to re-engage the depressed patient in activities that are both meaningful and necessary in daily living. This is done without any exploration of depressive thoughts. Patients become aware that their depressive cognitions are in conflict with their other needs and are of little or no value. The evidence that this may be effective only comes from one group at the University of Washington. Two trials have been carried out. The first compared CBT, behavioural activation combined with automatic thought medication, and behavioural activation alone. No differences were found between the three treatments either at the end of treatment (20 sessions) or at 6 months follow-up (Jacobson et al., 1996). The second study, carried out with 241 more severely depressed patients, compared antidepressant

therapy with behavioural activation and cognitive behavioural therapy. The response to behavioural activation was equivalent to that for antidepressants and superior to that for cognitive behavioural therapy (Martell et al., 2003; Dimidjian et al., 2006).

It is difficult to extrapolate from these studies to the treatment of depression in general, but the findings cannot be ignored and need investigating further. One of the problems in this area is that therapists who are enthusiastic about one form of treatment are often a little more effective than those who are just giving it as a routine treatment, and this may influence results in both trials and clinical practice.

Cognitive behavioural analysis of psychotherapy (CBASP)

This treatment has been introduced for people with more chronic forms of depression, probably including what is currently known as dysthymia, and is best thought of as a behavioural system of treatment since it emphasizes the function rather than the content of depressive thoughts and pays special attention to social problem-solving (McCullough, 2000). Patients are asked what their desired outcomes are from a specific situation and whether their thoughts and actions achieve these outcomes or undesirable ones. Social problem solving is introduced to aid the achieving of desired goals. The treatment also puts a great deal of stress on the therapeutic relationship to prevent or overcome the tendency for "depressogenic" relationships.

This treatment has been evaluated somewhat unusually in a very large trial before having its components tested previously in smaller ones. Six hundred and eighty-one people with depression were allocated to CBASP, nefazodone (an antidepressant now withdrawn from prescription), or combined CBASP and nefazodone. CBASP was as effective as nefazodone in the acute phase of treatment but the combination was more effective than either treatment alone (Keller et al., 2000). A further trial has now been published (Kocsis et al., 2009) in which CBASP was compared with brief supportive psychotherapy. This 12–week trial in chronically depressed patients initially compared continued pharmacotherapy and augmentation with CBASP with continued pharmacotherapy and augmentation with brief supportive psychotherapy, and continued (optimized) pharmacotherapy alone. Subsequently there were other combinations of these interventions but, disappointingly, none of the three interventions showed any advantage over the other. Although further long-term work is continuing on outcome these findings do not suggest that CBASP has a significant role in chronic depression.

Psychodynamic psychotherapy

Although classical psychodynamic therapy was probably the mainstay of treatment for depression for over 50 years it has not performed well in this evidence-based era. Several attempts have been made to subject it to randomized controlled enquiries, and most have foundered on the problem of randomizing people who have not been judged to be suitable for the treatment (Candy et al., 1972). A recently developed form of this treatment, psychodynamic interpersonal therapy, was roughly equivalent to the effects of cognitive behavioural therapy in a multicentre trial with only scores on the Beck Depression Inventory showing superiority for cognitive behavioural therapy (Shapiro et al., 1994).

Conclusions

The main message from the psychotherapy of depression is that treatment works and is competing strongly with antidepressants in

Table 21.1 Effectiveness of psychotherapies in depression

Treatment	Form of treatment	Psychiatric disorder	Level of evidence to test efficacy	Comments
Cognitive behavioural therapy	Individual	Mild to moderate depression	Ia	Highly effective and equivalent to antidepressant therapy
Cognitive behavioural therapy	Individual	Severe depression	IIb	Probably effective with experienced therapists
Cognitive behavioural therapy in combination with antidepressant drugs	Individual	Severe and resistant depression	Ia	Strong evidence of superiority over drug treatment alone
Cognitive behavioural therapy	Individual	Long-term remission	Ia	Good evidence of long-term benefits from CBT
Interpersonal psychotherapy	Individual	Mild to moderate depression	Ia	Effective and equivalent to antidepressant therapy
Interpersonal psychotherapy	Individual	Severe depression	Ia	Not as effective as antidepressants when given alone
Interpersonal psychotherapy and antidepressants	Individual	Relapse prevention	Ib	Some evidence of superiority of combined therapy over drugs alone
Mindfulness-based cognitive behavioural therapy	Group	Relapse prevention	Ib	Effective in people with repeated episodes but not with others
Behaviour therapy and activation	Group	Moderate depression	Ib	May have similar benefits to CBT
Psychodynamic psychotherapy	Individual	Moderate depression	IIa	Some slight evidence of efficacy
Cognitive behavioural analysis system of psychotherapy	Individual	Chronic depression	Ib	May be similar to antidepressant therapy in this special group

terms of efficacy. This is an important conclusion but has to be qualified in several ways. Firstly, we must not get too preoccupied with the individual names and theories of the different psychotherapies that are effective. The simple reason why so many of these are jostling with each other tightly in the treatment stakes is that they overlap in their theory and practice. Cognitive behavioural therapy, as the oldest and most established therapy, is like an old-fashioned drug such as chlorpromazine in the treatment of schizophrenia. All the new drugs want to compete against it successfully, and there is a tendency to load the odds so that the new ones come out on top. There is a similar tendency in studies of new psychotherapies. It is as though the aim of treatment is not to show that a new treatment is effective but that it is at least as good as CBT. This is easier to achieve than comparing the new treatment with a control intervention as the ethical aspects are more straightforward, but it is then easy to load a study with indifferent therapists in one arm of a trial and compare them with a new "treatment" given by enthusiasts. The results will invariably favour the new treatment but may not be a valid assessment of its value. Secondly, the benefits of antidepressant drug therapy in depression are far from dramatic and the achievement of equivalent efficacy is only the first stage in establishing a good evidence base for the treatment. Where psychological treatments persistently score better than drug ones is in their lower incidence of adverse effects and their more prolonged benefits after treatment has finished. In Chapter 19 we noted that the relapse rates after switching to placebo within 5 years of responding to an antidepressant are twice as high as those for patients who stay on treatment. When effective psychological treatments are given at the same time (or possibly just after) benefit has been shown then the relapse rates are much lower. We need to build on this in developing these treatments and also to try different approaches for chronic depression, where we now seem to be becalmed when trying to find a way forward in treatment. Thirdly, we need to ensure that effective psychological treatments are available when and where needed, and that the therapists who administer them are competent and committed, as for too long practitioners have had to rely only on what is available, not what is the best treatment for the patient.

Interventions discussed in this chapter are summarized in Table 21.1.

22

Alternative therapies for depression

Based on "Alternative therapies for mood disorder" by William H. Coryell in Effective
Treatments in Psychiatry, Cambridge University Press, 2008

Introduction

As depression is so common it is not
surprising that many sufferers seek
help from others who are outside the
conventional frame of medicine. The
evaluation of these is far from easy as
so many of the alternative treatments
available have many potential ingredients and it is often difficult to separate them. The following chapter
summarizes the evidence for those
approaches that are supported by at
least two prospectively randomized
and controlled, parallel-design studies, and this includes both drug studies and other interesting interventions.
Most phytotherapy (herbal remedies)
has been excluded on grounds of
limited evidence.

Light therapy

The observation that many persons
regularly experience depressive
symptoms during winter months,
and that the prevalence of this pattern
increases with latitude, led to the use
of light exposure as a treatment for
seasonal affective disorder. Many
controlled studies have followed
(Terman et al., 1989) and the results
support the conclusion that improvement following bright light exposure
far exceeds that following dim light
exposure, with greater benefits for
morning than for evening exposures.
Atypical depressive symptoms such
as hypersomnia, evening worsening,
and carbohydrate craving predict
response to light therapy while

melancholic symptoms such as psychomotor retardation, morning worsening, and terminal insomnia predict non-response (Terman et al., 1996). The amount of improvement with morning light appears to correlate with the degree to which melatonin onset is enhanced by the exposure, and is thought to be optimal when timed to begin 2½ hours after the sleep midpoint (Terman et al., 2001). There is an interesting finding from research in northern Norway, where in mid-winter there is no light during the day and where a much lower proportion of the population (around 1 in 5) have problems relating to sleep or mood during the winter months (Hansen et al., 1998). This suggest that when daylight is absent different mechanisms are operating.

Earlier studies applied 2500 lux of light for 2 hours in the morning but most recent trials have used 10 000 lux for 30 minutes. Still better compliance may be expected with dawn simulation, a gradual increase in ambient light to 2500 lux over a 1½ hour period beginning at 4:30 a.m. (Avery et al., 2001). Relatively few controlled studies have tested this dosing, and direct comparisons to conventional bright light exposure have had inconsistent results that, on balance, have favoured bright light exposure (Avery et al., 2001).

Though light treatment was first applied to seasonal affective disorder it may be no less effective for patients with a non-seasonal temporal pattern. Of six randomized studies that have compared bright light to dim light as monotherapy for non-seasonal depression, three showed a significant advantage for bright light (Kripke et al., 1992; Yamda et al., 1995; Beauchemin & Hays, 1997). A differential sensitivity has been revealed in a naturalistic study of inpatients in which those with bipolar depression assigned to rooms facing east (i.e., towards the dawn light in the northern hemisphere) had significantly shorter stays in the hospital than those given rooms facing west while no such difference emerged for patients with unipolar depression (Benedetti et al., 2001).

Sleep deprivation

Numerous studies have shown that the deprivation of sleep for a 36-hour period (total sleep deprivation or TSD), or for the second half of the night (partial sleep deprivation or PSD), leads to an immediate improvement in depressive symptoms in a substantial proportion of patients. Symptoms return at their previous severity after a night of sleep when sleep deprivation is used as monotherapy. The combined use of sleep deprivation with antidepressant drugs, however, appears to offer clear and practical advantages over either treatment alone.

Two prospectively randomized studies (Baxter et al., 1986; Colombo et al., 2000) have described bipolar I patients given sleep deprivation with or without lithium. One used partial sleep deprivation on two consecutive nights (Baxter et al., 1986), and the other used three TSDs over a 1-week period (Colombo et al., 2000). Despite these treatment differences, all described significantly lower depression scores after the final recovery night. The only study to provide follow-up data found that those who had received sleep deprivation while taking lithium had significantly lower depressive symptom scores 3 months later than did those who had received sleep deprivation without lithium even though the latter group had begun taking lithium following the TSD course (Benedetti et al., 1999). Only one report compared patients randomized to lithium with sleep deprivation to those given lithium alone. Outcome measured 5 days later significantly favoured the combined therapy (Baxter et al., 1986).

Similarly, sleep deprivation in conjunction with antidepressants has been shown in four trials with clomipramine and fluoxetine to improve depression to a greater extent with TSD than with the antidepressant alone, but this benefit disappeared after 1 to 3 weeks (Elsenga & van den Hoofdakker, 1982; Benedetti et al., 1997; Barbini et al., 1998).

There is thus substantial evidence that sleep deprivation can at least hasten antidepressant responses to lithium and to other antidepressants. This potential has particular applicability to inpatient settings. Evidence that the benefits of sleep deprivation combined with lithium may be sustained well beyond the first week in bipolar patients, together with findings that bipolar I patients are more likely than bipolar II or unipolar patients to have sustained improvement with TSD monotherapy (Barbini et al., 1998), suggest that bipolar I patients who develop depression despite lithium prophylaxis may be helped by sleep deprivation.

Omega-3 supplementation

Extensive evidence from epidemiological and case–control studies now exists to show that deficits in certain of the essential fatty acids (EFAs) both raise the risk of affective disorder and worsen its course. These findings have sparked numerous treatment trials that have assessed omega-3 supplementation in the treatment or prevention of depressive symptoms or episodes. There are two important omega-3 fatty acids, eicosapenta-enoic acid (EPA) and docosahexaenoic acid (DHA), which are involved in the synthesis of hormones, ageing and control of inflammation, and, more recently, in the control of mood.

A recent meta-analysis of 28 placebo-controlled trials showed the largest effect sizes for the treatment of major depressive episodes rather than symptoms, for therapeutic rather than preventive intervention, and for the use of EPA rather than DHA (Frangou et al., 2006; Martins 2009).

Exercise therapy

Carefully controlled trials have demonstrated the benefits of supervised exercise programmes for depressive symptoms, with the main gains being made for aerobic exercise for periods of several weeks (Blumenthal et al., 1999; Babyak et al., 2000; Mather et al., 2002).

One of these studies compared the exercise programme with sertraline, or a combination of the drug and exercise (Blumenthal et al., 1999). Although the decrease in depressive symptom scores was similar in the three groups at follow-up 6 months later, the two exercise groups had significantly lower recurrence rates than the sertraline group.

A recent controlled trial testing the biophilia hypothesis, that good health is maintained only by a positive relationship with the natural environment, compared the treatment of depression by swimming with dolphins with a control group having time-equivalent water-based therapy only. The results showed significantly greater benefit in the dolphin-assisted therapy group (Antonioli & Reveley, 2005). Exercise levels were roughly similar in both groups.

Oestrogen replacement in perimenopausal depression

A meta-analysis of the extensive literature on hormone replacement treatment and mood symptoms concluded that oestrogen replacement benefits mood symptoms in mixed samples of perimenopausal and postmenopausal women (Zweifel and O'Brien, 1997). Results varied considerably across studies, and drug–placebo differences were not significant for the 12 samples consisting entirely of postmenopausal women. The results leave quite unclear the ideal hormonal dose or delivery, or the duration of an adequate trial. In one study, improvement after 6 weeks was no greater than improvement after 3 weeks (Schmidt et al., 2000). In another, differences between oestrogen replacement and placebo increased throughout the 12-week trial (Soares et al., 2001), with the benefits of oestrogen replacement persisting after a 4-week washout.

Androgens

The previously mentioned meta-analysis also found that androgen replacement, with or without oestrogen, was associated with substantially more improvement in mood symptoms than hormone replacement therapy with oestrogen alone (Zweifel and O'Brien, 1997).

Numerous reports have demonstrated an association between depressive disorders in males and low testosterone concentrations (Margolese, 2000). In perhaps the earliest placebo-controlled study, depressed men who received the synthetic androgen, mesterolone, for 6 weeks had outcomes similar to placebo. The participants had a mean age of 43 and baseline testosterone concentrations were not assessed. Another more recent trial required a baseline testosterone concentration of 350 ng/ml or less and used weekly intramuscular injections of 200 mg testosterone for active treatment (Seidman et al., 2001), but, again, improvement with androgen treatment resembled that for treatment

with placebo. By contrast in another trial comparing placebo and 10 g of testosterone gel applied daily for 8 weeks in a sample of antidepressant-unresponsive men who had testosterone concentrations less than 300 ng/dl, the clinical response was significantly greater with testosterone (Rabkin et al., 2000). The difference in depression scores between testosterone and placebo increased throughout the 8-week trial, and responses were limited to those whose testosterone concentrations increased by more than 200 ng/dl. Another trial administered 400 mg testosterone or placebo in bi-weekly intramuscular injections to HIV-positive men with low baseline testosterone concentrations and clinical evidence of "hypogonadal mood symptoms" (Rabkin et al., 2000). Among the 26 with an Axis-I mood disorder at baseline, those who received testosterone were four times (58% versus 14%) more likely to be much, or very much, improved than were those given placebo. Yet another trial randomized HIV-positive men who had had clinical signs of hypogonadism and who had responded to a 12-week open trial of the same testosterone regime to either continue with testosterone, or to receive placebo injections instead, for an additional 6-week trial (Rabkin et al., 1999). Nine in ten of those switched to placebo lost their responses compared to only

Table 22.1 Summary of evidence base of alternative treatments (excluding dietary supplements) for mood disorders

Treatment	Form of treatment	Psychiatric disorder	Level of evidence for efficacy	Comments
Light therapy alone	2500 lux for 2 h to 10 000 lux for 30 min	Depression (mainly seasonal affective disorder)	Ib	Undoubtedly effective as an antidepressant treatment
Light therapy with antidepressant drugs	As above with antidepressants in conventional dosage	Depression (mainly seasonal affective disorder)	Ib	Undoubtedly effective and may be of greater superiority to antidepressants alone in this group
Sleep deprivation	Total sleep deprivation for 36 hours or partial sleep deprivation for 5 hours	Depression	IIa	Antidepressant effect short-lived
Sleep deprivation with mood stabilizers (lithium)	As above	Bipolar I	Ib	Effective but more information needed on persistence of benefit
Sleep deprivation with antidepressant drugs	As above with conventional doses of drugs	Depression	Ib	Effects short-lived and after 3 weeks no difference between treatments
Exercise therapy	Variable periods of mainly aerobic exercise (3–12 weeks) often with maintenance exercise	Depression	Ib	Undoubted efficacy with equivalent benefit to antidepressant drugs

Treatment	Indication	Duration	Evidence	Comments
Oestrogen replacement	Perimenopausal and postmenopausal women with depression	3–12 weeks	Ia	Limited evidence of efficacy with any benefits mainly in perimenopausal group (with possible gains from added androgens)
Testosterone and related compounds (e.g. mesterolone)	Depression	6–10 weeks	IIa	Very mixed results with no clear benefit
St. John's wort (Hypericum extract)	Depression	4–12 weeks	Ia	Early evidence of benefit thrown into doubt by recent larger studies

two of ten of those maintained on testosterone.

As three placebo-controlled trials found that testosterone supplementation benefited depressed men and two did not, no firm conclusions can yet be drawn about the value of testosterone therapy.

Hypericum extract (Saint John's wort)

A meta-analysis of 14 placebo-controlled studies concluded that hypericum extract, or St. John's wort, was significantly superior to placebo for depression with a responder-rate ratio of 2.67 (CI = 1.78–4.01) (Linde et al., 1996). Nearly all of the samples were comprised of fewer than 100 subjects, most of whom were thought to have "neurotic depression". Another recent meta-analysis using later studies by the same authors (Linde et al., 2005) was much less positive but since then there have been further reports in favour of the drug both against placebo and in comparison with SSRIs (Kasper et al., 2008).

Whether or not a clinician recommends St. John's wort to his patients, he or she should at least inquire whether they are taking it, or plan to do so. Because of its effects on cytokine p450 enzymes and on serotonin reuptake hypericum can lower blood levels of certain medications and can result in a serotonin syndrome when combined with other drugs (Izzo, 2004).

Summary

Depression is commonly treated by alternative approaches to standard drug and psychological therapy. The evidence (Table 22.1) shows that light therapy, sleep deprivation, and exercise therapy are all valuable treatments but probably not substitutes for other treatment. Eicosapentaenoic acid (EPA), one of the omega-3 fatty acids, also appears to have clear antidepressant properties and may be used without other treatments. Oestrogens and testosterone appear to have some value but the population that can be helped is still not completely clear. St John's wort (Hypericum and its extracts) remains a bit of an enigma but appears likely to have some therapeutic value.

Anxiety and neurotic disorders

23

Treatment of generalized anxiety and somatoform disorders

Based on "Treatment of generalized anxiety and somatoform disorders" by Peter Tyrer and David Baldwin in Effective Treatments in Psychiatry, Cambridge University Press, 2008

Introduction

These conditions are common and most are managed in primary care. Neither of these conditions has a good diagnostic base in the sense that they overlap with many other related disorders (see chapters on panic, agoraphobia, and social phobia) and also are intimately involved with depression. Because of this overlap it is not surprising that the treatments also overlap. The diagnostic grouping of somatoform disorders is one of the least useful in psychiatry (Mayou et al., 2005) and for many of the conditions within the group there are no clear effective treatments. 'Medically unexplained symptoms' has become a commonly used term to describe many of these disorders and health anxiety is gradually replacing the older, and somewhat pejorative, term, hypochondriasis, and consequently moving the condition closer to the anxiety disorders (Olatunji et al., 2009).

Drug treatment of generalized anxiety disorder

Acute treatment

Antidepressants

Both tricyclic antidepressants and selective serotonin reuptake inhibitors (SSRIs) have been evaluated in many randomized controlled trials. Most of the early trials with tricyclic antidepressants did not specifically assess those with generalized anxiety disorder because this condition was subsumed under the label of "anxiety neurosis" before it was abolished in DSM-III, but their benefits had by then been demonstrated (Casacalenda & Boulenger, 1998). Following introduction of the diagnosis of generalized anxiety disorder the results were very similar (e.g., Kahn et al., 1986), but in this era of new drugs there were many more studies with the selective serotonin reuptake inhibitors (SSRIs). All the common members of this group, including citalopram, escitalopram, paroxetine, sertraline, fluoxetine and fluvoxamine, have been found in randomized trials to be superior to placebo. Currently only escitalopram and paroxetine are licensed for the treatment of anxiety disorder. Recently pregabalin has also been tested in randomized controlled trials and found to be effective in this condition in both adults and older people (Montgomery et al., 2008). The onset of benefit with all these drugs tends to be delayed by between 1 and 3 weeks although with the tricyclic antidepressants the sedative effects are noted immediately and may also be of benefit. Generally the SSRIs are preferred for the treatment of generalized anxiety disorder rather than tricyclic antidepressants, but this view has been heavily influenced by drug marketing and the differences in value may have been overstated. The choice of antidepressant is an important clinical decision (see Chapter 21) and in the case of generalized anxiety disorder depends critically on the symptoms and nature of the disorder. If a patient is highly anxious and restless and has major problems with sleeping at night then a sedative antidepressant (e.g. amitriptyline) may be considered superior to an SSRI, not least because anxiety may be a prominent symptom initially with SSRIs. By contrast, an elderly depressed person prone to orthostatic hypotension is best treated with an SSRI as postural hypotension is a significant handicap of antidepressants.

There is also considerable concern about the withdrawal symptoms that follow reduction of SSRIs, particularly if this is done abruptly. This withdrawal syndrome (which as a good example of sophistry is usually called a discontinuation syndrome in case anyone might think that these drugs cause dependence) includes sudden changes in mood, sometimes amounting to suicidal feelings and behaviour, dizziness, insomnia, and a range of dysphoric symptoms that can be quite unpleasant but difficult to define easily (Price et al., 2009).

Related drugs such as the serotonin-noradrenaline reuptake inhibitors (SNRIs) venlafaxine and duloxetine, the 5-HT$_{1A}$ partial agonist buspirone, the antipsychotic drug trifluoperazine, and the antihistamine hydroxyzine, have all been shown to have some benefit in generalized anxiety (Ballenger et al., 2001; Baldwin et al., 2005; 2006). There are few head-to-head comparisons with other antidepressants and so it is difficult to evaluate the comparative value of these compounds, but they may be of value as second-line treatments.

Benzodiazepines and cyclopyrrolones

Benzodiazepines are still the most effective drugs for the treatment of generalized anxiety disorder in the short term. In therapeutic dosage they reduce the symptoms of anxiety within 30–45 minutes and in correct dosage do not lead to sedation. Because benzodiazepines are associated with significant problems of dependence after repeated dosage

(Tyrer et al., 1981; Hallstrom et al., 1981) they are not recommended for long-term use. Short-term regular prescriptions of benzodiazepines are of limited benefit and if suddenly stopped this benefit disappears (Tyrer et al., 1988) and so intermittent flexible dosage, which can be given long-term, is probably the best way of treating generalized anxiety. There is also some evidence that those without dependent or obsessional personality characteristics are much less likely to develop dependence (Tyrer et al., 1983).

Benzodiazepines are often used initially when combined with other drugs for the treatment of anxiety. This is because antidepressants have a longer latent period before beneficial effects are shown. This is a perfectly proper way of using benzodiazepines for this condition. The cyclopyrrolones, zolpiden, zopiclone and zaleplon, also bind to benzodiazepine receptors but are primarily prescribed for insomnia rather than anxiety. They too have a risk of tolerance in continued use and withdrawal symptoms after sudden cessation (see Chapter 6).

Recommendations

Most consensus guidelines and reviews suggest that tricyclic antidepressants, SSRIs, and SNRIs have similar overall efficacy (Baldwin et al., 2005; NICE, 2007). Although venlafaxine is licensed for generalized anxiety disorder in dosage ranging from 37.5 mg to 150 mg daily, and with some evidence that it is marginally more effective than other antidepressants (Thase et al., 2001), there have been concerns about its safety and it is generally recommended that specialist mental health practitioners only should prescribe these drugs.

Maintenance treatment

Most trial evidence concerns acute treatment yet generalized anxiety disorder is often a chronic condition. There is no simple answer to the problems of long-term therapy with any of the agents discussed earlier in this section. It would rarely be a problem to continue treatment if there were no risks but adverse effects are frequent and prominent. Tricyclic antidepressants have marked anticholinergic effects and weight gain can be a persistent problem with the danger of the development of secondary diabetes mellitus. SSRIs may provoke nausea and vestibular problems and a variety of unpleasant symptoms on withdrawal, and the benzodiazepine drugs and their analogues all are associated with tolerance and clear withdrawal phenomena. Buspirone is clearly non-addictive (Murphy et al., 1989) but is

not well liked by patients and appears to be particularly unhelpful in those who have previously had benzodiazepine dependence (Ashton et al., 1990). By comparison with cognitive behavioural therapy all drug treatments come out badly in comparisons of long-term treatment.

Second-line drug treatments

Beta-blocking drugs such as propranolol still account for a significant proportion of prescriptions in primary care and these are effective in reducing somatic symptoms of anxiety (Tyrer & Lader, 1974), so they also have a role in some somatoform disorders, and in combination with benzodiazepines (Hallstrom et al., 1981). Monoamine oxidase inhibitors (MAOIs) such as phenelzine and isocarboxazid may also have a place in the treatment of intractable generalized anxiety but should never be first-line treatments because of the concern over potential food and drug interactions. The evidence base for their efficacy is old but robust (Sheehan et al., 1980). The reversible MAOI, moclobemide, has some efficacy in social phobia (Versiani et al., 1992) but, despite its greater safety as it is free from the drug and food interactions of the irreversible MAOIs, it is not as effective.

Low-dose antipsychotic drugs and antihistamines have also been used for treatment of anxiety but these tend to be associated with marked sedation. Hydroxyzine is the most commonly used.

Psychological treatments

Acute treatment of generalized anxiety disorder

The most common treatments used for generalized anxiety disorder are cognitive behavioural therapy (CBT), various forms of dynamic psychotherapy, and behavioural-based treatments such as anxiety management training. CBT has the best evidence in its favour and its effect size is at least as great as that of drug treatment (Gould et al., 1997a). Adverse effects are almost zero, so the benefit–risk ratio supports its use in this condition and these are recommended in general guidelines (Kendall et al., 2011). By comparison dynamic psychotherapy and behavioural therapy have much less evidence supporting them. The best example is anxiety management training (Butler et al., 1991). There is evidence in all these studies that the effects of cognitive behavioural therapy persist much longer after treatment finishes than do drug treatments and significant withdrawal problems do not occur.

Somatoform disorders

These conditions include the dissociative disorders (formerly subsumed under hysteria), somatization disorder, hypochondriasis, and a variety of undifferentiated somatoform, including pain, disorders. Chronic fatigue syndrome also comes under this group, although there is a vociferous group who have campaigned for years for this condition to be regarded as a neurological disorder. Although many of these patients are seeking medical answers for their problems they do not, in general, respond to drug treatments. Pharmacological treatments are generally ineffective, with only one randomized study supporting fluoxetine, and this only to a limited extent (Fallon et al., 2008). One of the problems in this group of patients is that they are more sensitive than most to changes in their autonomic and physiological status (colloquially they have "noisy bodies") and so they are much more sensitive to the adverse effects of drugs.

Psychological treatments of somatoform disorders

Cognitive behavioural therapy has also been shown to be effective in the treatment of somatoform disorders, particularly chronic fatigue syndrome (Kroenke & Swindle, 2000). It has also been found in adapted form

Table 23.1 Effectiveness of treatments for generalized anxiety disorder (GAD) and somatoform disorder (SD)

Treatment (and diagnosis)	Form of treatment	Duration of treatment	Level of evidence for efficacy	Comments
Benzodiazepines (e.g. diazepam, alprazolam, clonazepam) (GAD)	Tablets, liquid, or IM/IV injection	Acute and long term	Ia	Clinically effective in short term and also in long term, but dangers of dependence in long term tend to preclude usage (but see Chapter 13
Tricyclic antidepressants (best evidence with clomipramine) (GAD)	Oral (IM preparations available but no evidence of value)	Medium and long term	Ib	Effective but preferred less than others because of adverse effects and toxicity
Selective serotonin reuptake inhibitors (GAD) (and SD – fluvoxamine only)	Tablets	Medium, long term, and relapse prevention	Ia	Demonstrably effective in both acute and long-term treatment
Serotonin-noradrenaline reuptake inhibitor (SNRI) (e.g. venlafaxine) (GAD and SD)	Tablets	Medium and long term	Ia	Concern over potential cardiotoxicity has blunted strong evidence of efficacy
Azaspirodecanediones (e.g. buspirone) (GAD)	Tablets (10–60 mg)	Medium to long term	Ib	Effective but not well liked by patients, lack dependence risk
Antihistamine (e.g. hydroxyzine) (GAD)	Tablets	Medium to long term	Ib	Definite evidence of efficacy but comparative studies lacking

Treatment	Form	Timing	Evidence	Comment
Low-dose antipsychotic drugs (e.g. trifluoperazine) (GAD)	Tablets or IM injections (not indicated for this disorder)	Medium term	Ib	Certainly effective and not addictive, but dangers of movement disorders in prolonged dosage
Anticonvulsants (pregabalin) (GAD)	Tablets	Medium term and relapse prevention	Ib	Certainly efficacious but have some advantages early in treatment
St John's wort (Hypericum) (SD)	Extract in tablet form	Acute treatment	Ib	Some value
Cognitive behavioural therapy (GAD and SD)	Individual treatment	Acute and medium-term treatment	Ia	Highly efficacious for GAD, health anxiety, chronic fatigue and pain symptoms
Self-help and bibliotherapy (GAD)	Personal choice	Acute and long term	Ia	Effective with particular value in those with no personality disturbance
Relaxation training (and hypnosis) (GAD)	Group or individual	Acute	IIa	Some evidence of benefit but not as strong as for other therapies
Counselling (GAD)	Individual	Acute	Ib	Only works in short term, effect probably lost later
Internet and computerized cognitive behavioural therapy	Individual	Acute	IIa	Increasing evidence of efficacy but more information needed in clinical populations

to be helpful in hypochondriasis, or health anxiety (Barsky & Ahern, 2004; Seivewright et al., 2008). In these disorders a course of 6–10 treatments is often sufficient to change the course of the disorder fundamentally and such benefit can be maintained over the longer term with very little in the way of additional therapy. The groups of patients who do not do particularly well with any form of treatment are those with medically unexplained symptoms and somatization disorder. Although there is some evidence that psychological treatments may be helpful here, comparison with well-structured care with at least some psychological input shows no specific benefit of focused therapy (Sumathipala et al., 2008). Reattribution of symptoms (from a physical to a psychological cause) has been found to be possible in primary care but does not lead to better outcomes (Morriss et al., 2007).

Combined drug and psychological treatments

In practice a large number of patients take both drug and psychological treatments for these disorders but there is little evidence that either supports or refutes their value.

Summary

In generalized anxiety disorder both psychological treatments in the form of cognitive behavioural therapy and antidepressants in the form of SSRIs are regarded as roughly equal in merit for the short-term treatment of generalized anxiety disorder (Kendall et al., 2011), but in the longer-term cognitive behavioural therapy may be superior to drug treatment (Tyrer and Baldwin, 2006). For somatoform disorders psychological treatments, preferably those based on cognitive behaviour therapy, should be preferred as first line treatments. Although cognitive behaviour therapy is rarely available in some settings for both generalised anxiety and somatoform disorders it should be preferentially chosen when available. Drug treatments are best used intermittently but may be condoned if all other treatments have failed.

Interventions discussed in this chapter are summarized in Table 23.1.

24

Panic disorder

Based on "Panic disorder" by Stacy Shaw Welch, Michelle Craske, Murray B. Stein, Phil Harrison-Read and Peter Roy-Byrne in Effective Treatments in Psychiatry, Cambridge University Press, 2008

Introduction

Panic can be part of all anxiety disorders, but when present in primary form is a disabling mental disorder that affects up to 5% of the population at some point in their lives, and around 3% in any given year (Kessler et al., 2005a; 2005b). Its costs are high and people with the disorder suffer from both an individual and public health perspective, including reduced quality of life, increased healthcare utilization, reduced workplace productivity, and absenteeism (Greenberg et al., 1999).

Panic attacks need to be differentiated from panic disorder. *Panic attacks* are characterized by sudden,

paroxysmal bursts of severe anxiety, accompanied by a range of physical (cardiorespiratory, autonomic, gastrointestinal, and/or otoneurological) as well as cognitive (fears of losing control, dying, or going crazy) symptoms. The diagnosis of formal panic disorder requires the presence of recurrent panic attacks accompanied by either (1) worry about the possibility of future attacks or (2) development of phobic avoidance or other change in behaviour due to the attacks. These attacks often have a dramatic initial presentation, as well as an unexpected quality, with onset unaccompanied by an obvious trigger. Panic disorder is traditionally differentiated from the experience of panic attacks by the experience of the attacks as unexplained, as though they appear "out of the blue". The anxiety about recurrence of future attacks is also an important difference between panic disorder and panic attacks (Kessler et al., 2006). However, recent evidence suggests that a substantial proportion of panic attacks in patients with panic disorder are not unexpected or unanticipated but have clear cut, identifiable cues (Norton et al., 1992). In clinical settings, panic disorder is almost always accompanied by comorbid conditions, especially major depression, bipolar affective disorder, other anxiety disorders, and alcohol abuse. Both separation anxiety and childhood panic are linked to adult panic disorder (Aschenbrand et al., 2003).

Most treatments for panic disorder are preventive rather than of immediate benefit; panic attacks reach a crescendo so quickly that very few treatments could be effective in this time scale. The important aim is to prevent anxiety escalating to panic.

Treatment

Pharmacotherapy

The selective serotonin reuptake inhibitors (SSRIs) have the best evidence base for efficacy in panic disorder. Six different agents have been shown to be effective in randomized clinical trials – fluoxetine, fluvoxamine, sertraline, paroxetine, citalopram, and escitalopram. Meta-analyses have indicated medium to large effect sizes compared to placebo for several SSRIs (Otto et al., 2001; Bakker et al., 2002) but there is no evidence of differential efficacy between them (Bakker et al., 2002). The most important distinctions between them are in their relative costs, with the generic forms being the cheapest. Efficacy has been confirmed up to 1 year using placebo-controlled discontinuation designs (Pollack et al., 2003). Placebo-controlled trials also support efficacy for an extended-release form of venlafaxine (Bradwejn et al., 2005). Other second generation antidepressants such as duloxetine, mirtazapine, trazodone, or bupropion have either no evidence for efficacy or apparent lack of efficacy. The older class of tricyclic antidepressants and monoamine oxidase inhibitors are less commonly used because of their adverse effects, but they are equally effective and less expensive, and should be considered either as first-line treatments in patients who prefer them (and want sedation) or, in cases of lack of response to SSRIs, as second-line treatments. Because of their different mechanism of action they can be effective when all other drugs fail. Imipramine, desipramine, clomipramine, nortriptyline and amitriptyline, and MAO inhibitors, particularly phenelzine, were effective in six studies that preceded the DSM-III classification of panic disorder and subsumed many cases under the previous label of "phobic anxiety" (Roy-Byrne & Cowley, 2002).

Benzodiazepines may also be used. They have a number of advantages: they are very effective, work rapidly, may be even better tolerated than the SSRI class of agents (though systematic comparisons are lacking), and are widely available generically (Bruce et al., 2003). Limitations of benzodiazepines include the risk of physiological dependence and withdrawal, and the risk of abuse. This profile has made benzodiazepine use in panic disorder controversial; the recent NICE guidelines make it clear to patients that long-term use is contraindicated (National Collaborating Centre for Mental Health 2004a, 2007) whereas the equivalent US guidelines suggest that fears about abuse and dependence are exaggerated (American Psychiatric Association, 1998). Because many anxious patients do not fully respond to, or become more anxious initially after therapy with, SSRIs, it is common to co-prescribe benzodiazepines with antidepressants initially (Bruce et al., 2003).

Numerous studies show clearly that discontinuation of medication results in relapse in a significant proportion of patients, with placebo-controlled discontinuation studies showing rates between 25% and 50% within 6 months, depending on study design (Roy-Byrne & Cowley, 2002), and a somewhat greater rate is found for the benzodiazepines (Rickels et al., 1993), which either suggests the presence of a withdrawal syndrome or resetting of the benzodiazepine receptors that may promote or contribute to panic disorder relapse.

A course of cognitive behavioural therapy (see below) appears to be the best option for non-responders to pharmacotherapy; a recent study found that nearly two-thirds of non-responders who received a course of CBT met remission criteria. Significant benefits were sustained for up to 1 year and were associated with reductions in medication use (Heldt et al., 2006). In the case of cognitive behavioural therapy non-response, one controlled study indicated a better response to paroxetine than placebo (Kampman et al., 2002) and another showed paroxetine superior to placebo in augmenting the impact of brief cognitive behavioural therapy (Stein et al., 2000).

Psychological treatments

By far the most extensively validated psychotherapeutic treatment for panic disorder is cognitive behavioural therapy (CBT) in its various forms. Other psychotherapeutic treatments frequently used in clinical practice, such as insight-oriented therapies, supportive therapies, relaxation training without exposure, hypnosis, eye movement desensitization, and reprocessing therapy (EMDR, and stress management), have not received good empirical support, and are not discussed further here. There is no reason to consider them for panic disorder on grounds of either effectiveness or cost. Two large meta-analyses of cognitive behavioural therapy for panic disorder found large effect sizes for the treatment of 0.90 and 1.55 (Craske, 1999; Mitte et al., 2005) with gains maintained up to 8 years after treatment (Kenardy et al., 2005). The treatment appears to be well tolerated and is associated with relatively low dropout rates. Other commonly associated aspects of this treatment include psychoeducation and breathing retraining. Some studies have found this to be useful regardless of whether patients actually hyperventilate or not (Garssen et al., 1992) but others have questioned the necessity of breathing retraining (de Beurs et al., 1995). Behavioural experiments (now considered to be an essential part of cognitive behavioural therapy) are also used frequently in the course of treatment.

Comparative and combination treatments

A recent review of the literature found clear evidence for cognitive behavioural therapy linked to exposure in extending the treatment effects of medication. However, only modest support appears for adding pharmacotherapy to comprehensive cognitive behavioural therapy (Smits et al., 2006). It appears that some medications may initially augment the effects of CBT but later detract from them. For instance, a study of the benzodiazepine, alprazolam, alone or in combination with exposure in patients with panic disorder and agoraphobia, revealed that alprazolam marginally improved the effects of exposure in the short term but that, following taper and discontinuation, patients who had received alprazolam with their exposure had worse outcome than patients receiving exposure with a placebo (Marks et al., 1993). Another major multicentre study compared imipramine, cognitive behavioural therapy, or placebo with combinations of CBT, imipramine, and placebo (Barlow et al., 2000). At 6 months, the combination of imipramine and cognitive behavioural therapy was marginally superior to either treatment alone at 6 months (consistent with prior reports of the superiority of combined treatment in more complicated panic). Following discontinuation, however, patients receiving the cognitive behavioural therapy plus imipramine combination were somewhat worse (Barlow et al., 2000). One hypothesis is that attributions and state- (or context)-dependent learning when treatments are combined might attenuate the new learning that would otherwise cause sustained benefit in cognitive behavioural therapy (Smits et al., 2006).

Once active treatment is discontinued, the beneficial effects of cognitive behavioural therapy effects are generally more durable than those of medication, and this is reflected in recent NICE guidelines (National Collaborating Centre for Mental Health, 2004a). Meta-analyses show that cognitive behavioural treatments yield larger mean effect sizes (averaging over all dependent variables) (ES = 0.88–0.90) than either antidepressants (ES = 0.40–0.55) or benzodiazepines (ES = 0.40). It is fair to add that patient samples might not be comparable across these studies.

Cognitive behavioural therapy is still not generally available, except in the UK following the recent initiative (Improved Access to Psychological Therapies; IAPT) where it is being focused on delivery in primary care. Emerging evidence indicates that models of emphasizing a primary role for the primary care physician but adding support from a mental health provider to either deliver medications, manage care in general, and/or provide cognitive behavioural therapy specifically adapted for that setting are both effective (Bower & Gilbody, 2005) and cost-effective (Katon et al., 2002). Other promising approaches include a range of self-help approaches using Internet-driven or computer-assisted cognitive behavioural therapy discussed in the other chapters in this section.

Several reports of computer or Internet-assisted treatments for panic disorder have emerged in the past few years, including several comparisons with traditional cognitive behavioural therapy. One randomized trial compared 10 weekly sessions of cognitive behavioural therapy with 10 modules of a web-based self-help programme which included email interactions with a therapist (Carlbring et al., 2005). Results indicated that the treatments were comparable in efficacy, although there were slight advantages to the live CBT programme. Marks and colleagues (2004) compared patients with phobia or panic disorder who were randomized to exposure therapy guided by a clinician or mainly by a computer system, with a computer-guided relaxation condition (included as a placebo). In this study, the two exposure treatments showed comparable improvement and satisfaction post-treatment and at follow-up 1 month later, while the relaxation

Table 24.1 Summary of evidence base of treatments for panic disorder

Treatment	Form of treatment	Psychiatric disorder	Level of evidence for efficacy	Comments
Drug treatments	Selective serotonin reuptake inhibitors (SSRIs) Standard doses but it is usual to start with lower doses to avoid initial increase in anxiety	Panic disorder with and without agoraphobia	Ia	Undoubtedly effective. First-line treatment, but relapse frequent when drug discontinued
Drug treatments	Tricyclic antidepressants (TCAs) Standard antidepressant doses but starting with lower doses	Panic disorder with and without agoraphobia	Ia	Undoubtedly effective. Increased and more uncomfortable side effects compared to SSRIs
Drug treatments	Benzodiazepines	Panic Disorder with and without agoraphobia	Ia	Undoubtedly effective. Some risk of physiological dependence/withdrawal/abuse. Greater chance of abuse in those with substance abuse history and personality disorder. Cognitive impairment can occur
Psychological treatments	Cognitive behavioural therapy (10–16 sessions) with some studies demonstrating efficacy with fewer sessions	Panic disorder with and without agoraphobia	Ia	Undoubtedly at least as effective as drug treatments. Probably more effective in long-term as relapse less common after treatment discontinued. First-line treatment

Psychological plus drug treatments	Combined cognitive behavioural therapy and SSRIs	Panic disorder with and without agoraphobia	Ia	Undoubtedly effective but more information needed on persistence of benefit compared to cognitive behavioural therapy alone
New psychological treatments	Computer-assisted delivery of cognitive behavioural therapy; recommended dose not yet established	Panic disorder with and without agoraphobia	Ib	Probably efficacious; efficacy compared to therapist-delivered cognitive behavioural therapy needs further study

treatment was associated with low efficacy and satisfaction. However, it had lower dropout rates than the clinician-assisted or computer-assisted exposure treatments (6, 24, and 43%, respectively). The authors estimate that the computer condition cut clinician time per patient by 73%. In a multisite, randomized trial Kenardy and colleagues (2003) compared standard (12 sessions) and brief (6 sessions) therapist-delivered cognitive behavioural therapy, a computer-augmented CBT protocol (6 sessions), and a wait-list control condition. Unlike a previous report (Clark et al., 1999), the outcome for the 12-session cognitive behavioural therapy was significantly better than the 6-session CBT. While the outcomes for the computer-augmented treatment were in between the 12- and 6-session therapist-delivered conditions, it did not differ statistically from either. At a 6-month follow-up, none of the active treatments were statistically different. While more research is clearly needed, these trials are a very promising beginning and point to the possibilities of adding computer or Internet-assisted treatment to primary care.

Summary

The treatments for panic disorder and agoraphobia have good evidence generally (Table 24.1) and the initial treatment effects of antidepressants and cognitive behavioural therapy are almost identical. In the longer-term cognitive behavioural therapy improves its performance because of reduced relapse rates. Internet and related self-therapies appear likely to improve outcome generally in less severe cases and should have a major influence on population health.

25

Specific phobias and agoraphobia

Based on "Specific phobias and agoraphobia" by Sonya B. Norman and Ariel J. Lang in
Effective Treatments in Psychiatry, Cambridge University Press, 2008

Introduction

Specific phobias (also called simple phobias) are common, affecting nearly one in ten of the population. People with these disorders have a persistent, excessive, and unreasonable fear of an object or well circumscribed situation. The most common types of phobias are animal, natural environment (e.g. heights, lightening), situational (e.g. air travel, enclosed spaces), and blood-injury. The feared object, because it is specific, can normally be avoided, but may cause distress or interfere with functioning. An individual may also spend a great deal of time and energy preparing in case the feared stimulus is encountered, even when the likelihood of encountering the stimulus is

extremely low. Agoraphobia describes the fear of being in situations that would be difficult to escape or in which help might not be available in the event of panic or panic-like symptoms. Agoraphobia is most commonly associated with panic disorder and is included with panic in this book (Chapter 24), but new evidence suggests that agoraphobia not only occurs in many people without any history of panic (Andrews and Slade, 2006) but also predicts the development of panic disorder (Bienvenu et al., 2006). For this reason it could be argued that agoraphobia should be viewed as a single stand-alone diagnostic entity. Even without the coexistence of panic, agoraphobia carries considerable morbidity and is costly as agoraphobia patients have higher than average rates of medical consultation (Swinson et al., 1992).

Both these conditions often remain untreated and this chapter illustrates why such inaction is dilatory. Perhaps not surprisingly, people often prefer to work around the fears by a combination of avoidance and enterprise rather than face them. As for these conditions we have genuinely curative therapies we must try harder to make them available.

Pharmacotherapy

This is one group of disorders in which drug treatment has no established formal role. The previous chapter discusses the treatment of agoraphobia with panic and this includes drug treatments. However, for agoraphobia alone there is no good evidence that drug treatment is necessary or carries any benefit. There is also no good evidence that combined drug and psychological treatments are effective in this condition (Furukawa et al., 2007), but there is one trial that showed that p-cycloserine (DCS), a partial N-methyl-D-aspartate receptor agonist, enhanced the value of virtual reality exposure therapy in 28 patients compared with exposure therapy alone (Ressler et al., 2004). However, a subsequent study in spider phobia did not confirm this benefit (Guastella et al., 2007).

Psychological treatments

Exposure therapy

The theory behind exposure therapy is very simple. If an object or situation provokes fear then it tends to be avoided, and if experienced again, fear and immediate avoidance are the natural consequences. If the subject is encouraged, trained, or educated into facing up to the situation that provokes the fear, and if they can stay in that situation long enough, they will typically find that the feared consequence does not occur and the phobia will be conquered. There are now many systematic reviews and meta-analyses that confirm the value of this treatment in specific phobias (Horowitz et al., 2005). This treatment can be given in as little as one session with long-term success (Öst et al., 1991; 1997; 2001). It may be easier or more tolerable to carry out exposure therapy according to a hierarchy in which the person has to be exposed to minor forms of the situation before moving up the hierarchy. For example, a person with a fear of large dogs might be exposed to small dogs earlier in the treatment. Even in such situations the treatment can usually be completed successfully within five sessions.

Exposure treatment in virtual reality

Virtual reality exposure therapy (VRET) involves exposing patients to their feared stimuli using an integrated combination of computer graphics, body tracking devices, visual displays, and other forms of sensory input that immerses the patient in a virtual environment that simulates the feared situation (Gros and Antony, 2006). Studies that compare exposure therapy with and without virtual reality show comparable results for both conditions in acrophobia and spider phobia (Garcia-Palacios et al., 2002; Krijn et al., 2004; Pull, 2006); it is therefore up to a clinician to decide when the expense of virtual reality technology is warranted. There is no doubt that this treatment has potential but its exact place is uncertain.

Applied tension

Blood-injury phobia is unique in that the main reaction to the sight of blood for those with these phobias is a sudden drop in blood pressure leading to fainting or loss of consciousness. "Applied tension" is a technique of raising the blood pressure to prevent this reaction. The patient in applied tension therapy is instructed to tense the muscles of the arms, chest, and the legs until there is a feeling of warmth rising to the face (which usually takes 15–20 seconds). The patient is then instructed to release the tension to return to the starting level, pause, and then repeat the procedure five times (Öst and Sterner, 1987).

Unlike other specific phobias, exposure therapy is not the treatment of choice in this condition (Öst et al., 1991). Applied tension has been shown in one randomized trial to be superior to in vivo exposure therapy. In another study, five sessions of applied tension incorporating a hierarchy of exposures, a single session of applied tension and a single session of tension only (learning the technique without practice in encounters with blood or injury) had equivalent efficacy in treating blood-related phobias (Hellstrom et al., 1996). As similar efficacy is shown with smaller numbers of sessions the longer course of treatment may be unnecessary.

Cognitive behaviour and exposure therapy

The addition of cognitive techniques to behavioural therapy is common to CBT for most conditions. It is not considered to be essential to all forms of behavioural treatment for specific phobias. A meta-analysis of 35 randomized trials has shown that exposure therapy is by far the most superior (Horowitz et al., 2005). Although there is evidence that avoidance need not be addressed directly in treatment (Craske et al., 2003) this does not mean that cognitions should be avoided. Supplementation with cognitive techniques to counter beliefs that underlie avoidance may be helpful in increasing compliance with or tolerability of exposure.

Treatment of agoraphobia in the absence of panic

Very little evidence about the successful treatment of this condition is available as patients with this disorder seldom present for treatment (Andrews & Slade, 2006). There is considerable clinical overlap between this condition and avoidant or anxious personality disorder, in which patients develop a preferred life-style that allows their avoidance but puts pressure on relatives and friends. Often this leads to a different, but harmonious, relationship that can be disturbed by successful treatment (Marcaurelle et al., 2003). It has been suggested that the addition of problem solving and communication skills might be necessary in the treatment of this group (Daiuto et al., 1998) but this remains to be tested.

Treatment delivery challenges

One of the biggest problems in delivering treatment to those with specific phobia or agoraphobia alone is that patients often do not present for treatment, either because of avoidance or because of barriers to receiving care (e.g. living in a rural setting). Because of this there is considerable interest in treatment over the Internet, which allows access to well-qualified therapists in home settings. It seems increasingly likely that Internet-based treatments will become more widely used, not least as the Internet is becoming so widely available for all kinds of daily activity. Internet-based treatment may eventually become the treatment of choice for many people with specific phobias and agoraphobia alone. The consensus of evidence seems to be that when guided help is given, either with telephone support or Internet help lines, the outcome is better (Kenwright & Marks, 2004; Andrews et al., 2010). In one recent trial there was no difference between exposure treatment and Internet-based self-help together with Internet support, in the treatment of spider phobia (Andersson et al., 2009).

Table 25.1 Summary of treatments for specific phobias and agoraphobia

Treatment	Form of treatment	Psychiatric disorder	Level of evidence to test efficacy	Comments
Exposure therapy in vivo	Individual treatment	Specific phobias apart from blood phobia	Ia	Unequivocal evidence of benefit – even after single session of treatment
Exposure therapy in virtual reality	Individual treatment with virtual reality technology	Specific phobias	Ib	
Applied tension	Individual treatment	Blood phobias	Ib	
Cognitive behavioural and exposure therapy	Individual treatment	Agoraphobia	III	
Cognitive behaviour and exposure therapy	Self-directed	Agoraphobia	III	
Cognitive behaviour and exposure therapy	Internet	Specific phobias and agoraphobia	II	A growing branch of therapy that is particularly effective in this group

Summary and guidelines

Specific phobias and agoraphobia are highly prevalent conditions that may create considerable distress and impairment and yet much less often present for therapy. Exposure treatments, whether or not they are linked to other components of cognitive behavioural therapy, are highly effective in specific phobias (Table 25.1) but very little is known about their effects in agoraphobia alone, and we have been unable to find any evidence of successful treatment for this latter condition. The growth of self-directed and computer driven treatments over the Internet constitutes the most promising development of recent years, and the most optimal way of improving access to, and delivery of, this treatment is one of the main challenges that lies ahead.

26

Social phobia

Based on "Social phobia" by Laura Campbell-Sills and Murray B. Stein in Effective
Treatments in Psychiatry, Cambridge University Press, 2008

Introduction

Social phobia, also known as social anxiety disorder, is a common mental disorder with an estimated lifetime prevalence of 12% (Kessler et al., 2005a). Individuals with social phobia strongly fear social or performance situations in which they might be exposed to unfamiliar people or scrutinized by others (American Psychiatric Association, 2000). The discomfort provoked by social situations leads many people with the disorder to avoid interactions with others. Such avoidance can lead to disruptions in occupational, academic, interpersonal, and other areas of functioning.

Social phobia can present in many different ways and with varying levels of severity. Some individuals fear and avoid just one or two highly specific social situations, commonly performance situations such as public speaking or job interviews. By contrast, other individuals with this diagnosis fear and avoid a broad range of situations (from casual social interactions to performance situations), and are described as having generalized social phobia (GSP). In extreme cases, individuals with GSP may only be comfortable interacting with close family members. GSP is highly overlapping with another DSM-IV diagnosis, avoidant personality disorder. These conditions are challenging to discriminate and may be alternative conceptualizations of the same condition, with avoidant personality disorder simply representing a more severe version of GSP (Chavira and Stein, 2002).

Social phobia has high rates of comorbidity with other mental disorders (Kessler et al., 2005a). In many cases, onset of social phobia precedes the onset of other disorders and there is some evidence that social phobia increases risk for developing other problems such as mood disorders (Kessler et al., 1999). Individuals suffering from social phobia experience impairment in major life roles and report high levels of dissatisfaction (Stein & Kean, 2000).

While it is clear that social phobia negatively affects individuals and the community, it should also be noted that the boundary between the diagnosis of social phobia and personality traits such as "shyness" or "introversion" is not always clear. To minimize the likelihood of overpathologizing shyness, clinicians must carefully consider whether each of the diagnostic criteria for social phobia is met. In particular, clinicians must establish that the levels of functional impairment and/or distress associated with the social fears are at a level that meets or exceeds the threshold for clinical diagnosis.

Pharmacological treatments

Serotonin reuptake inhibitors (SSRIs)

Selective serotonin reuptake inhibitors (SSRIs) are generally considered to be first-line pharmacotherapy for social phobia. Randomized controlled trials (RCTs) support the efficacy and tolerability of citalopram, escitalopram, fluvoxamine, paroxetine (including its controlled release formulation), and sertraline for treatment of social phobia. The positive results of individual trials are also supported by meta-analytical studies (Gould et al., 1997b; Blanco et al., 2003).

Several RCTs support the efficacy of venlafaxine extended-release, a dual serotonin–noradrenaline reuptake inhibitor (SNRI) for treatment of social phobia (Liebowitz et al., 2005; Stein et al., 2005), making it a suitable first- or second-line choice.

Dosing of SSRIs for treatment of social phobia is similar to that used in the treatment of major depression. Effects of SSRIs can be slow to accrue and a period of 12 weeks has been recommended to ensure an adequate trial of these drugs (Stein et al., 2002). If treatment is stopped too early after apparent response then relapse may occur (Stein et al., 2003; Montgomery et al., 2005). Evidence suggests that treatment with SSRIs should be continued for 3 months or longer after remission of social phobia (and expert clinicians would argue for 6 months or longer), to decrease the risk of relapse (Stein et al., 2002; Montgomery et al., 2005). Although these studies offer some evidence regarding the need to continue treatment beyond the time of remission, more investigation is needed to determine how long most patients with social phobia should be treated with SSRIs.

Monoamine oxidase inhibitors (MAOIs)

Several RCTs support the efficacy of irreversible MAOIs such as phenelzine for the treatment of social phobia (e.g. Liebowitz et al., 1992; Versiani et al., 1992; Heimberg et al., 1998; Blanco et al., 2010). The main disadvantage of these drugs is the risk of food and drug interactions leading to a hypertensive crisis, although such adverse outcomes are avoidable if precautions are taken with regard to diet and medication, and concerns about adverse effects have considerably limited their use. Reversible selective inhibitors on monoamine oxides (RIMAs) such as brofaromine and moclobemide are considered safer and have demonstrated efficacy in RCTs; however,

they have not proven as effective as phenelzine (Versiani et al., 1992; Fahlen et al., 1995; Stein et al., 2002).

Other antidepressants

Mirtazapine has been shown to be superior to placebo in one trial (Muehlbacher et al., 2005). Tricyclic antidepressants have not been properly tested in this population and are seldom recommended.

Benzodiazepines

Clonazepam has proven effective for reducing symptoms of social phobia in two RCTs (Davidson et al., 1993; Otto et al., 2000). Other benzodiazepines have not been well tested apart from alprazolam which was less effective than phenelzine in one study (Gelernter et al., 1991).

Other drugs

Other drugs have been used in the treatment of social phobia but most have not been evaluated in RCTs. However, a number of drugs that have been compared to placebo have shown superiority. This includes the anticonvulsant, gabapentin (Pande et al., 1999), the anxiolytic pregabalin (Pande et al., 2004), and, in a small trial, the antipsychotic drug, olanzapine (Barnett et al., 2002). None of these would be considered first-line treatments, and would typically be used only after more standard treatments had failed.

For patients with social phobia specific to performance situations, the beta-blocking drugs may be of particular value because they reduce tremor in addition to their effects on anxiety (Tyrer & Lader, 1973). Some patients see added value in decreasing tremor, or in reducing tachycardia (which beta-blockers also do), because they are focused on the potential negative impact of these symptoms in performance situations. It should be noted that the reduction of tremor may give an unfair advantage to some individuals (e.g. archers or snooker players) and so these drugs are now banned for participants in these competitive activities.

A recent meta-analysis of 51 pharmacotherapy trials (Ipser et al., 2008) showed that 55% of participants responded to medication for social phobia, with approximately four participants having to be treated for an average of 12 weeks before an additional person responded to medication, relative to placebo (number needed to treat (NNT) of 4.2). This represents a significant clinical benefit of these pharmacological agents.

Psychological treatments

Cognitive behavioural therapy (CBT)

CBT is also first-line treatment for social phobia. It is tailored to the symptoms and concerns associated with the disorder; for example, efforts are made to modify cognitions focused on being evaluated negatively by others and to decrease avoidance of social situations. The evidence base is strong with numerous RCTs and several meta-analyses supporting the efficacy of CBT (Rodebaugh et al., 2004; Butler et al., 2006). There is also evidence that the effects of CBT are durable, persisting for 1 year or more after treatment is completed (Heimberg, 2002; Clark et al., 2003).

Most RCTs demonstrating the efficacy of CBT for social phobia have delivered the treatment in a group format. Assumed benefits of the group modality for socially phobic patients have included the normalization of social concerns, social support, and opportunities for naturalistic exposure to social situations inherent in the group format. However, meta-analyses suggest that individual and group CBT produce at least equivalent effects (Rodebaugh et al., 2004), and in one head-to-head study individual treatment produced stronger effects than group treatment (Stangier et al., 2003).

Exposure therapy

Exposure to feared social situations is a core component of most CBT programmes and can be the sole focus of treatment – in which case the treatment is called "exposure therapy". Exposure therapy is effective in treating social phobia (e.g. Hope et al., 1995; Hofmann et al., 2006). However, some recent investigations have shown subtle advantages of CBT that combines cognitive techniques with exposure. For instance, one study showed continued improvement after treatment withdrawal in patients treated with CBT but not in those treated with exposure therapy (Hofmann, 2004).

Internet CBT

CBT requires significant time and effort on the part of the patient, and it is not readily available in all settings (e.g. rural areas). Some investigations have focused on developing CBT programmes that can be completed without frequent in-person visits to a therapist. RCTs have shown Internet-based CBT to be effective; however, there appear to be advantages to having some therapist contact via telephone or email (Andersson et al., 2006; Titov et al., 2008). A recent meta-analysis of internet CBT for patients with diagnoses of major depression, panic disorder, social phobia, or generalized anxiety disorder (Andrews et al., 2010) showed an effect size of 0.88 (NNT = 2.2) compared with control conditions. To what extent the participants in these trials can be regarded as similar to those presenting in clinical practice is difficult to determine, and there are likely patients who require a higher-intensity intervention to overcome their social phobia.

Social skills training (SST)

The theory underpinning SST is that people with social phobia have deficits in social skills that contribute to their anxiety in social situations. There is some evidence that SST augments the effects of CBT, specifically for patients who have avoidant personality disorder as well as social phobia (Herbert et al., 2009).

Comparison of drug and psychological treatments

In general, CBT compares favourably with drug treatments when direct comparisons are made between them. In most RCTs, CBT has been shown to be at least as effective as drug treatments such as fluoxetine (Clark et al., 2003; Davidson et al.,

Table 26.1 Effectiveness of treatments for social phobia

Treatment	Form of treatment	Psychiatric disorder	Level of evidence for efficacy	Comments
Pharmacological	Selective serotonin reuptake inhibitors (SSRIs)	Generalized social phobia	Ia	Highly effective in many patients but around half do not show significant benefit – allow 12 weeks for this to be shown
Pharmacological	Irreversible monoamine oxidase inhibitors (MAOIs) (e.g. phenelzine)	Generalized social phobia	Ia	Highly effective but dietary and drug restrictions limit use
Pharmacological	Reversible monoamine oxidase inhibitors (RIMAs) (e.g. moclobemide)	Generalized social phobia	Ib	Safer, but not as effective as irreversible MAOIs
Pharmacological	Serotonin–noradrenaline reuptake inhibitors (SNRIs) (e.g. venlafaxine)	Generalized social phobia	Ia	Probably equivalent to SSRIs in efficacy
Pharmacological	Tricyclic antidepressants	Generalized social phobia	III	Not properly evaluated
Pharmacological	Benzodiazepines (e.g. clonazepam)	Generalized social phobia	IIa	Less evidence of efficacy than SSRIs and venlafaxine but may be useful as adjunctive therapy; use as monotherapy possible but not extensively studied

Pharmacological		Specific social phobia	II	Effective in reducing anxiety associated with performance (public speaking, violin playing) as reduces tremor and tachycardia
Beta-adrenergic blocking drugs (e.g. propranolol)				
Cognitive behavioural therapy (CBT)	Individual treatment	Generalized social phobia	Ia	Excellent evidence of effectiveness maintained over a long time period
Cognitive behavioural therapy (CBT)	Group treatment	Generalized social phobia	Ia	Results similar to those of individual treatment
Social skills training	Individual and group	Generalized social phobia	IIb	May be useful to combine with CBT for patients with avoidant PD
Combined CBT and pharmacotherapy	Individual	Generalized social phobia	Ib	Marginal evidence of superiority of combined treatment versus monotherapy
Computerized CBT	Self-administered via Internet	All types of social phobia	Ia	Effective but some patients need or prefer interventions with therapist contact

2004), phenelzine (Gelernter et al., 1991; Heimberg et al., 1998), and clonazepam (Otto et al., 2000). One study found the drug phenelzine to have a faster and more robust effect than CBT (Heimberg et al., 1998); however, participants treated with phenelzine had a 50% relapse rate after treatment withdrawal (compared with 17% relapse in the CBT group (Liebowitz et al., 1999). Other studies have also found that CBT is associated with a lower rate of relapse after treatment withdrawal compared to drug treatments (e.g. Haug et al., 2003). Meta-analyses that have attempted to compare the effects of pharmacotherapy and CBT for social phobia have yielded mixed results (Gould et al., 1997b; Fedoroff & Taylor, 2001).

Combination therapy with CBT and drug treatment

Although it would seem that combining first-line pharmacological and psychological treatments could enhance treatment efficacy (both modalities are effective, but they have different mechanisms of action), the limited clinical research on this topic suggests that there is little difference between single and combination therapy (Davidson et al., 2004), although a more recent study did find an advantage of combination phenelzine pharmacotherapy and CBT over either treatment modality alone (Blanco et al., 2010). One challenge to this type of research is that large sample sizes are needed to demonstrate superiority of the combined treatment, and it is possible that most trials to date have been underpowered.

Conclusions

Both drug and specific psychological treatments have demonstrated unequivocal efficacy for treatment of social phobia, and their effects are roughly equivalent in magnitude (Table 26.1). Existing research suggests that drugs may act more quickly but psychological treatments such as CBT may have more enduring effects after treatment discontinuation.

Despite this, only about 50% of patients derive significant benefit from the first treatment for social phobia they receive, and virtually nothing is known about treatment sequences that should be applied to increase overall response rates. Preliminary studies of combining CBT and SSRIs have failed to show additional benefits of the combination (although one study has suggested additional benefits of combining CBT and phenelzine (Blanco et al., 2010)), but such studies have not been conducted in subjects who fail single treatments. We need more studies of "stepped-care" approaches that would provide information about the best sequences of treatment application.

27

Obsessive compulsive disorder

Based on "Obsessive compulsive disorder" by Helen Blair Simpson and Phil Harrison-Read in Effective Treatments in Psychiatry, Cambridge University Press, 2008

Introduction

Obsessive compulsive disorder is a relatively common (12-month prevalence of 0.6–1.0% (Kessler et al., 2005)) disorder that is classified with the anxiety disorders but which has the distinctive features of obsessions – recurrent and persistent ideas, images, or impulses – and compulsions – intentional repetitive behaviours or mental acts (rituals) that are carried out as a response to, or a way of avoiding, obsessions. These include repetitive checking, washing, repeating, ordering and reordering, arranging, or hoarding of objects. Because OCD usually has a chronic waxing and waning course, treatment often has to be prolonged, and relapse is common.

Pharmacological treatments

Clomipramine

This is a tricyclic antidepressant that is both a serotonin and norepinephrine reuptake inhibitor. It is an old drug, and the value of old drugs is sometimes forgotten, but over the past 40 years it is the drug with the most consistent evidence of efficacy in obsessive compulsive disorder. A series of randomized controlled trials and systematic reviews have shown that it is unequivocally more effective than placebo (Katz et al., 1990; Clomipramine

Collaborative Study Group, 1991) and a meta-analysis suggests that the number needed to treat (in a dose of 50 to 300 mg daily) to show evidence of efficacy is only 2 (Kobak et al., 1998). It is also superior to other tricyclic antidepressants that are primarily norepinephrine reuptake inhibitors (Thoren et al., 1980) and at least as good, if not better, than other SSRIs (Mundo et al., 1997; Bergeron et al., 2002).

Selective serotonin reuptake inhibitors (SSRIs) and other drugs

The SSRIs (e.g. fluoxetine, paroxetine, fluvoxamine, sertraline, citalopram) are also superior to placebo in the treatment of obsessive compulsive disorder with over 2500 patients being assessed in placebo-controlled studies (Montgomery et al., 1993, 2001; Greist et al., 1995; Pigott & Seay, 1999). Because of their tolerability, they are usually tried before clomipramine. Venlafaxine also appears to be an effective drug in obsessive compulsive disorder in open label and active comparison trials, although venlafaxine was not superior to placebo in the one small placebo-controlled trial (Yaryura-Tobias & Neziroglu, 1996). The choice of SSRI is really left to the clinician and in most cases is determined by the adverse effect profile rather than by any intrinsic merits of the drug with regard to efficacy.

Adjuvant drugs

Only about half of all patients with obsessive compulsive disorder make a good response to clomipramine or SSRIs and so it is not surprising that other treatments have been tested as 'add-on' therapies. Most other treatments that alter mood, such as lithium, electroconvulsive therapy and benzodiazepines, are ineffective in resistant obsessive compulsive disorder (Fineberg & Gale, 2005), but there is some evidence that augmentation with antipsychotic drugs may be of value. Haloperidol (McDougle et al., 1994), risperidone (Hollander et al., 2003; Erzegovesi et al., 2005), and olanzapine (Bystritsky et al., 2004) have all been tested in randomized studies and shown to augment the benefits of SSRIs in up to half of patients. It is not known for how long such additional medication should be given but in view of the potential problems with regular antipsychotic medication, it is advisable to only maintain this treatment if it is clearly effective (Marder et al., 2004).

Cognitive behaviour therapy (including exposure and response prevention (ERP))

A large number of controlled trials have been carried out into the efficacy of cognitive therapy and CBT in the treatment of obsessive compulsive disorder and the evidence for their efficacy is strong but not dramatic, with only a minority of patients showing improvement that could be regarded as recovery (Abramowitz, 1997; Tolin et al., 2004; Huppert & Franklin, 2006).

As CBT commonly includes behaviour therapy, often in the form of behavioural experiments, it could be argued that the separation of the cognitive from the behavioural aspects, including exposure and response prevention, is artificial. The experienced therapist would probably agree; all these aspects are commonly involved during the care of an individual patient, but as the evidence base has developed the individual components of treatment have been evaluated separately.

Cognitive therapy alone involves the identification of, the subsequent challenging, and later modification of faulty beliefs that lie behind the obsessions and rituals. If the disorder is shown almost entirely in the form of obsessions then the collaborative approach of cognitive therapy alone may be sufficient, but this is relatively uncommon and normally it has to be combined with a behaviour element in which changes in thinking are tested out by experiments with behaviour (Freestone et al., 1997). So a patient who has apparently overcome ruminations about fear of contamination may continue to wash his hands repeatedly almost as a safeguard, and this will have to be addressed if therapy is to be fully successful.

Computerized cognitive behavioural therapy

The practice of cognitive behavioural therapy is increasingly being computerized or reformulated in the form of self-help guides as its essential elements do not always have to be administered by a face-to-face therapist (Greist et al., 2002; Mataix-Cols & Marks, 2006). The evidence from recent controlled studies is now becoming clear; this treatment is both effective and cost-effective (as it is so much cheaper than direct therapist contact) (Tumur et al., 2007), but its value is increased by having additional guidance from a real life therapist, even if this is only available from a distance in the form of a telephone call.

Neurosurgery

Obsessive compulsive disorder can become an intractable condition that completely dominates and prevents any reasonable form of existence. Under such circumstances neurosurgery, mainly in the form of cingulotomy, capsulotomy, and subcaudate tractotomy (all procedures that reduce neurotransmission from the prefrontal parts of the cortex to other parts of the brain), has been attempted. As might be expected, no randomized controlled trials have been carried out with these procedures but there are some reported gains (Jenike, 1998). There are more recent updates.

Transcranial magnetic stimulation

This treatment is discussed fully in the book linked to this guide (Mantovani et al., 2008). Repetitive transcranial magnetic stimulation has been found in short-term controlled studies to be effective in reducing obsessional symptoms when administered to the right and left prefrontal cortex (Greenberg et al., 1997; Sachdev et al., 2001) and more studies are needed to determine the relative value of this treatment compared with other therapies.

Combined psychological and pharmacological treatments

Common sense suggests that combined treatments would be most helpful in obsessive compulsive disorder. The data support this contention when there is comorbid depression (Cottraux et al., 1990;

Hohagen et al., 1998). However, in the absence of significant depression, exposure and response prevention can be highly effective on its own if delivered intensively by skilled therapists (Foa et al., 2005). Because of the delay in onset of benefit with antidepressant drug therapy it is sometimes preferable to add the psychological therapies later, particularly exposure and response prevention, in order to get maximum benefit (Tenneij et al., 2005).

Recommended guidelines

In standard guidelines (National Collaborating Centre for Mental Health, 2006a; Koran et al., 2007) both SSRIs and CBT are prominent. The NICE guidelines suggest a step-wise approach where initially patients are treated with low intensity CBT with up to 10 therapist hours per patient, and this may include treatment in groups, self-help, or computerized treatment. If people are not able to engage in low intensity CBT then a course of SSRIs (no specific drug mentioned) is recommended or more intensive CBT involving between 10 and 30 hours per patient. This can also be given in the form of combined CBT and antidepressant therapy. If after this treatment there is little sign of progress, referral to a specialist multidisciplinary clinic is

Table 27.1 Effectiveness of treatments for obsessive compulsive disorder

Treatment	Form of treatment	Psychiatric disorder	Level of evidence to test efficacy	Comments
Psychosocial	Cognitive behaviour therapy (CBT)	OCD	Ib	Some evidence of efficacy when CT contains behavioural experiments. Little evidence supporting CT in the absence of behavioural experiments
Psychosocial	Computerized CBT	OCD	Ia	Similar level of efficacy to other forms of CBT and as this is cheaper it is more cost-effective in those who find this form of treatment acceptable
Pharmacotherapy	SSRIs (mainly sertraline, paroxetine, fluoxetine, fluvoxamine, and citalopram)	Obsessive compulsive disorder	Ia	Unequivocal superiority over placebo
Pharmacotherapy	Clomipramine (50–300 mg daily)	Obsessive compulsive disorder	Ia	Best evidence for efficacy overall, at least as effective as SSRIs
Pharmacotherapy	Antipsychotic drugs	Obsessive compulsive disorder	Ia	Some value as adjuvant therapy

Psychological treatments	CBT adapted for OCD	Obsessive compulsive disorder	Ia	Some evidence of efficacy but no clear placebo-controlled trials
Psychological treatments	Computerized CBT (either self-help or therapist guided)	Obsessive compulsive disorder	Ia	Definite evidence of efficacy but usually better with some guidance
Psychological treatments	Exposure and response prevention (ERP)	Obsessive compulsive disorder	Ia	Good evidence of short- and long-term efficacy
Psychological treatments	Cognitive therapy alone	Obsessive compulsive disorder	Ib	Efficacy good but less acceptable for some people than CBT
Somatic	Psychosurgery	Obsessive compulsive disorder	III	
Somatic	Transcranial magnetic stimulation	Obsessive compulsive disorder	III	
Psychopharmacology	SSRIs	OCD	Ia	Effectiveness shown across all the SSRIs. May need higher doses than for depression. About 65% of patients have symptoms reduced between 40% and 50%
Psychopharmacology	Clomipramine	OCD	Ia	Effective as well. Many RCTs to support it. Unclear whether it is more or less effective than the SSRIs. Has more side effects than the SSRIs

Table 27.1 (cont.)

Treatment	Form of treatment	Psychiatric disorder	Level of evidence to test efficacy	Comments
Psychopharmacology	Typical and atypical antipsychotics	OCD	Ia	Are effective as augmentation in helping up to 50% of patients further diminish OCD symptoms
Psychosocial	CBT	OCD	Ia	Numerous studies support its effectiveness. Two versions of CBT have been examined in OCD: one focused on behavioural techniques (ERP) and one focused on cognitive techniques (CT)
	ERP	OCD	Ib	Effective as monotherapy. Unclear whether more effective when formally combined with CT but difficult to test because ERP contains some cognitive components
	CT	OCD	Ib	Some evidence for efficacy when CT contains behavioural experiments. Little evidence supporting CT in the absence of behavioural experiments

| Psychopharmacology and psychosocial treatments (combination) | ERP and SSRIs | | Combination treatment is highly effective. Available data suggest that there are specific clinical situations where it is preferable to SSRIs or ERP alone | Ia |
| Somatic | Psychosurgery, transcranial magnetic stimulation | OCD | May be somewhat effective in the most difficult cases. Subject pool remains small and definitive studies have yet to be conducted | IIb |

suggested or combining CBT with another SSRI or with clomipramine. The final stage in the stepped programme is to give more intensive CBT or to add an atypical antipsychotic drug to the antidepressant.

This advice illustrates that response to treatment in obsessive compulsive disorder is far from guaranteed. Reduction in symptoms achieved by SSRIs is between 20 and 40% overall (Pigott & Seay, 1999). Therefore, when these drugs are recommended as first-line treatments, as they are in the American guidelines (American Psychiatric Association, 2007) it is clear that this is often only the first stage in treatment (and will often have been initiated in primary care before psychiatric assessment). The recommendation to change to another SSRI or to clomipramine, to add antipsychotic drugs, or to add psychological therapies, if response is not made to the SSRIs alone, is based as much on the availability of treatments as their efficacy. Unfortunately the psychological treatments are not readily accessible in many places, although the recent initiative to improve access to psychological treatments (IAPT) in the United Kingdom has made the NICE guidance more realistic.

There is much variability in the treatment progress and planning of patients with obsessive compulsive disorder. Firstly, dosages of antidepressants may need to be higher than in the conventional treatment of depression (Tollefson et al., 1994) and so the first change in management if a patient fails to respond is an increase in dosage. Once improvement has begun, and this may be delayed for several weeks, it is wise to continue on treatment for at least a year. The value of longer-term continuous treatment has yet to be determined. There is also a great deal to be said for the treatment of obsessive compulsive disorder to be carried out by the same therapist (or multi-disciplinary team in more complex cases) rather than have a series of separate referrals for different therapies. The knowledge of an individual patient's clinical profile is very helpful in deciding how the effective treatments (Table 27.1) can be integrated most appropriately.

28

Post-traumatic stress and adjustment disorders

Based on "Post-traumatic stress disorders and adjustment disorders" by Randall
D. Marshall, Steven B. Rudin, and Peter Tyrer in Effective Treatments in Psychiatry,
Cambridge University Press, 2008

Introduction

Post-traumatic stress and adjustment disorders are on a continuum of conditions all precipitated by external stress but otherwise highly variable in key clinical aspects such as severity, symptom presentation, chronicity, comorbidity, and treatment approach. Acute stress and adjustment disorders are by definition time-limited, and despite being very common in clinical practice are among the least studied conditions in psychiatry (Stirman et al., 2003). Adjustment disorders are defined as clinically significant (but non-specific) emotional or behavioural symptoms in response to

an identifiable stressor. In contrast, acute stress disorder and PTSD are specifically defined symptom clusters that occur in response to a traumatic stressor. Traumatic events (operationally defined) typically involve actual or threatened death or serious injury, or a threat to the physical integrity of self or others, together with a powerful negative emotional reaction such as fear, helplessness, or horror. It is fair to add that the introduction of the nature of the traumatic event (Criterion A in DSM-IV) as a diagnostic feature has come under heavy criticism and this, together with other controversial criteria, has led to the suggestion that this condition should be relegated to the appendices of international classification systems (Rosen et al., 2010).

The prevalence of adjustment disorders ranges from 11 to 18% in primary care and from 10 to 35% in liaison psychiatry (Casey, 2009). Post-traumatic stress disorder is also common (e.g. 6.8% lifetime preva-lence in the US; Kessler et al., 2005a) and highly associated with comorbid-ity including suicide. It follows severe stressors with certain characteristics that define them as trauma.

Course and treatment of acute stress and adjustment disorder

Acute stress disorders in the ICD-10 classification are defined as condi-tions that resolve within 8 hours, so specific treatments are not consid-ered necessary. If any intervention is conducted it should be time-limited and focused on providing support and quickly returning the patient to their previous level of functioning. Adjustment disorders can persist in chronic form, and despite their prev-alence there is only one randomized trial (Klink et al., 2003) published to date for treatment of these condi-tions. Persons on sick leave in a Dutch company (Royal KPN) were randomized either to treatment as usual by occupational physicians, or to a new 5–6-session intervention based on stress inoculation training (a form of cognitive behavioural ther-apy). Stress inoculation training led to superior functioning at 3 and 12 months, with a 30% superiority in work return time but no difference in symptoms. Adjustment disorders are generally associated with rela-tively good functioning (Casey et al., 1985) and a good outcome.

Psychopharmacology is not gener-ally recommended in the treatment of adjustment disorders (Anderson et al., 2000) though benzodiazepines may occasionally be used in a mod-erately dosed, time-limited fashion when anxiety is paralyzing.

Acute stress disorder in the DSM-IV is essentially an early-onset form of PTSD with dissociative symptoms. Several studies show that brief trauma-focused cognitive behaviour-al models can accelerate recovery and possibly reduce long-term risk. A recent study found that exposure therapy was superior to cognitive restructuring in preventing PTSD (Bryant et al., 2008).

Post-traumatic stress disorder

Antidepressants

Selective serotonin reuptake inhibi-tors (SSRIs) have the best published evidence base for the treatment of post-traumatic stress disorder, with multiple single and multisite trials attesting to their efficacy, as well as clear evidence of increased relapse when treatment is discontinued in double-blind conditions after 6 months (Davidson et al., 2001). SSRIs are rated as either first- or second-line treatment in most guidelines (Bisson et al., 2010; Forbes et al., 2010). Sertraline (Brady et al., 2000) and paroxetine (Marshall et al., 2001) are approved by the United States FDA for this condition, and other similar drugs are generally assumed to be effective also. The serotonin-noradrenergic reuptake inhibitor, venlafaxine, is also effective in chronic post-traumatic stress disorder (Davidson et al., 2006a; 2006b).

When symptoms have proven refractory to both evidence-based psychotherapy and SSRIs or SNRIs, other medications are sometimes used, but these practices are based on small controlled trials and case series and so should be considered and presented to the patient accordingly.

Irreversible monoamine oxidase inhibitors (phenelzine and tranylcypromine) may be used but care has to be taken with a special diet and avoidance of specific drug interactions. In one trial phenelzine was superior to both imipramine and placebo (Kosten et al., 1991). Reversible monoamine oxidase inhibitors such as brofaromine (Katz et al., 1995) and moclobemide (Neal et al., 1997) may also be considered but are probably not as effective as the irreversible MAOIs (Baker et al., 1995). Mirtazepine may also be valuable with equivalent efficacy to sertraline (Chung et al., 2004). Mood stabilizers (valproate, carbamazepine, topiramate, lamotrigine) are sometimes used in refractory PTSD based on no more than preliminary evidence and a few small controlled trials. Antipsychotic drugs also have a limited evidence base, with only one randomized trial showing that risperidone was superior to placebo in reducing intrusive thoughts and heightened arousal in chronic PTSD (Reich et al., 2004). Adrenergic modulators such as the beta-blocker propranolol (Kolb et al., 1984) and the alpha$_2$-agonist clonidine (Harmon & Riggs, 1996) are sometimes used to address hyperarousal symptoms such as severe startle and intrusive memories and nightmares in particular. Tricyclic antidepressants have been shown to be effective (Davidson et al., 1990; Kosten et al., 1991) but are currently not first-line treatments because of cardiovascular risks.

Benzodiazepines are generally avoided in PTSD because they have not been studied and found ineffective, and also can lead to disinhibited aggressive reactions (Risse et al., 1990) and potential addiction.

SSRIs and SNRIs remain the drug treatments of choice. A systematic review of alternatives to SSRIs covering 63 articles found that none reached the top level of evidence of effectiveness, with risperidone showing the best evidence of value (Berger et al., 2009). Drug therapy is currently not recommended for children and adolescents with PTSD (Strawn et al., 2010) even though there is some slight evidence of value (see Chapter 49).

Psychological treatments

Cognitive behavioural therapy adapted for PTSD (i.e. trauma-focused CBT) has a strong evidence base (Cloitre et al., 2002) and is a first-line treatment in virtually all guidelines, including those of NICE (Bisson et al., 2010; Forbes et al., 2010; National Collaborating Centre for Mental Health, 2006b). Of its various forms, trauma-focused exposure therapy has the largest evidence base. This literature, however, is lacking in large multisite studies, which could evaluate the effectiveness of these treatments on a broader scale and outside academic centres of excellence.

Trauma-focused CBTs involve specific techniques and require specialized training, and should be distinguished from general counselling and from debriefing, which can aggravate the symptoms of post-traumatic stress disorder (Rose et al., 2003), especially if given improperly. Exposure therapy is the best studied, involving both imaginal exposure and in vivo exposure to feared and avoided but low-risk trauma reminders (Foa et al., 1999), and similar therapies such as cognitive processing therapy (Resick et al., 2002) and stress inoculation training have all been demonstrated to be effective. All include the strategy of helping the patient confront disturbing thoughts, situations, beliefs, and sometimes people that are anxiety-provoking because they are reminders of some aspect of the trauma, but are not in reality inherently harmful. The clinician helps the patient draw a clearer distinction between the trauma as a frightening and dangerous experience and the memory of the trauma. Eye movement desensitization and reprocessing (EMDR), a multi-stage treatment that incorporates several different therapeutic techniques (e.g. cognitive restructuring, desensitization, coping and reframing strategies), has also been shown to be effective in multiple randomized trials and is rated a first-line treatment in most but not all guidelines (e.g. Rothbaum et al., 2005; Forbes et al., 2010).

Choice of treatment in post-traumatic stress disorder

Both psychosocial and pharmacological treatments have been shown effective for PTSD in dozens of randomized controlled trials, and

Table 28.1 Efficacy of treatments for adjustment and stress disorders

Treatment	Form of treatment	Psychiatric disorder	Level of evidence to test efficacy	Comments
CBT	Stress inoculation training	Adjustment disorder	IIb	Better functional outcome compared with control, no difference in symptoms
Trauma-focused CBT	5 sessions	Acute post-traumatic stress	Ib	Significantly reduced rates of PTSD at 6 months (30% vs. 67%)
Pharmacotherapy	SSRIs (mainly sertraline (50–100 mg) and paroxetine (20–40 mg))	PTSD	Ia	Unequivocal superiority over placebo
Pharmacotherapy	Tricyclic antidepressants (imipramine and amitriptyline) (150–300 mg)	PTSD	Ib	Fewer trials but no clear differences in efficacy compared with SSRIs
Pharmacotherapy	Monoamine oxidase inhibitors (phenelzine, brofaromine)	PTSD	IIb	Old (irreversible) MAOIs have better evidence base than reversible ones
Pharmacotherapy	Other antidepressants (mirtazepine, venlafaxine)	PTSD	IIa	Some evidence of efficacy but no clear placebo-controlled trials
Pharmacotherapy	Benzodiazepines	PTSD	III	Potential adverse effects suggest they should be avoided apart from occasional brief use
Pharmacotherapy	Mood stabilizers	PTSD	III	Insufficient evidence to recommend

Table 28.1 (cont.)

Treatment	Form of treatment	Psychiatric disorder	Level of evidence to test efficacy	Comments
Pharmacotherapy	Antipsychotic drugs	PTSD	IIa	Risperidone of some value
Pharmacotherapy	Autonomic nervous system stabilizers (propranolol, clonidine)	PTSD	IIb	Some evidence that specific symptoms may be helped
Psychological treatments	Trauma-focused CBT	PTSD	Ia	Good evidence of short- and long-term efficacy
Psychological treatments	Exposure therapies and other cognitive therapies	PTSD	Ia	Efficacy good but less acceptable for some people than CBT
Psychological treatments	Eye movement desensitization and reprocessing (EMDR)	PTSD	Ia	Similar to drug treatments in that many of the most positive studies are by product champions

guidelines generally recommend a cognitive behavioural treatment as first-line, with medications as second-line or for use when such treatments are unavailable, or when symptoms are particularly severe (Forbes et al., 2010). In addition, available research suggests that the majority of PTSD patients may have a preference for psychotherapy over medication. There is also overwhelming evidence that PTSD involves profound neurobiological alterations, also supplying the rationale for a biological treatment, in addition to multiple randomized trials.

Both treatments in the forms studied to date leave many patients with residual symptoms when provided alone, and thus combination treatment is often provided in clinical practice when a first treatment is not fully effective, or when there is considerable comorbidity (e.g. severe depression and suicidal thoughts). Only a handful of studies to date have studied combination therapy (Hetrick et al., 2010). Combination studies to date suggest that CBT added to medication treatment can further increase response. Since clinical need far outstrips our evidence base at present, clinicians must always exercise sound judgement when going beyond the relatively sparse literature on what to do if the first- or second-line treatments are not completely effective.

Summary

The subject of stress and adjustment disorders illustrates the problems of matching treatments to diagnoses in psychiatry. Diagnoses that are clear cut and well defined, such as obsessive compulsive disorder discussed in Chapter 27, allow a substantial body of knowledge to be applied to that condition over a long time period. The stress disorders suffer from uncertainties in their definition, in both current and forthcoming classifications (Rosen et al., 2010), and differences between ICD and DSM, as acute stress disorders are defined differently in the two systems. Adjustment disorders, probably the most common disorders in mental health, are rarely studied because very few practitioners use the diagnosis, so there is almost no evidence base. Post-traumatic stress disorder attracts by far the most interest, but this is also a diagnosis that is notoriously comorbid with other diagnoses, so one can never be quite sure that a successful treatment has acted on the primary disorder or a concurrent one. In spite of this concern there is a range of useful therapies that is being built up for effective management (Table 28.1) which suggests that early intervention (but not debriefing) with well-focused aims, can yield substantial benefit.

Eating disorders

29

Psychopharmacology of eating disorders

Based on "Psychopharmacology of eating disorders" by Andrew Bennett, Rishi Caleyachetty, and Janet Treasure in Effective Treatments in Psychiatry, Cambridge University Press, 2008

Introduction

There is a great deal written about the use of medication in the treatment of eating disorders, including good systematic reviews leading to guidelines in Australia, the United States, and the UK (Beumont et al., 2004; American Psychiatric Association 2000; National Collaborating Centre for Mental Health, 2004b; Treasure et al., 2010). Unfortunately, for a variety of reasons, they are not generally followed in practice. One of the problems is that for several indications, including the emergency treatment of anorexia nervosa, it is very difficult to carry out randomized trials

of treatment for what is a potentially fatal condition. Despite this we have good islands of evidence that should aid practice.

Anorexia nervosa

The use of drugs in the treatment of anorexia nervosa depends greatly on the form in which the illness presents. This ranges from presentation in childhood to late in adult life and from severe life-threatening illness to relatively minor daily dysfunction. Most of the trials of drugs in the treatment of anorexia nervosa have been carried out in adults. It would be unwise to extrapolate to their use in children or adolescents. It is also worth noting that the QT interval of the electrocardiogram is prolonged by starvation and electrolyte imbalance (Cooke et al., 1994) and thus there is the potential for adverse interactions with drugs which have an independent effect on cardiac rhythmicity. ECG monitoring is recommended for high-risk patients. There is no strong evidence to support medication use either in the acute or maintenance phases of the illness (Claudino et al., 2006; Crow et al., 2009).

It might be expected that these drugs, many of which have weight gain as an adverse effect, would be valuable in this disorder but in clinical practice many people with anorexia nervosa do not adhere to medication as they are fearful of the loss of control inherent in drug treatment, the additional calories in the coating of drugs, and the threat of weight gain itself.

Patients with high medical risk

In the most acute form of anorexia nervosa patients may require admission to hospital because of threat to life and here medication may be considered for many other reasons apart from that of weight gain. In this phase it may be appropriate to give a low dose of antipsychotic drugs to reduce anxiety and agitation. The older antipsychotic drug, chlorpromazine, has some advantages because it has anxiolytic and anti-emetic properties. There have been recent case series and small randomized trials with the new generation of antipsychotic medication (e.g. olanzapine, quetiapine) but their place in therapy is not yet established (Cochrane Review, in preparation; Claudino et al., submitted for publication).

Cyproheptadine is both an antihistamine with sedative properties and also an appetite stimulant. In one of three controlled trials it has been shown to have some benefit in hospitalized patients in promoting weight gain in the restricting subtype of anorexia nervosa (Halmi et al., 1986). However, this small evidence is not sufficient to recommend this drug formally in official guidelines (National Collaborating Centre for Mental Health, 2004b; Beumont et al., 2004).

Patients with moderate medical risk

There is little firm guidance that can be given in this population because most of the studies of medication are open studies which are not open to satisfactory conclusion (Ruggiero et al., 2006). Antidepressants, particularly SSRIs, are commonly given in this stage, partly because they are regarded as valuable in treating the accompanying obsessional behaviour, but there is no clear evidence of their benefit. Some argue that SSRIs should be started only after the patient has undergone nutritional rehabilitation and attained oestrogen levels within the normal range. In the acute anorexic state nutritional deficiencies (e.g. tryptophan or the secondary consequences of malnutrition such as oestrogen deficiency) may render medication ineffective. However, in an interesting study which addressed this hypothesis in part it was found that nutritional supplements (tryptophan, vitamins, minerals, and essential fatty acids) did not enhance the effectiveness of fluoxetine in underweight patients with anorexia nervosa (Barbaric et al., 2004). In addition, little is known about how people with anorexia nervosa absorb and metabolize antidepressants or any medications, raising the possibility that there may be inadequate penetration to the brain. Thus more research into the use of medication in ambulatory care is needed.

Relapse prevention

There are two roles for psychopharmacological treatment after the anorexic patient has restored weight. The first is to treat those psychiatric symptoms associated with anorexia

nervosa that persist after weight restoration. In the USA guidelines it is recommended that because symptoms associated with anorexia nervosa, such as depression or obsessive compulsive disorder may remit with weight restoration, the practitioner should, if possible, defer decisions over the use of medications until the person with anorexia nervosa has reached an appropriate weight. This includes depressive and obsessive compulsive symptoms and both SSRIs and the partial SSRI, clomipramine, are used in this group. However, these are best thought of as treatments for comorbid conditions rather than for the anorexia nervosa itself. There is insufficient evidence to suggest that atypical antipsychotic drugs such as aripiprazole and ziprasidone are effective in preventing weight loss and a practitioner has to be aware of the bias in promoting these drugs while they are under patent.

Bulimia nervosa

There is a better evidence base for the drug treatment of bulimia nervosa but most of this has to be accompanied by the caveat that studies have been mainly in adults and may not generalize to children or adolescents. The results of recent reviews suggest that tricyclic antidepressants and SSRIs and monoamine oxidase inhibitors

(MAOIs) are superior to placebo in promoting remission from binge eating and purging (McCann & Agras, 1990; Mitchell et al., 2001; Carruba et al., 2001; National Collaborating Centre for Mental Health, 2004b). There is also evidence that the frequency of binge eating is helped by antidepressants, both tricyclic antidepressants and SSRIs, and a number of positive trials demonstrate that this is a robust finding with a high proportion reducing the frequency of binge eating by over 50% (Laederach-Hofmann et al., 1999; McElroy et al., 2000; Arnold et al., 2002). There is also evidence that the drug treatments are superior to psychotherapy in the acute treatment of binge eating and purging. Interestingly enough, there are no good studies comparing tricyclic antidepressants but because the SSRIs are more recent and heavily promoted they tend to be used more often.

The main drug used in clinical practice is fluoxetine and this is the only one approved by the US FDA for the treatment of bulimia nervosa. This is used in higher dosage than normally used in depression, usually in a dose of 60 mg daily. The recommended course of treatment is between 6 months and 1 year and it is generally recommended that the drug be stopped when symptoms have been in remission for several months. There is also some evidence that switching

between antidepressants may sometimes aid response (Mitchell et al., 2001). Tricyclic antidepressants may be less often used because of their propensity to cause weight gain and this may be highly relevant in bulimia. Because depressive symptoms and suicidal acts are sometimes quite common in bulimia nervosa there is also concern about prescribing the more toxic tricyclic antidepressants in this population.

Three recent systematic reviews found strong evidence for the use of antidepressants to treat bulimia nervosa in the short term (around 8 weeks) (Shapiro et al., 2007; Hay & Bacaltchuk, 2008; Treasure et al., 2010). However, this conclusion has to be moderated by the evidence that the effect sizes and overall acceptability of antidepressant treatment are relatively low (Treasure et al., 2010).

Fluoxetine is the main drug tested in trials and approved for use in bulimia nervosa by health regulatory agencies; it is recommended in a dose (60 mg/day) that is higher than usually necessary to treat depression (20–40 mg/day) (Treasure et al., 2010). There is less evidence of efficacy for other SSRIs (citalopram, sertraline, fluvoxamine) (Milano et al., 2005; Hay & Bacaltchuk, 2008). It is also not known yet whether antidepressant treatment can prevent relapse in bulimia nervosa, as the existing few trials were limited by their high attrition rates. Topiramate can be effective in reducing bulimic and purging symptoms, but the safety profile of this drug still needs to be established in this disorder (Hay & Bacaltchuk, 2008).

New approaches

Two randomized controlled studies have shown that topiramate, an anticonvulsant, reduced binge eating and purging in patients with bulimia nervosa when compared with placebo (Hedges et al., 2003; Hoopes et al., 2003). Its side-effect profile, however, may limit its use. Paraesthesias and cognitive impairment are the most common side effects, and because of this a slow titration is recommended (e.g. 25–50 mg increase per week). Caution is advised, especially when using topiramate with those bulimics who are below normal weight, even if they do not meet criteria for anorexia nervosa, as weight loss is a common side effect. The mechanism of weight loss following topiramate is unknown.

Rarely used approaches

The use of the opiate antagonist naltrexone is not common. One small study, however, did show some efficacy when used in higher doses of 200–300 mg/day, which is higher than the doses used to prevent alcohol relapse and opiate addiction

(Marrazzi et al., 1995). The risk of nausea, however, may preclude use at such doses for most patients. There are some case reports of using naltrexone to augment SSRIs. It is more likely to be used when a history of self-injurious behaviour, such as cutting, is present. Liver function tests must be monitored because of the risk of hepatotoxicity in high doses.

Irreversible MAOIs are rarely used because of the dietary restrictions necessary to avoid tyramine reactions, although weight gain can be very marked with these drugs.

Binge eating disorder (atypical eating disorder)

Sibutramine, a specific reuptake noradrenaline and serotonin inhibitor (SNRI), has been used in the treatment of obese patients with binge eating disorder and was found to reduce both weight and binge frequency. Dry mouth and constipation were side effects (Appolinario et al., 2003). NICE guidelines suggest it is only given to those who have seriously tried to lose weight by other methods and who are being carefully monitored. It is only licensed for use for 1 year, and rebound weight gain may follow its cessation.

Systematic reviews and meta-analyses of treatments for binge eating disorder suggest that drug

Table 29.1 Effectiveness of drug treatments for eating disorders

Treatment	Form of treatment	Psychiatric disorder	Level of evidence for efficacy	Comments
Tricyclic antidepressants (TCAs)	(e.g. amitriptyline, clomipramine) Conventional treatment (up to 6 weeks' acute treatment and then maintenance dosage)	Anorexia nervosa	IIIa	No incremental value when combined with full multimodal treatment Care to be taken with very emaciated patients with electrolyte disturbance or suicidal risk
Selective serotonin reuptake inhibitors (SSRIs)	(e.g. fluoxetine)	Anorexia nervosa (particularly in restricting subgroup)	Ib	Evidence generally weak
Typical antipsychotic drugs	(e.g. chlorpromazine) May be useful as anti-nausea drug	Anorexia nervosa	IV	No firm evidence of efficacy
Atypical antipsychotic drugs	(e.g. aripiprazole, ziprasidone)	Anorexia nervosa	IV	Possible use to maintain weight gain or to modify additional psychopathology
Anti-anxiety drugs	(e.g. diazepam)	Anorexia nervosa	IV	Use as required at times of great distress but not regularly
Monoamine oxidase inhibitors	Up to 8 weeks initially	Bulimia nervosa	Ib	Evidence favouring MAOIs in remission from binge eating
		Bulimia nervosa	Ia	

| Tricyclic antidepressants | (e.g. clomipramine) in conventional dosage up to 1yr | Bulimia nervosa | Ia | Significantly superior to placebo in reducing binge eating |
| Selective serotonin reuptake inhibitors (SSRIs) | (e.g. fluoxetine in higher than conventional dosage) 40–60 mg daily for up to 8 weeks and subsequent maintenance treatment up to 1yr | | | Significantly superior to placebo in reducing binge eating and maintaining remission. Paroxetine avoided because of weight gain |

Conclusions

treatments show, at least, a moderate effectiveness in reduction of binge frequencies and promotion of binge remission in the short term, with a remission rate of 48.7% reported with pharmacotherapy (including antidepressants, anticonvulsants, and obesity drugs) compared with 28.5% with placebo (Treasure et al., 2010). Several guidelines recommend short-term treatment with anti-depressants (mainly SSRIs) as an alternative first approach to CBT. Although antidepressants are usually effective in reducing binges, negative findings have also been reported and there is less confidence in their impact on depressive symptoms and on weight (Stefano et al., 2008).

Modest weight loss as well as binge remission have been reported with drugs approved for use in obesity (Reas and Grilo, 2008), such as sibutra-mine (Appolinario et al., 2003;Wilfley et al., 2008) and orlistat, and with drugs associated with weight loss, such as topiramate, zonisamide, and atomoxetine (McElroy et al., 2007). Sibutramine and topiramate have both been tested in multisite trials and showed binge remission rates greater than SSRIs compared to placebo (see Treasure et al., 2010 for review). Although all these drugs may be con-sidered as having sufficient evidence to be suitable for treating binge eating disorder, the short-term duration of tri-als (12–24 weeks) and high dropout and high placebo response rates limit recommendations over their use (Brownley et al., 2007; Vocks et al., 2010). In addition, the risk–benefit balance is uncertain as adverse effects may be prominent (Hay and Bacaltchuk, 2008; Treasure et al., 2010).

Conclusions

In the main, psychotherapeutic approaches have been both more effec-tive and acceptable in the management of eating disorders than drug treat-ments, but the evidence base is increas-ing to such an extent (Table 29.1) that medication will increasingly be used also. However, it is possible that tailor-ing medication to the type, severity, and duration of the illness, and combining it with psychological treatments, may improve both outcome and clinical util-ity. Thus research with new drugs such as sibutramine and others specifically marketed for these disorders, each with a more comprehensive risk–benefit profile, and more trials in which both the type and severity of the disorder is characterized more carefully, may widen their use in this patient popula-tion. There is very limited evidence, and no controlled trials, comparing pharmacological and, psychotherapeu-tic approaches in the treatment of eat-ing disorders and, despite the common use of combined therapy, no clear rec-ommendations can be made here.

Somatic treatments for eating disorders

Based on "Other somatic physical treatments and complex interventions for eating disorders" by Philippa Hugo and Scott Crow in Effective Treatments in Psychiatry, Cambridge University Press, 2008

Introduction

None of the treatments in this chapter have a very strong evidence base but deal with an important part of management of eating disorders and are commonly used in practice in one form or another. Potential somatic treatments for eating disorders include: drugs (discussed in Chapter 29), intensive feeding, heat and light treatments, exercise, electroconvulsive therapy, and psychosurgery. Randomized controlled trial evidence is very difficult to obtain in this population and explains the relative lack of good data.

Intensive feeding

Refeeding is clearly an important component of the treatment of anorexia nervosa. Although it is a critical part of treatment there is no really clear evidence about whether the different methods, setting and rate of refeeding are preferred options and so there is relatively little to guide clinical practice. Having said this, it is very important to stress that most patients can be fed orally with the skilled support that is available in eating disorder units or even in general psychiatric settings. The minority who do need other forms of refeeding put themselves at risk to their physical health if they continue to starve and for this group specialized staff are required. Many of these patients develop serious metabolic complications such as severe hypophosphataemia if they receive too much in the way of concentrated calories given by parenteral nutrition, and expert advice is needed to prevent this "refeeding syndrome" (Solomon & Kirby, 1990). There are also ethical issues involved here in forcibly feeding patients who may be considered to have full mental capacity and these need to be considered before any form of coercion is involved (Goldner et al., 1997).

Nasogastric and other forms of tube feeding

Nasogastric tube feeding is the preferred route for invasive refeeding. It has few medical complications and can be easily halted so this means a return to normal eating can occur as soon as possible. It is also possible to deliver nutrients directly into the stomach (gastrostomy) or jejunum of the small bowel (jejunostomy) (Pesenti et al., 1999; Neiderman et al., 2000), and, to guarantee that all food given goes directly into the body, total parenteral nutrition (TPN) (Mehler and Weiner, 1993) has also been recommended. In this treatment all nutritive components are given in exactly the right proportions. The latter treatment

has been shown to produce significantly more rapid weight gain when compared to a match group receiving behaviourally orientated inpatient therapy (Pertschuk et al., 1981), but as complications are common this treatment is now rarely recommended.

Although nasogastric feeding is often used there have been very few studies examining its efficacy and acceptability. Although there is a general view that this form of feeding prevents a good therapeutic relationship from developing there is no good evidence that this is true (Serfaty and McCluskey, 1998), and in fact, the opposite may be the case. Two retrospective studies have recently been published in which nasogastric feeding plus oral feeding has been compared with oral feeding alone. These both showed that there is greater weight gain with the nasogastric feeding group compared with oral feeding (Robb et al., 2002; Zuercher et al., 2003). There was no difference between the groups in the length of hospital stay. There is, by contrast, little evidence about long-term outcome with nasogastric feeding.

Exercise

Anorexia nervosa

There have been several reports describing the use of exercise as an additional treatment for patients with eating disorders. Most of these are merely descriptive and of limited value. Much is written about exercise being one of the aims of patients wishing to reduce weight in anorexia nervosa and restricted exercise is often part of standard treatment programmes. In spite of this, physical therapies such as dance movement therapy, yoga, tai chi, and horse riding may be used in management, and, whilst there is little evidence that they lead to greater weight gain, they are associated with reports of greater satisfaction (Beumont et al., 1994; Szabo & Green, 2002).

Binge eating disorder

Binge eating disorder is often treated with exercise programmes, but most of these are descriptive only. However, Levine et al. (1996) compared 44 patients in an active treatment group receiving exercise with 33 in a delayed treatment control group, and at the end of treatment there were significantly greater increases in exercise frequency and overall calorie expenditure in the active treatment group in patients with binge eating disorder. Those who became abstinent from binges had significant increases in exercise frequency after treatment compared with those who continued to binge. Pendleton et al. (2002) also evaluated the effects of

adding exercise to cognitive behavioural therapy for binge eating disorder. There was a significant decrease in frequency of binge eating and an increase in abstinence rates from binging in the exercise group at the end of treatment, and this was maintained at follow-up at 16 months. There was also an improvement in mood as well as weight loss.

Bulimia nervosa

Patients with bulimia nervosa tend to adopt dramatically different approaches to exercise, varying between excessive activity and none at all. Beumont et al. (1994) have suggested that regular exercise, both aerobic and non-aerobic, may help patients to reach a more healthy weight and reduce anxiety and depression. This has been tested further in a randomized controlled trial of cognitive behavioural therapy and nutritional advice compared with an exercise regimen (Sundgot-Borgen et al., 2002). Sixty-nine patients were included in the trial, and though it was handicapped by not having a control group, the results suggested a slight advantage for physical exercise compared with cognitive behavioural therapy in reducing the frequency of binge eating, purging, and laxative abuse.

Whilst the evidence for benefit of exercise therapy is too limited to make a specific recommendation for its use, the finding that it may aid therapeutic programmes by improving satisfaction and engagement lend it some credibility.

Heat treatment

William Gull, the discoverer of anorexia nervosa, was the first to note the therapeutic effect of heat treatment. There have been several reports of the value of this approach and two small trials have been published (Bergh et al., 2002; Birmingham et al., 2004). The first of these compared the combination of heat and a computerized eating monitor with a waiting list control. Higher remission rates were found in the experimental group and the authors suggested most patients recover with this treatment. However only 16 patients were treated (a mixture with both anorexia nervosa and bulimia nervosa) and physical activity was restricted.

Although in a larger group of 168 patients the estimated rate of remission was 75% (with time to remission of 14.7 months) it is difficult to know to what extent heat treatment was essential to this programme. The second study (Birmingham et al., 2004) treated 21 patients and found no difference in BMI between the two groups after treatment.

Light therapy

Light therapy is now a recommended treatment for a seasonal affected disorder and as mood disturbances are common in eating disorders it is not surprising that this treatment has been given also. However, the effects of bright light therapy have also been tested specifically in binge eating disorder, in which purging and mood were also assessed (Lam et al., 1996; Blouin et al., 1996; Braun et al., 1999). In a crossover design (not ideal for this population) with 17 women there was a significant improvement in binge eating, purging, and depressive symptoms after light therapy, but only one patient was abstinent from binge eating after 2 weeks' treatment (Lam et al., 1996). These results contrasted with those for a similar study of 18 patients in which light therapy was associated with improvement in mood but not in binge eating or purging (Blouin et al., 1996).

The last trial of 34 patients (only a quarter of whom were depressed clinically) showed some improvement in binge eating but not in purging or mood. The variation in these results was explained to some extent by an additional study in which 22 patients with bulimia nervosa and seasonal affective disorder were treated with bright light therapy. In this population both mood and binge eating frequency

Table 30.1 Effectiveness of other somatic treatments for eating disorders

Treatment	Form of treatment	Psychiatric disorder	Level of evidence	Comments
Refeeding	Nasogastric tube feeding	Anorexia nervosa	III	Supplementary nasogastric (NG) feeding produces significant weight increases in the short term. The impact of NG feeding on long-term outcome is unknown
Refeeding	Total parenteral nutrition	Anorexia nervosa	III	Complications are common
Exercise	Graded prescribed physical exercise	Anorexia nervosa	III	Inconclusive
Exercise	Graded prescribed physical exercise	Bulimia nervosa	Ib	One small RCT found a physical exercise regime to be more effective than CBT in reducing bulimic symptoms. Abstinence rates were not reported
Exercise	Graded prescribed physical exercise	Binge eating disorder	Ib	Adding exercise to treatment of BED enhances outcome and contributes to reductions in binge eating and BMI
Heat treatment	e.g. sauna, heating vests, or heated environment	Anorexia nervosa	Ib	Evidence inconclusive
Light therapy		Bulimia nervosa	Ib	Some effects on mood or eating disorder symptoms. Evidence inconclusive
Electroconvulsive therapy		Anorexia nervosa	IV	Case reports only

improved (Lam et al., 2001). The synthesis of these findings suggests that those who have binge eating disorder and depression (a common combination) are likely to improve with light therapy but the effect of the therapy on binge eating is not primary. Because of this current recommendations are that light therapy should not be considered to be a main-line treatment for any form of eating disorder. Nevertheless, this is an interesting subject that deserves further study.

Electro-convulsive therapy

Electro-convulsive therapy was often used in a wide range of psychiatric disorders when it was a popular treatment. Almost all the reports referred to the treatment of anorexia nervosa and were published over 20 years ago; most of these are of historical interest only. In those cases in which a good response has been suggested it appears that most of the patients concerned had additional depressive symptoms (e.g. Bernstein, 1964; Morgan et al., 1983). There have been no published reports on the use of ECT for the treatment of bulimia nervosa apart from one case report describing the development of myoclonic jerks after this treatment (Dibble & Tandon, 1992). It is therefore not possible on the basis of current evidence to recommend this treatment for any form of eating disorder.

Psychosurgery

There have been occasional reports on the use of leucotomy in the treatment of anorexia nervosa (e.g. Kelly and Mitchell-Heggs, 1973; Crisp and Kalucy, 1973), including a long-term follow-up of the last series of four patients (Morgan and Crisp, 2002). In the short term these patients showed some improvement but although weight gain had been restored, there were still disordered cognitions about eating. Despite this the authors concluded that leucotomy may be "a justifiable recommendation of last resort". In the present state of knowledge and with the concerns about psychosurgery, including the attraction of reversible forms of electrical simulation and ablation (see Chapter 20), even the "last resort" may be one step too far.

Conclusions

The level of evidence for each of these treatments is summarized in Table 30.1. None of these could be regarded as primary treatments for eating disorders and their value as adjunctive treatments is limited, but is certainly worthy of further investigation. Of the treatments available, exercise appears to be the one that is most likely to be valuable.

31

Psychological treatments for eating disorders

Based on "Psychological treatments for eating disorders" by Roz Shafran, Pamela K. Keel, Alissa Haedt, and Christopher Fairburn in Effective Treatments in Psychiatry, Cambridge University Press, 2008

Introduction

The strength of the evidence-base for the treatment of anorexia nervosa (AN), bulimia nervosa (BN), binge eating disorder (binge-eating disorder) and remaining eating disorders not otherwise specified (EDNOS; or atypical eating disorders (AEDs)) varies across disorders, despite considerable overlap that needs diagnostic attention (Fairbairn & Cooper, 2011), so the evidence for each will be considered separately. This has already been done in the UK by the National Institute for Health and Clinical Excellence (NICE) (National Collaborating Centre for Mental

Health, 2004b), the primary source of information on which this chapter is based. In the USA, the *American Psychiatric Association Practice Guidelines for the Treatment of Psychiatric Disorders Compendium* (2004) provides recommendations for the treatment of eating disorders in a second edition, but there have been many recent developments that affect the evidence base.

Anorexia nervosa

Primary care

The lack of research into anorexia nervosa in general applies to the

investigation of the optimal treatment setting for this disorder
(Fairburn & Bohn, 2005) (see also
Chapter 30). It is far from clear
what proportion of patients are treated in primary care, although clinical
guidelines exist on their management (e.g. Powers & Santana, 2002;
Waller & Fairburn, 2004). In England
and Wales, it is recommended that
general practitioners should pay
attention to a global clinical assessment that is repeated over time
(National Collaborating Centre for
Medical Health, 2004, p. 64) that
includes BMI, the rate of weight
loss in adults or growth rates in children, objective physical signs, and
relevant laboratory tests. The guidelines state that patients with chronic
anorexia nervosa who are not being
treated in specialist care should be
offered an annual physical and mental health review.

There is no evidence suggesting strict
behavioural programmes are superior
to more flexible ones (Vandereycken &
Pieters, 1978; Touyz et al., 1984) and
expert opinion suggests that rigid inpatient behaviour modification programmes should not be used in the
management of anorexia nervosa
(National Collaborating Centre for
Medical Health, 2004, p. 65). Instead, a
structured symptom-focused intervention with an expectation of weight gain
is warranted and wider psychosocial
issues should also be addressed.

Outpatients

Six studies have compared outpatient
treatment in adults. Nutritional counselling has been compared with psychotherapy in 30 adolescent and adult
outpatients (Hall and Crisp, 1987) and
with cognitive behavioural therapy in
35 adolescent and adult outpatients
(Serfaty et al., 1999). In the latter
study, all 10 patients randomized to
the nutritional counselling dropped
out. Differences in treatment completion may be attributable to differences
in mean age between treatment
groups. The mean age of participants
randomized to cognitive behavioural
therapy was 22.1 years while the
mean age of patients randomized to
nutritional counselling was 17.9 years
(Serfaty et al., 1999). Despite the
dramatic differences in treatment
completion between conditions,
there were no significant outcome differences between groups on BMI, total
EDI score, or body dissatisfaction.
Behaviour therapy has been compared
with cognitive behavioural therapy
and a low-contact control condition
in 24 adult patients (Channon et al.,
1989) and with cognitive analytical
therapy in 30 adult patients (Treasure
et al., 1995). No consistent statistically
significant findings of note were found
in any of these studies.

The largest study comprised 84
patients (mean age 26.3 years; mean
duration of the disorder = 6.3 years)

(Dare et al., 2001). The patients were randomized to focal psychoanalytical psychotherapy, cognitive analytical therapy, family-based treatment, or routine outpatient treatment involving brief sessions with a trainee psychiatrist. Approximately one-third of patients improved significantly, and all three psychotherapies were more effective than the routine treatment for weight gain, although there were no significant differences across the four conditions. In addition, no specific psychotherapy was superior to the others. The superiority of the psychotherapies could either be attributed to the potency of the interventions or to the fact that the routine treatment involved less than half the therapist–patient contact and was delivered by trainees.

The study of Russell and colleagues (1987) also included adults and compared treatment conditions in adults with early-onset anorexia nervosa (N = 15) and late-onset anorexia nervosa (N = 21). No statistically significant differences emerged between treatments within these adult groups.

In a more recent study, 33 patients whose weight had been restored with inpatient treatment were randomized to receive 12 months of CBT or nutritional counselling (Pike et al., 2003). CBT was superior to nutritional counselling in terms of the proportion remaining in treatment, relapse rates, and meeting criteria for a good

outcome. In this study, the superiority of CBT over nutritional counselling could have been partially attributable to antidepressant medication since more patients in the CBT group were receiving antidepressants, and antidepressants have been associated with decreased risk of relapse following weight recovered in patients with anorexia nervosa (Kaye et al., 2001).

Anorexia nervosa is usually treated in outpatient, day patient, or inpatient settings. There has only been one study in which patients have been randomized to different treatment settings (Crisp et al., 1991). Ninety patients were randomized to inpatient treatment, two forms of outpatient treatment or detailed single assessment with advice regarding further management. The study was limited by small numbers but no important differences were found between the four types of management. There is no evidence that suggests that strict behavioural programmes are superior to more flexible ones (Vandereycken and Pieters, 1978; Touyz et al., 1984) and treatment guidelines suggest that rigid inpatient behaviour modification programmes should not generally be used in the management of this condition (National Collaborating Centre for Mental Health, 2004, p. 65).

This data has led to recommendations that those family interventions that directly address eating disorders should be used in the treatment of anorexia nervosa (National Collaborating Centre for Mental Health, 2004, p. 65) and that nutritional counselling is much less effective than a structured, focused psychological treatment.

Bulimia nervosa

Primary care

Much more is known about the treatment of bulimia nervosa than anorexia nervosa and over 70 RCTs have been conducted (Wilson & Fairburn, 2002; National Collaborating Centre for Mental Health, 2004). Most studies have been conducted on outpatients in specialist settings and only one has been conducted in primary care. In this recent study, Walsh and colleagues compared the psychological and pharmacological treatment of BN in two primary care clinics in the USA (Walsh et al., 2004). Of the 91 female participants, 15 did not meet full DSM-IV criteria in terms of the frequency or size of the episodes of binge eating. Patients were randomly assigned to receive either 60 mg fluoxetine alone, placebo alone, fluoxetine plus guided self-help, or placebo plus guided self-help. The guided self-help was an adaptation of cognitive behavioural therapy based on previous studies (Palmer et al., 2002).

The main finding from this study was that almost 70% of participants dropped out. Some participants reported leaving the study as it was too demanding whilst others felt that it was not demanding enough. Overall, compared to placebo those who received fluoxetine attended more physician visits, had a greater reduction in binge eating and vomiting, and had a greater improvement in psychological symptoms. There was no evidence of benefit from guided self-help. These findings contrasted with a smaller previous study in primary care using guided self-help. In this case series of 11 patients, 6 did well (Waller et al., 1996).

In secondary care, there is a large body of evidence demonstrating the efficacy of a range of psychological treatments for bulimia nervosa (Wilson and Fairburn, 2002; National Collaborating Centre for Mental Health, 2004). The results of these treatments have been remarkably robust even though not all trials have been as consistent (Hay et al., 2009). This has led to NICE recommending that cognitive behavioural therapy (CBT) should be offered to adults with bulimia nervosa as the first-line treatment (National Collaborating Centre for Mental Health, 2004, p. 128). This specific form of CBT is based on a theory of the maintenance of bulimia nervosa (Fairburn, 1981; Fairburn, 1997) and is tailored to changing the mechanisms hypothesized to be responsible for the persistence of the disorder. The duration of treatment is 16 to 20 sessions over 4 to 5 months. Although it is not exactly clear whether adding antidepressants to CBT results in an improved outcome (Wilson & Fairburn, 2002), the APA Practice Guidelines recommend a combination of antidepressant medication and psychosocial treatment for bulimia nervosa with "moderate clinical confidence". In summary, CBT is not a panacea but it can benefit a substantial proportion of patients and it is clearly superior to the other interventions currently available.

The question of how best to help those patients who fail to respond to CBT or do not want it is a pressing one, since no evidence-based guidelines can be formulated at this time. The leading alternative psychological intervention to CBT is interpersonal psychotherapy (IPT). The results from two treatment trials, one of which was large, suggest that this focal psychotherapy is eventually as effective as CBT but takes 8 to 12 months longer to achieve results comparable to CBT (Agras et al., 2000; Fairburn et al., 2003).

There has been much attention given recently to the possibility of giving CBT using a book format (e.g. Cooper et al., 1996), via the telephone or Internet (Palmer et al., 2002). These have generally shown positive results and it is now suggested that patients with bulimia nervosa should initially be encouraged to follow a self-help programme with one of the evidence-based psychological treatments (National Collaborating Centre for Mental Health, 2004, p. 128). However, a recent randomized trial (Schmidt et al., 2008) did not provide good evidence of benefit.

Summary

Cognitive behavioural therapy is the universal first-line treatment of choice for bulimia nervosa and has been endorsed as such. There is no clear second line of treatment, but both interpersonal therapy and behaviour therapy may have some value.

Atypical eating disorders and binge eating disorder

Atypical eating disorders (or EDNOS) are the most common eating disorder diagnosed in clinical practice (see Fairburn and Bohn, 2005), and epidemiological data support the preponderance of EDNOS among individuals with clinically significant eating disorders (Keel et al., 2004). The absence of research evidence to guide the management of such disorders, other than binge eating disorder, means that clinicians are recommended to treat these patients following the principles advocated for treating the eating disorder that their eating problem most closely resembles. Thus, for conditions resembling anorexia nervosa in adolescent patients, a symptom-focused family-based therapy may be beneficial. For conditions resembling bulimia nervosa in adult patients, cognitive behavioural therapy, behaviour therapy, and interpersonal therapy may prove useful. A recent study by Fairburn et al. (2009) compared "transdiagnostic" CBT that addressed mood intolerance, clinical perfectionism and low self-esteem with standard CBT and a wait-list control in a group of patients with eating disorders that included all diagnoses apart from anorexia nervosa. Both CBT treatments were more effective than wait-list control and for the more complex disorders the transdiagnostic approach had advantages.

There is a body of evidence, however, about the treatment of binge eating disorder although none addresses the best service setting. The research on the treatment of binge eating disorder has focused mainly on patients with comorbid obesity. The results show that both CBT and IPT help reduce the frequency of binge eating. In the largest study 20 weekly sessions of group CBT and group IPT were compared for 162 overweight patients with binge eating disorder (Wilfley et al., 2002). Binge eating recovery rates were equivalent for CBT and IPT at post-treatment and at 1-year follow-up, with approximately 60% of patients reporting remission from binge eating at follow-up. The treatments were also equivalent in terms of their reductions in associated eating disorders and psychiatric symptoms. There was only a slight decrease in patients' weight and clinicians are suggested to inform patients that interventions for binge eating disorder will only have a minimal impact on their weight (National Collaborating Centre for Mental Health, 2004). The conclusion from this and other studies is that there is a range of efficacious interventions for binge eating disorder, and there is little consistent evidence to favour one treatment over another (National Collaborating Centre for Mental Health, 2004). Reflecting this doubt, the APA guidelines remain silent on the issue of treating binge eating disorder or any other form of EDNOS.

These findings should be considered in light of natural history studies in the USA and UK (Cachelin et al., 1999; Fairburn et al., 2000) and drug trials (Dingemans et al., 2002) that all suggest that there is a high spontaneous remission rate from binge eating disorder at least in the short term. There is also a relatively high response to placebo (Dingemans et al., 2002).

Summary

There is now a range of effective psychological treatments for eating

Table 31.1 Summary of effective psychological treatments for eating disorders

Treatment	Form of treatment	Psychiatric disorder	Level of evidence for efficacy	Comments
Cognitive behavioural therapy	Individual	Anorexia nervosa	Ib	Limited evidence of efficacy but some positive evidence
Cognitive behavioural therapy	Individual	Bulimia nervosa	Ia	Excellent evidence of efficacy supported by controlled trials and meta-analyses
Cognitive behavioural therapy	Individual	Binge eating disorder	Ia	Growing evidence of value but still not secure
Cognitive behavioural therapy	Internet delivered	Anorexia nervosa	IV	Unlikely to be effective in established illness
Cognitive behavioural therapy	Internet delivered	Bulimia nervosa	IIb	Variable results from trials and so remains of uncertain value
Cognitive behavioural therapy	Internet delivered	Binge eating disorder	IV	Not yet fully tested
Interpersonal therapy	Individual	Anorexia nervosa	Ib	Some value, but limited evidence
Interpersonal therapy	Individual	Bulimia nervosa	Ib	Undoubtedly of value, but usually as second-line treatment

Table 31.1 (cont.)

Treatment	Form of treatment	Psychiatric disorder	Level of evidence for efficacy	Comments
Interpersonal therapy	Individual	Binge eating disorder	Ia	Increasing evidence of efficacy
Family therapy	Family and patient	Anorexia nervosa	Ib	Some evidence of value in younger people
Family therapy	Family and patient	Bulimia nervosa	Ib	Some evidence of value in younger people
Family therapy	Family and patient	Binge eating disorder	III	Not yet properly tested
Behaviour therapy alone	Patient	Anorexia nervosa	IV	Not recommended
Behaviour therapy alone	Patient	Bulimia nervosa	III	Not recommended
Behaviour therapy alone	Patient	Binge eating disorder	IV	Not evaluated
Nutritional counselling alone	Patient	Anorexia nervosa	II	Insufficient evidence to recommend
Nutritional counselling alone	Patient	Bulimia nervosa	II	Not recommended
Nutritional counselling alone	Patient	Binge eating disorder	IV	Not tested but unlikely to be of value
All treatments	All forms	EDNOS	II	Some evidence that "transdiagnostic" CBT may be of value here as it treats additional pathology

disorders, but most of the evidence has accumulated around CBT for bulimia nervosa, and other eating disorders have much less evidence to support any psychological treatments. However, now that binge eating disorder is becoming accepted as a diagnostic grouping early results suggest that this too will respond to CBT. These data indicate that a range of interventions may be efficacious but they do not impact greatly on patients' weight. Moreover, there is no first or second line of treatment for binge eating disorder, but a recent large trial showed both CBT with guided self-help and IPT to have better results than behavioural weight loss treatment (Wilson et al., 2010),

so both CBT and IPT can be recommended as effective (Table 31.1).

Unfortunately there is little information on the treatment of other atypical eating disorders and this is a research priority (Table 31.1). In a recent Cochrane Review the size of the task ahead to improve the evidence base was summarized as: "there is a small body of evidence for the efficacy of CBT in bulimia nervosa and similar syndromes, but the quality of trials is very variable and sample sizes are often small. More and larger trials are needed, particularly for binge eating disorder and other EDNOS syndromes" (Hay et al., 2009). With better diagnostic descriptions this should be possible.

32

Educational interventions for eating disorders

Based on "Educational interventions for eating disorders" by Mima Simic, Pauline S. Powers, and Yvonne Bannon in Effective Treatments in Psychiatry, Cambridge University Press, 2008

Introduction

Educational interventions in medicine involve providing information about risk factors, causes, symptoms, or implications of a disorder, as well as focusing on psychosocial pressures that might influence development or maintenance of a disorder. Psycho-education aims to prevent, or improve, the symptoms of a mental disorder, engage people in treatment, or improve their adherence to treatment. This involves teaching people about their illness, how to treat it, and how to recognize signs of relapse. The postulated mechanism of action of these strategies is that not only knowledge will be improved, but also attitudes and beliefs, so motivating the recipient to alter behaviours that might lead to the development of a disorder or serve to maintain or worsen it. Such interventions may also promote engagement in and adherence to treatment (Andersen, 1999; Powers and Bannon, 2004).

Educational interventions form the basis of recently developed Expert Patient and Carer Programmes (Lorig and Holman, 2003) that teach people with chronic disorders and their families the knowledge and essential disease management skills to the point at which they can manage the disorder themselves.

Ignorance or misconceptions about eating disorders may provoke and maintain symptoms. For example, a person with anorexia nervosa who experiences a sense of fullness after eating only a small amount of food may believe that she needs to reduce her food intake further. Upon learning that eating little slows gastric emptying and 'makes food sit in your stomach like a lump of concrete' and that this is reversible with the gradual introduction of larger amounts of food, she may be willing to increase her portions. A person with bulimia nervosa may believe that taking laxatives or inducing vomiting may help her "get rid of all calories ingested" and this can be readily contradicted.

The families of people with eating disorders are often very involved in their care, yet lack essential information on how best to support the sufferer. Indeed one of the most common unmet needs identified by families was the lack of appropriate information at an early stage in the illness (Haigh and Treasure, 2003). Parents may alternate between different extreme and unhelpful beliefs. Beliefs such as that their daughter's disorder may just be a passing phase may lead them to ignore the problem. Similarly, the view that it is a self-inflicted problem that can be overcome by will-power is likely to lead to unhelpful confrontation.

Thus, given the chronicity, severity, and complexity of eating disorders psychoeducational interventions should play a prominent role in their management, both targeting patients and their families. Indeed, these strategies are recommended as valuable in recent eating disorder guidelines from both sides of the Atlantic (NICE, pp. 7–8, 2004; American Psychiatric Association (APA), 2000, pp. 9–13), and such interventions form an integral part of eating disorder treatments of different theoretical orientation, including cognitive behavioural therapy, family therapy, and multifamily group therapy. Yet psychoeducation interventions are rarely used as a stand-alone treatment in eating disorders and evidence for the efficacy of these approaches in eating disorders whether used on their own or in combination with other treatment components is sparse. There are hazards as well as benefits of education that need to be mentioned also.

Psychoeducation packages for patients with eating disorders

So far only five studies have explored the effect of psychoeducational packages on the outcome of patients with eating disorders. Most of these were small, non-randomized, and used quasi-experimental designs. The exception is a randomized controlled study by Andrews and colleagues (1996) who compared a computerized health education package with a computer-based placebo programme for patients with bulimia or anorexia nervosa and found benefits in terms of improving knowledge about and attitudes towards eating disordered behaviour. The effect of this intervention on symptoms was not studied.

Ricca et al. (1997) compared cognitive behavioural therapy (CBT) with a combination of group psychoeducation and fluoxetine in outpatients with bulimia nervosa. Combined group psychoeducation and fluoxetine was as effective as CBT in reducing the number of binge episodes and compensatory behaviours as measured on the Eating Disorder Examination (EDE) 6 months after the beginning of treatment. Both treatments reduced depressive and anxiety symptoms on self-report questionnaires, but only CBT yielded a significant improvement of overall EDE scores.

In a small cohort of 41 women with bulimia nervosa Davis and colleagues (1990) assessed the clinical significance of change after five sessions of brief group psychoeducation. Between 29% and 56% of subjects showed significant change on instruments measuring bulimic symptoms, drive for thinness, dietary restraint, and body dissatisfaction. By contrast, only a small number of subjects (6–19%) reported clinically

significant change on measures of personality dysfunction and associated psychopathology. In a second study by the same authors (Davis et al., 1997) the outcome of the previous cohort of patients was compared with that of patients who had received seven sessions of group psychotherapy with integrated CBT interventions in addition to the psychoeducation. Both treatments yielded comparable levels of change on measures of specific and non-specific psychopathology. The third study by the same group (Olmsted et al., 1991) compared a cohort of 29 bulimic patients who received the brief group educational programme with a cohort of 30 bulimic patients who received 19 sessions of the CBT. Overall, CBT was superior treatment to the educational programme, but on several important post-treatment outcome measures, both treatments appeared to be equally effective for the subgroup of subjects with less severe symptomatology. Interestingly, educational interventions were found to be significantly more cost-effective than CBT.

Psychoeducation for family members of patients with eating disorders

Psychoeducation is an integral component of family interventions for anorexia nervosa in adolescents and adults, for example in Behaviour Family System Therapy (Robin et al., 1998) and the Multifamily Group Day Treatment (Eisler et al., 2000; Treasure et al., 1999). Here, psychoeducational interventions serve to explain the facts about eating disorders, their physical risks, and psychological consequences as well as giving encouragement to families to expand their coping and problem-solving skills in order to manage the illness more effectively.

Two studies have used psychoeducation for parents as a stand-alone intervention. In a small randomized controlled trial Geist and colleagues (2000) compared the effects of family therapy to the effects of family group psychoeducation in 25 newly diagnosed adolescents with anorexia nervosa requiring hospitalization (see also Chapter 50 on adolescent eating disorders). Weight gain following the 4-month period of treatment was equivalent in both groups but no significant change was reported in psychological functioning by either adolescents or parents. Unfortunately the cost-effectiveness of these interventions was not examined although the authors claim the educational treatment was cheaper.

Uehara and colleagues (2001) explored the effect of the five monthly sessions of multifamily psychoeducation on changes in expressed emotion (EE) in a small cohort of families of people with eating disorders. The rates of high-EE relatives tended to decrease at the end of the intervention, especially for high emotional overinvolvement and families' assessment of symptoms. This study provided only preliminary evidence that needs further enquiry.

Psychoeducation for the prevention of eating disorders

In contrast to the paucity of evidence concerning the efficacy of psychoeducation in full-blown eating disorders, a large number of studies has focused on the use of education for their prevention. Two systematic reviews have been conducted. Pratt and Woolfenden (2002) found eight randomized controlled studies in children and adolescents. Meta-analysis showed only one significant effect for two eating disorder programmes based on a media literacy and advocacy approach (Kusel, 1999; Neumark-Sztainer et al., 2000). Both prevention programmes were effective in reducing internalization and promoting acceptance of societal ideas relating to appearance at 3 to 6 months follow-up. The reviewers concluded that due to the insufficient evidence of the effectiveness of other programmes, no firm conclusion about the impact of prevention programmes for eating disorders in children and adolescents can yet be drawn.

A second larger review (Stice and Shaw, 2004) included 38 prevention programmes evaluated in 53 separate controlled trials. These authors distinguished between three generations of prevention programmes: (1) universal didactic psychoeducational material about eating disorders, (2) a similar universal didactic format that also included components focusing on resistance of sociocultural pressures for thinness and healthy weight control behaviours, and (3) selective programmes that target high-risk individuals with interactive exercises that focus on risk factors that have been shown to predict onset of eating pathology. The average effect size for the outcomes of all trials ranged from 0.11 to 0.38 at termination of the programme and from 0.05 to 0.29 at follow-up. The meta-analysis showed that more selective programmes provided to high-risk populations produced significantly larger intervention effects than did (the older) universal programmes. Interactive programmes were more effective than didactic programmes and effects were significantly larger for multi-session programmes offered solely to females over age 15. These factors seemed more important than the actual content of the programmes, although programmes with psychoeducational content were less effective than those without this content for four out of seven outcome measures.

One further prevention study not included in the meta-analysis by Stice and Shaw deserves mentioning. Olmsted and colleagues (2002) studied a population of 85 young women with type I diabetes mellitus who had disturbed eating attitudes and behaviour. Patients were randomly assigned to either a 6-week psychoeducation programme or treatment as usual. The intervention group had significant reductions on the Restraint and Eating Concern subscales of the Eating Disorder Examination and on the Drive for Thinness and Body Dissatisfaction subscales of the Eating Disorder Inventory, but no improvement in frequency of purging by insulin omission or in haemoglobin A1c levels.

Negative effects of education/information about eating disorders

The equivocal results of some educational efforts to prevent eating disorders has led to speculation that they may actually cause harm. Anecdotal reports suggest that among some groups, efforts to educate may introduce the recipients to maladaptive eating practices and weight control behaviours. However, both the Cochrane Review (Pratt & Woolfenden, 2002) and the meta-analysis by Stice and Shaw (2004) concluded that there was no real evidence to suggest potentially

Table 32.1 Summary of evidence base of educational interventions in eating disorders

Treatment	Form of treatment	Psychiatric disorder	Level of evidence for efficacy	Comment
Psychoeducation	Computerized education	Anorexia or bulimia nervosa	Ib	The package was superior to placebo computer programme in terms of improving knowledge about and attitudes towards eating disordered behaviour
Psychoeducation	Group psychoeducation	Bulimia nervosa	III	No firm evidence yet
Psychoeducation	Group psychoeducation	Parents of adolescents with anorexia nervosa	Ib	In one small RCT parental group psychoeducation produced similar improvements as family therapy in patients' weight (but this does not indicate effectiveness)
Psychoeducation	Prevention programmes	Prevention of eating disorders	Ia	The evidence from two systematic reviews suggests that focused interventions targeting high-risk individuals, with emphasis on specific risk factors and an interactive format, do reduce eating disorder risk

harmful effects from eating disorder prevention programmes.

In the last few years there has been a proliferation of so-called "pro-anorexia" sites on the Internet (see position statement of the Academy for Eating Disorders; http://www.aed.org). Although it is widely agreed that these sites promote dangerous and deadly eating practices and efforts have been made to curb access, the sites are still easy to locate. One study (Chesley & Kreipe, 2003) found that these pro-anorexia sites were more organized than traditional sources of information about eating disorders. The danger of the proliferation of these pro-anorexia sites lies in reinforcing the denial that is often a part of the clinical presentation of anorexia nervosa. They may also demotivate people with anorexia nervosa from actively seeking treatment.

Eating disorder curriculum for primary care providers

Primary care providers could be valuable if they were able to detect and intervene early with eating disorder patients. A pilot study by Gurney and Halmi (2001) suggests that brief intensive training can increase primary care providers' knowledge resulting in increased rates of screening and detection of eating disorders, but we need more knowledge of the long-term outcome.

Conclusions

Psychoeducational strategies are generally recommended as valuable in treatment guidelines from both the UK and the USA but this recommendation is based on clinical consensus, not the evidence base, which is generally slim. Consequently psychoeducation interventions are not recognized as either first- or second-line treatment for eating disorders (National Collaborating Centre for Mental Health, pp. 7–8, 2004; American Psychiatric Association (APA), 2000, pp. 9–13) although they form an integral but ancillary part of eating disorder treatments with proven efficacy such as cognitive behavioural therapy and family therapy. Eating disorder prevention programmes are more extensively researched, and the evidence shows that they are more effective if they are multi-session, interactive, and delivered to high-risk female populations over age 15 (Table 32.1).

The research evidence implies rather than indicates clearly that educational interventions are of value in eating disorders, and what is needed now is to establish what models of intervention might be most relevant and effective for whom, and at what stage of the illness.

33

Alternative treatments for eating disorders

Based on "Alternative treatments for eating disorders" by Pauline S. Powers, Yvonne Bannon, and Adrienne J. Key in Effective Treatments in Psychiatry, Cambridge University Press, 2008

Introduction

Both the lay public and identified specialists/practitioners have practised alternative medicine strategies for the treatment of numerous maladies for centuries. Unfortunately most treatments in use today for eating disorders would be considered complementary or alternative treatments, including weight restoration programmes and individual psychotherapy for adult anorexia nervosa patients. Another odd consequence of the popularity of alternative treatments is that some interventions that have been found to be at least marginally effective in randomized controlled trials, have,

nonetheless, not found general acceptance. Examples would include cyproheptadine in hospitalized anorexia nervosa patients (Goldberg et al., 1979) and naltrexone in the outpatient treatment of anorexia or bulimia nervosa (Marrazzi et al., 1995).

NCCAM

In the United States, the National Centre for Complementary and Alternative Medicine (NCCAM) is one of 27 institutes and centres that make up the National Institutes of Health (NIH). It was founded in 1998 and funding for that fiscal year was

277

19.5 million dollars; in 2004 funding had risen to 117.7 million dollars. This federal agency defines complementary and alternative medicine as a group of diverse medical and health care systems, practices and products not presently considered part of conventional medicine. Complementary medicines are defined as those added to conventional treatments and alternative medicines are those used instead of conventional treatments.

Certain celebrity figures have promoted the use of complementary and alternative treatments and fuelled both their popularity and possibly the quest to test them by more stringent or acceptable methods. Many patients report the successful use of complementary treatments in a wide spectrum of disorders, usually where conventional medicine has proven limited or ineffective or frequently as an adjunct to accepted treatment. Eating disorders are an example of this, in which a whole plethora of suggestions have been made. The scientific evidence of clinical effectiveness can, however, remain elusive. In this chapter the nature and extent of various alternative and complementary treatments used by eating disorder patients will be outlined. The results of a literature search will be used to describe the extent of the evidence to support their use. Finally, examples of treatments considered to have promise and in use in some eating disorder treatment facilities but not yet validated will be described.

Complementary and alternative treatments for eating disorders

Following a standard database search we found the complementary and alternative treatments listed below are judged to be useful in the treatment of eating disorders in descending order of level of scientific evidence: massage, hypnosis, meditation, yoga, and herbal remedies. Finally we have commented on anecdotal and patient reports on each treatment type based on the authors' knowledge as practitioners in the field of eating disorders.

Massage

The only randomized controlled trial identified in the search, by Field et al. (1998), studied the use of massage therapy in conjunction with standard treatment versus standard treatment alone in 24 adolescents with bulimia nervosa. Patients receiving the massage treatment showed improvement on several behavioural and psychological measures, including reductions in anxiety and depression. The same authors (Hart et al., 2001) also described the use of massage in anorexia nervosa and again found reduced stress levels in the group receiving massage. Taken together these findings provide preliminary evidence of the utility of massage as an adjunct treatment for eating disorders. A review of the use of massage therapy in many types of conditions, including eating disorders, offers some hypotheses on potential underlying mechanisms (Field, 2002). Many eating disorder treatment facilities report the use of massage. Anecdotally, patients report beneficial effects including anxiety reduction and a reduction in body dissatisfaction but there are some negative reports including a heightening in fears of being physically touched, feeling intruded upon, and embarrassment.

Mind–body medicine

The field of meditation and hypnosis falls under the heading of mind–body medicine. Barrows and Jacobs (2002) provide a useful introduction and general review of the literature in this field.

Hypnosis

Griffiths et al. (1996) compared hypno-behavioural therapy with standard CBT for bulimia nervosa in a clinical trial and found no superiority of either treatment. Two case reports describe the use of hypnosis as an adjunct to standard treatment as "effective" but without definition

(Segal, 2001), and the use of "ego-state" treatment with hypnosis for the treatment of binge eating disorder (Degun-Mather, 2003). The treatment was associated with a reduction in eating-related behaviours when other previously attempted therapies had been unsuccessful. The paper reports the patient then successfully returning to CBT.

Meditation

There are many different types of meditation and certain elements are now incorporated into standard treatments; the use of "mindfulness" is an example of this. A review of Buddhist philosophy and addictive behaviours (Marlatt, 2002), which has included eating disorders in this addictive umbrella, outlines the theoretical underpinning of the philosophy. It examines several concepts in more detail, with mindfulness being one example. Marlatt theorizes how these concepts may relate directly to cognitive behavioural therapy.

No randomized controlled trials have been identified in the search directly related to eating disorders. A cohort study by Kristeller & Hallett (1999) followed 18 obese women with binge eating disorder through a 6-week meditation-based group intervention using standard group treatment plus eating-specific mindfulness meditation. There were significant reductions in scores on the binge eating scale (BES) and depression and anxiety scores. Time using the eating-related meditations predicted decreases on the BES. A case study (Morishita, 2000) from Japan examined the treatment of a woman with anorexia nervosa with Naikan therapy, an ancient form of psychological treatment involving self-reproach, self-reflection, and meditation. A reduction in eating behaviours and an improvement in mood was reported.

Many eating disorder centres report the use of yoga with or without meditation as part of standard care packages. Only one trial was identified comparing Hatha yoga to aerobics and another unspecified body-orientated exercise group. Hatha proved more beneficial than the comparison treatment and a number of hypotheses about mechanisms were proposed (Daubenmier, 2003). Some studies focusing on the narratives of individuals who have recovered from eating disorders highlight the spiritual nature of this process as defined by the patients. Their definitions included connection of the many aspects of the self, especially of body and spirit/self/mind; also a connection with others and a connection with nature (Garrett, 1997). It may be that certain core elements of meditation and yoga are useful in CBT/psychological therapies and warrant closer exploration. In one qualitative study, women perceived an overall reduction in the quantity of food they consumed (not confirmed independently), decreased eating speed, and an improvement in their choice of food during treatment (McIver et al., 2009).

Herbalism/homeopathy

Patients and clinicians report multiple uses and abuses of non-prescription drugs. In an interesting case series Yager and colleagues (1999) described a patient with anorexia nervosa who sought conventional treatment at a university eating disorder centre after being referred by her naturopath, general internist, and psychologist. She brought with her a large shopping bag of natural remedies that she had been taking and wanted to continue these remedies during her treatment on the inpatient ward. The authors utilize this case to discuss some of the dilemmas around caring for patients who seek both conventional and non-conventional treatments and provide a series of recommendations regarding alternative/complementary treatments. These recommendations include: (1) routinely question patients about alternative and complementary treatments; (2) discuss safety and efficacy; (3) discuss merits of alternative treatments; (4) provide information; (5) learn about alternative therapies; and (6) determine characteristics of proposed alternative treatments and practitioners.

Two recent studies have evaluated the use of alternative treatments by patients with eating disorders. In a study of 39 consecutive bulimia nervosa patients seeking treatment, Roerig and colleagues (2003) found that 64% of patients used diet pills and 31% of patients utilized diuretics. In the preceding month, 18% had used diet pills and 21% had used diuretics. These investigators found that a wide range of products had been used and that many which were used had potential toxicities.

In the second study by Trigazis and colleagues (2004), 46 patients with anorexia nervosa, bulimia nervosa, or eating disorder not otherwise specified were given a questionnaire to determine their use of herbal remedies: 37% (17 patients) used herbal remedies. The major reasons for the use of herbal remedies were to decrease appetite and induce vomiting. One-fourth (24%) of patients reported their physicians had asked if they used herbal remedies. Interestingly, the patients were generally satisfied with the traditional health care system and used herbal remedies as complementary rather than alternative treatments.

Ephedra

Ephedra (ephredrine alkaloids) containing products are among the best known herbs used as dietary aids. In April 2004, in the USA, the Food and Drug Administration (FDA) rule banning the sale of dietary supplements containing ephedra became effective. The rule was passed due to concerns over the cardiovascular side effects of ephedra including hypertension and cardiac arrhythmias. Although ephedra may result in short-term weight loss, the hazards, especially when combined with other stimulants such as caffeine, are significant and have resulted in a number of deaths. Despite the rule, however, ephedra-containing products are still available over the Internet.

Other alternative and complementary treatments reported to be in use by patients but not apparent in the literature review include acupuncture, osteopathy, and spiritual or faith healing.

Frequently used treatments not considered mainstream medicine

Although there are many treatments in this category, only art therapy, dance and movement therapy, and psychodrama will be considered here. The use of these treatments rests on the theory that patients with eating disorders, particularly patients with anorexia nervosa, are delayed or regressed in their ability to describe or express emotions (sometimes described as alexithymia; Smith et al., 1997). Based on these

Table 33.1 Effectiveness of treatments listed in NCCAM website possibly related to eating disorders

Treatment	Form of treatment	Psychiatric disorder	Level of evidence for efficacy	Comments
Massage		Bulimia nervosa	Ib	One small study supports the use of massage as an adjunct to inpatient treatment
Hypnosis	Hypnobehavioural therapy	Bulimia nervosa	Ib	One small RCT found no difference between hypnobehavioural therapy and CBT
Psychodrama	Adjunctive to standard treatments	Anorexia and bulimia nervosa	IV	No evidence for effectiveness
Meditation	Includes mindfulness, Naikan therapy, Hatha yoga	Different eating disorders	IV	No evidence of effectiveness
Herbalism/ homeopathy		Different eating disorders	IV	Eating disorder sufferers frequently use herbal remedies to decrease appetite and help them purge
Ephedra		Different eating disorders	IV	The FDA has banned the sale of dietary supplements containing ephedra

observations, the uses of various non-verbal therapies have been recommended by a number of authors. Although randomized controlled trials have not been done, many of the case reports and case series are poignant and suggest that these methods may help patients access emotions otherwise unavailable to them (Diamond-Raab and Orrell-Valente, 2002).

Conclusions

The definition of complementary and alternative treatments is controversial, but it is clear that many patients utilize various treatments considered outside mainstream medical practice. Surprisingly, this does not seem to be related to distrust of traditional medicine, but rather these strategies are often used in addition to conventional treatments. Since there are actually so few evidence-based treatments for eating disorders that meet the strict criteria of having been demonstrated effective in randomized controlled trials, it is not surprising that alternative and complementary treatments are widely used. Some alternative treatments used by patients with eating disorders are dangerous and/or ineffective, including the herbal dietary aid, ephedra. Until more effective treatments are found that are easily accessible, it is likely that the use of dangerous alternative treatments will continue.

Interventions discussed in this chapter are summarized in Table 33.1.

34

Complex treatments for eating disorders

Based on "Complex treatments for eating disorders" by Scott Crow and Ulrike Schmidt in Effective Treatments in Psychiatry, Cambridge University Press, 2008

Introduction

This chapter is focused primarily on the complex interventions of inpatient and day care in the treatment of anorexia nervosa. Other eating disorders are also included; most of these involve day care. Because the setting in which a treatment takes place is a multi-faceted one these studies are the hardest to execute and this will become apparent in evaluating the results.

Inpatient treatment of eating disorders

There is general agreement that inpatient care of anorexia nervosa is at times medically necessary and may indeed be life-saving in severe cases. Indicators of high medical risk in anorexia nervosa requiring inpatient care have been identified (APA, 2000; Winston and Webster, 2003; National Collaborating Centre for Mental Health, 2004).

However, the need for and role of more prolonged inpatient treatment aimed at helping the patient to progress towards full weight recovery by providing a combination of refeeding, physical monitoring, and psychosocial interventions is much more controversial (Vandereycken, 2003). The threshold for initiating inpatient treatment for anorexia nervosa varies widely across different health care systems. In some European countries such as Germany and Austria, inpatient care is still the norm as a first-line treatment (Kächele et al., 2001), and even a proportion of people with bulimia nervosa are treated as inpatients. In the USA the threshold for inpatient care is relatively low, i.e. a body mass index of less than 16 kg/m^2 (Garner and Needleman, 1997) or 20% weight loss (American Psychiatric Association, 2000). In contrast, in the UK inpatient care is typically reserved for the severely ill with a body mass index of less than 13.5 kg/m^2 (Winston and Webster, 2003) with little or no restriction on the duration of care.

Where should inpatient care of eating disorder patients take place?

A survey of child and adolescent inpatient provision (aged 12 to 18) in England and Wales (O'Herlihy et al., 2003) identified that 20.1% of all beds were occupied by eating disorder patients. About half of these were in general child and adolescent units, the other half in specialist eating disorder units. No comparable figures for adults exist.

There is very little hard evidence on the comparative outcomes produced by specialist or non-specialist inpatient treatment. A cohort study by Crisp et al. (1992) compared patients from an area without specialist inpatient provision with those admitted to a specialist eating disorder centre. The long-term mortality of patients treated in the specialist centre was significantly lower.

The impact of different types of inpatient programmes

A number of small studies of limited quality have compared different inpatient treatment regimes in randomized controlled trials or clinically controlled studies. There is some evidence from these that an inpatient programme with an explicit focus on changing eating disorder symptoms and weight is more likely to lead to short-term weight gain (Herzog et al., 1996).

Duration of inpatient care

Patients requiring admission for eating disorders often stay a long time. In England a survey of all inpatients found those with eating disorders to have the greatest median duration of admissions (36 days) and the highest proportion of patients with a length of stay of greater than 90 days (26.8% of admissions) (Thompson et al., 2004). In Germany, Krauth (2002) found the mean length of inpatient stay to be 49.8 days for anorexia nervosa and 45.5 days for bulimia nervosa. Striegel-Moore et al. (2000) in the USA found that 21.5% of women with anorexia nervosa were hospitalized per year with an average length of stay of 26 days, with very much lower hospitalization rates found for bulimia nervosa and EDNOS. Patients who are discharged early tend to have much higher readmission rates (Willer et al., 2005).

In one large prospective German study (Kächele et al., 2001) it was found that most of the between hospital variance in duration of treatment was explained by organizational factors. The same study found an interaction between duration of illness, duration of treatment, and outcome. At 2.5 years' follow-up people with a longer duration of anorexia nervosa had a higher likelihood of good outcome with longer rather than with briefer duration of inpatient treatment. In contrast, those with a shorter duration of illness had a higher likelihood of good outcome with briefer inpatient treatment.

Acceptability and potential harms of inpatient treatment

Patients generally report greater levels of satisfaction with outpatient than with inpatient care (Rosenvinge and Klusmeier, 2000). The lower treatment uptake of inpatient therapy in the study by Crisp et al. (see above) suggests that this was a less acceptable option to a proportion of patients than outpatient psychological treatment. Moreover, dropout from inpatient treatment for anorexia nervosa seems to be higher than that reported for general psychiatric patients (Kahn and Pike, 2001).

It has also been suggested that outpatient programmes may lead to better long-term outcomes than inpatient programmes (Beumont et al., 1993).

Day care treatments for eating disorders

Day care treatments represent an important piece of the continuum of care for individuals with eating disorders. They can either be used as an alternative to admission, or as "step-down" care from the structure and support of inpatient treatment with the aim to afford patients the chance to continue their recovery in what is increasingly their own environment. Indeed, there is evidence at least in the United States that use of day care following on from inpatient care is increasing, as early discharge from the hospital necessitated by managed care predicts rehospitalization (Wiseman et al., 2001).

Outcome studies of day care programmes

A number of the existing reports in the literature describe efforts at developing day hospital programmes. However, remarkably little is known at present about the efficacy or effectiveness of day hospital, or about the predictors of success or failure in such treatment (Zipfel et al., 2002). The existing literature on the use of day care programmes in six different centres for eating disorders is summarized in the parent book of this volume (Crow & Schmidt, 2008).

Results for both anorexia nervosa and bulimia nervosa patients are promising and several authors suggest that day care may be a cost-effective alternative to inpatient care (Williamson et al., 2001) but no formal examinations of the cost-effectiveness of day care versus other treatments of eating disorders have been carried out.

Special considerations in day care treatment

Franzen et al. (2004) studied reasons for dropout from day care treatment. In a sample of 125 patients with bulimia nervosa, 19 (15%) dropped out, and, in general, these had more severe bulimic symptoms, more aggression, more extraversion and more impulsivity.

Tasca and coworkers (2002) examined the nature and role of group climate in eating disorder day hospital groups as compared to non-eating disorder psychiatric day hospital groups. In comparing 61 eating disorder patients with 67 non-eating disorder female psychiatric day hospital patients, these investigators found higher levels of engagement in the eating disorder cohorts but also higher levels of avoidance; they set forth suggestions for how these factors may be useful in facilitating treatment.

Woodside and colleagues described the experience of treating males in the day hospital setting as compared to females (Woodside & Kaplan, 1994). This report described outcome for 334 women and 15 men treated during the same period of time. The authors concluded that in general the males and females looked quite similar in terms of characteristics and outcome, and concluded that treating women and men together in mixed gender day hospital programmes was quite feasible.

Direct comparison between inpatient, day patient, and outpatient care

There have only been two randomized controlled trials (RCTs) addressing this question. In the first of these, 90 people with anorexia nervosa were randomized to four treatment groups:

inpatient treatment, outpatient treatment (individual and family therapy), outpatient group therapy, and assessment interview only (Crisp et al., 1991; Gowers et al., 1994). Adherence to allocated treatment differed significantly among groups (adherence rates: inpatient treatment 18/30 (60%), outpatient treatment (individual and family therapy) 18/20 (90%), outpatient group (psychotherapy) 17/20 (85%), and assessment interview only 20/20 (100%)). Treatment adherence differed significantly between outpatient and inpatient treatment (RR 1.5, 95% CI 1.1 to 2.0). Average acceptance of treatment also varied among groups (20 weeks inpatient treatment, 9 outpatient sessions, and 5 group sessions).

In the assessment interview only group, six people had no treatment of any kind in the first year and the others had treatment elsewhere (6 had inpatient treatment, 5 had outpatient hospital treatment, and 3 had at least weekly contact with their general practitioners). Six people in this group spent almost the entire year in treatment. There were no significant differences in mean weight or in the Morgan Russell scale global scores among any of the four groups at 1, 2, and 5 years. The proportion of people with a good outcome was similar in all four groups (Crisp et al., 1991; Gowers et al., 1994).

The second trial was a multicentre RCT which compared inpatient psychiatric treatment, specialist outpatient treatment, and general outpatient treatment by a child and adolescent team in 167 adolescents with anorexia nervosa (Byford et al., 2007; Gowers et al., 2007). Outcomes and costs were assessed at baseline, 1 year, and 2 years. Adherence to inpatient treatment was poor, with only 50% of people randomized to this condition taking it up. In the intention-to-treat analysis there was no difference in clinical outcomes between the three groups. Inpatient treatment (randomized or after outpatient transfer) predicted poor outcomes. The specialist outpatient group was the least costly over the 2-year follow-up (mean total cost £26 738) and the general outpatient treatment the most costly, with the inpatient treatment in between, but this result was not statistically significant.

The conclusion that can be drawn from this evidence is that for patients with a degree of anorexia nervosa of such severity as not to require emergency intervention, specialist outpatient care may be the best alternative.

One study compared inpatient analytical therapy (2 months) with systemic outpatient therapy (15 sessions over 1 year) in patients with bulimia nervosa. Both therapies improved symptomatic behaviour as well as other psychosocial outcomes, with no differences between treatments (Jäger et al., 1996).

Table 34.1 Summary of evidence base of complex treatment in eating disorder

Treatment	Form of treatment	Psychiatric disorder	Level of evidence for efficacy	Comments
Inpatient treatment	Multimodal treatment involving refeeding; treatment in specialist eating disorders unit	Anorexia nervosa	Ib	No difference in outcomes between inpatient, day patient, and outpatient treatment in those not so severe as to require emergency treatment
Inpatient treatment	Explicit focus on changing eating disorder symptoms and weight	Anorexia nervosa	IIa	Superior to treatment without focus on eating disorder symptoms, in terms of short-term weight gain
Inpatient treatment	Operant conditioning regimes	Anorexia nervosa	IIa	A strict regime had no advantages over a more lenient one
Inpatient treatment	Inpatient psychoanalytical therapy	Bulimia nervosa	IIa	No difference to outpatient systemic therapy
Day care treatment	Multimodal treatment in specialist eating disorders unit	Anorexia nervosa	III	Whilst day treatment has shown promise, it is not clear what precisely its status is in the treatment of anorexia nervosa
Day care treatment	Multimodal treatment in specialist eating disorders unit	Bulimia nervosa	III	Whilst day treatment has shown promise, it is not clear what precisely its status is in the treatment of bulimia nervosa

Differences in UK and US guidance on inpatient and day care treatments for eating disorders

The UK NICE guideline (National Collaborating Centre for Mental Health, 2004b) recommends that most adults with anorexia nervosa should be managed on an outpatient basis. Where inpatient treatment is necessary a structured symptom-focused approach with the expectation of weight gain should be provided in order to achieve weight restoration during inpatient treatment. A weekly weight gain of 0.5–1 kg is regarded as optimal. The guideline specifically cautions against the use of strict behaviour modification programmes. It suggests that psychological treatment should be available during and after inpatient treatment as patients are very vulnerable to post-hospitalization weight loss. No recommendation is made about the kind of psychological treatment to be made available posthospitalization as the competitors – supportive individual therapy, CBT, nutritional counselling, family therapy – have roughly similar outcomes. The duration of psychological treatment posthospitalization should be at least 12 months. The APA Practice Guidelines for treatment of eating disorders acknowledge that selected individuals with AN do well in outpatient treatment but describe a wider variety of clinical situations in which hospitalization is recommended. Psychological treatments are strongly advocated, but these are non-specific; the use of medication as a major focus of treatment is discouraged.

Guidelines recommend day care as part of the spectrum of treatment, particularly for anorexia nervosa (APA, 2000; National Collaborating Centre for Mental Health, 2004). Other complex treatment such as home treatment and intensive outreach are in their infancy.

Conclusion

Some conclusions can be drawn based on the existing literature, and these are summarized in Table 34.1. Different health care systems have different thresholds for inpatient admission and the duration of such admissions for anorexia nervosa. These decisions are not usually evidence-based and depend mainly on issues such as cost-considerations and how risk-averse a particular health care system is (e.g. what is the potential for being litigated against). Whilst it is difficult at the best of times to mount sufficiently powered treatment trials on anorexia nervosa future research studies into the relative merits of inpatient, outpatient, and day care for this condition are urgently needed and are currently under way.

Personality disorders

35

Personality disorder

Based on "Personality disorder" by Anthony Bateman and Mary Zanarini in Effective Treatments in Psychiatry, Cambridge University Press, 2008

Introduction

Though there are insufficient levels of agreement between them, both DSM-IV and ICD-10 currently take a categorical approach to personality disorder (PD) diagnosis. DSM-V may change this categorical approach because there is little evidence that categories are helpful in determining treatment response or have predictive value. In an attempt to address lack of diagnostic specificity, specific trait-related personality disorders are clustered into three DSM-IV groupings (the odd-eccentric (type A), the impulsive-erratic (type B), and the anxious-avoidant (type C)). The three groupings have only face validity.

Assessment of treatment

Personality disorder is a multifaceted condition that can be influenced in many different ways and justifies use of what are described as "complex interventions". Requirements to determine the effectiveness of a PD treatment are to:

- Define target population carefully
- Consider comorbidity
- Define and specify treatment
- Ensure treatment is superior to no treatment since personality disorders can gradually improve over time
- Demonstrate that treatment impacts personality and not merely Axis I symptoms
- Have adequate follow-up

- Address the treatment's cost-effectiveness

We only review treatments for personality disorders subject to systematic study.

Psychotherapy and psychosocial treatments

Meta-analyses

Perry et al. (1999) examined 15 studies for evidence of psychotherapy effectiveness. All reported improvement with mean pre–post effect sizes quite large: (1.11 self-report; 1.29 observer measures). Recovery was defined as no longer meeting the full criteria for personality disorder. A recent review of 14 psychodynamic therapy and 11 CBT studies found psychodynamic studies yielding a large overall effect size (1.46) and CBT a value of 1.00. The authors concluded that there is evidence that both are effective modalities (Leichsenring & Leibing, 2003).

Schizotypal personality disorder (STPD)

Psychological treatment

Because of STPD's relationship to schizophrenia, it is one of the few personality disorders investigated from a preventive perspective. Eighty-three children were assigned to an experimental enrichment programme when aged 3 to 5 years. Compared with a matched control group, they showed lower scores for STPD and antisocial behaviour at age 17 and for criminal behaviour at age 23 (Raine et al., 2003).

Pharmacotherapy

The one randomized trial of STPD patients utilizing low-dose risperidone showed significantly greater declines in negative and general symptoms by week 3 and in positive symptoms by week 7 with active treatment (Koenigsberg et al., 2003). Other STPD pharmacotherapy studies involving thiothixene, amoxepine, fluoxetine, and haloperidol included subjects with additional borderline pathology (Silk & Jibson, 2010).

Borderline personality disorder (BPD)

Psychotherapy and psychosocial treatment

Most research on personality disorder has been with BPD. Psychotherapy is the primary treatment modality recommended in both US (Oldham et al., 2001) and UK guidelines (National Collaborating Centre for Mental Health, 2009a). No specific therapy was recommended but therapy should have a clearly stated and integrated theoretical approach shared and delivered by a team with supervision provided to the treaters and with session frequency up to twice a week. Brief interventions (< 3 months) were not recommended either for BPD or its symptoms (National Collaborating Centre for Mental Health, 2009a).

Dynamic psychotherapy

Mentalization-based therapy and transference-focused therapy

Support for a psychoanalytically based therapy comes from RCTs of the effectiveness of mentalization-based treatment (MBT), as well as from studies of transference-focused psychotherapy (TFP). Mentalization entails "teaching" the patient through group and individual therapy to make sense of the actions of oneself and others on the basis of intentional mental states such as desires, feelings, and beliefs by learning to recognize what is in one's own mind and appreciating and understanding the mental states of others, capacities thought to be enfeebled in borderline patients. Two RCTs, one of 38 patients in a partial hospital programme and one of 134 outpatients compared to general psychiatric care, showed statistically significant decreases on all measures when compared with general psychiatric care. The treatment, now fully manualized, has been found to be cost-effective (Bateman & Fonagy, 1999, 2009).

TFP, in an RCT of three treatments, TFP, DBT and supportive treatment, has been shown to be effective. All three groups showed improvements in depression, anxiety, global functioning, and social adjustment. TFP and DBT resulted in improvement in suicidality; TFP and supportive therapy, improvements in anger and impulsivity; TFP alone, improvements in irritability and verbal and physical assaults (Clarkin et al., 2007). A recently published randomized trial showed TFP superior to community-based psychotherapy for BPD (Doering et al., 2010).

Group psychotherapy

Non-controlled studies of day hospital stabilization followed by outpatient dynamic group therapy support use of these groups in BPD (Wilberg et al., 1998). Marziali and Monroe-Blum (1995) found equivalent results between group and individual therapy in an RCT and concluded group therapy is preferred for cost-effectiveness.

Cognitive analytical therapy (CAT)

CAT, manualized for BPD treatment, has some data suggesting effectiveness. Chanen et al. (2008) compared CAT with "good clinical care" in 86 patients aged 15–18 years old who met DSM-IV

BPD criteria and found no differences in general psychopathology, global functioning, and parasuicidality, though the CAT group appeared to improve more rapidly.

Cognitive and behavioural therapies

Dialectical behaviour therapy (DBT)

DBT, a manualized special adaptation of CBT, originally used for treatment of repeatedly parasuicidal BPD female patients, includes techniques at the level of behaviour (functional analysis), cognitions (e.g. skills training), and support (empathy, teaching management of trauma). DBT's main aim is to decrease emotional dysregulation thought to be at the core of BPD and involves both group and individual therapy. A number of RCTs reveals DBT's benefit for suicidal BPD patients at the end of DBT (1 year) vs. TAU (Linehan et al., 1991). At naturalistic 6-month follow-up, DBT patients continued to show less parasuicidal behaviour, though this difference disappeared at 1 year.

Widespread adoption of DBT has taken place. Its numerous RCTs establishes it as the best validated BPD treatment. A replication of the original study with TAU performed by therapists thought to be experts in their non-DBT therapy practice found, in most respects, results very similar to the original study (Linehan et al., 2006). An additional RCT of 58 DSM-IV BPD Dutch women randomly assigned to either 1 year of DBT or TAU supports these findings (Verheul et al., 2003). But a recent well-conducted trial found that DBT was no more effective than general psychiatric management on any measure including suicide attempts and self-harm (McMain et al., 2009).

Schema therapy (ST)

Schemas, patterns of social, motivational, and cognitive-affective processes, are, in schema-focused therapy (ST or SFT), thought to be cornerstones of cognitive formulations of BPD patients (Young, 1990). "Schema coping behaviour" is the best adaptation to living that BPD patients employ. ST was evaluated against TFP by Giesen-Bloo et al. (2006) and found more effective than TFP. Farrell et al. (2009) added an 8-month, 30-session ST group to TAU among 32 randomly assigned subjects and found significant reductions in BPD symptoms, global severity, and global functioning in the ST enhanced treatment (94% compared to 16% of controls no longer meeting BPD criteria).

Cognitive behavioural therapy

Davidson et al. (2006) conducted a 30-session (27 sessions average) RCT of CBT (CBT plus TAU vs. TAU alone) in 106 subjects. They found the CBT group had less inpatient hospitalizations, and less significant suicidal acts but greater emergency room contacts. These benefits were maintained long-term (Davidson et al., 2010).

STEPPS

An RCT (N = 124) of systems training for emotional predictability and problem solving (STEPPS) which combines cognitive behavioural elements and skills training with a systems component was added to ongoing TAU. Compared to TAU alone, STEPPS enhanced treatment resulted in greater improvement in impulsivity, negative affectivity, mood and global functioning, and fewer emergency room visits. Differences yielded moderate to large effect sizes. There were no group differences for suicide attempts, self-harm acts, or hospitalizations (Blum et al., 2008). Discontinuation rates were high in both groups.

Bateman and Fonagy (2000) outlined the characteristics of effective treatment as follows:

- Well-structured
- Concentrates on enhancing compliance
- Clearly focuses on a behavioural or interpersonal problem
- Is theoretically coherent to both patient and therapist
- Is relatively long term
- Encourages a strong attachment between patient and therapist

- Has a relatively active therapist
- Is integrated with the rest of treatment

Pharmacotherapy

A high percentage of borderline patients take psychotropic medications. Many are subjected to intensive polypharmacy (40% of BPD patients take three or more medications concurrently, 10% take five or more; Zanarini et al., 2004).

There are about 27 placebo-controlled RCTs of psychotropic medication effectiveness in BPD, but limitations of this book format prevent detailed review. Early emphasis was primarily on use of SSRIs in the treatment of mood, affective lability, emotion dysregulation, and anger and aggression (Oldham et al., 2001). Current meta-analyses and systematic reviews found greater support for antipsychotic (both typical and atypical) as well as mood stabilizer medications for many of these symptoms with decreasing support for SSRIs (Nosé et al., 2006; Stoffers et al., 2010) except perhaps if a current comorbid major depressive episode exists. NICE guidelines National Collaborating Centre for Mental Health, 2009a find little or no evidence for psychotropic medication value in BPD. APA and NICE guidelines suggest that medications are primarily adjunctive to psychotherapy (Oldham et al., 2001; National Collaborating Centre for Mental Health, 2009a).

SSRIs

The SSRIs studied in blinded RCTs are fluoxetine and fluvoxamine. The best evidence for SSRI effectiveness for affective symptoms in BPD is when a comorbid depressive episode is present. Evidence for effectiveness with impulsivity, aggression, and anxiety is inconsistent. Fluvoxamine in has revealed effectiveness with mood lability (Herpertz et al., 2007; Ingenhoven et al., 2010).

Atypical antipsychotics

Clozapine, risperidone, quetiapine, and zisprasidone have been studied in open-label trials with placebo-controlled RCTs for olanzapine and aripiprazole. The best evidence is for aripiprazole with more extensive but contradictory evidence for olanzapine. Atypical antipsychotic medication appears to work most consistently (across trials) for the symptoms of cognitive-perceptual distortions, impulsivity and aggression, and somewhat for affective lability and anxiety, as well as global functioning and overall psychopathology (Silk & Jibson, 2010).

Mood stabilizers

There are open as well as placebo-controlled studies that support the use of divalproex sodium as well as placebo-controlled trials for topiramate and lamotrigine. Mood stabilizers seem most effective against impulsivity, aggression, anger/hostility, and interpersonal sensitivity (Nose et al., 2006;

Herpertz et al., 2007). RCTs involving lithium had methodological problems.

Other agents

An open-label trial of naltrexone (for dissociative symptoms) as well as a placebo-controlled trial of omega-3 fatty acids (for aggression and depression) showed positive results in BPD.

Most classes of psychotropic medication appear somewhat effective for different symptoms or dimensions of BPD. While there seems to be a shift towards using antipsychotic and/or mood stabilizers over SSRIs, using SSRIs in BPD remains active and popular. More research with larger populations of subjects and more consistency in outcome measures and what constitutes a positive outcome, needs to be undertaken.

ECT

Patients with BPD were found to be less likely to remit from major depression after ECT than those in comparison groups.

Antisocial personality disorder (ASPD)

People with ASPD show a pervasive pattern of disregard for and violation of the rights of others with irresponsible and aggressive behaviour beginning in childhood that commonly leads to trouble with the law in adulthood.

Table 35.1 Effectiveness of treatments for personality disorder

Treatment	Form of treatment	Psychiatric disorder/target audience	Level of evidence for efficacy	Comments
Psychotherapeutic	Non-specific	Personality disorders in general	Ia	All studies (including RCTs) reported improvement with psychotherapy, whether the therapy was psychodynamic, interpersonal, cognitive behavioural, or supportive. Specific personality disorders or specific treatments were not identified
Psychotherapy	Individual dynamic	Borderline personality disorder	Ia	A number of naturalistic follow-up studies support effectiveness of psychodynamic therapy and there is good evidence for mentalization-base treatment (MBT) and transference-focused psychotherapy
Psychotherapy	Group dynamic	Borderline personality disorder	Ib	Equivalent results when compared with individual psychotherapy but more cost-effective
Psychotherapy	Systems training for emotional predictability and problem solving (STEPPS)	Borderline personality disorder	Ib	Decreased impulsivity, negative affectivity, improved mood and global functioning
Psychotherapy	Cognitive analytical	Borderline personality disorder	IIb	Improvement but equal to other psychological treatments. Patients with BPD may show better adherence to this therapy than to others

Table 35.1 (cont.)

Treatment	Form of treatment	Psychiatric disorder/target audience	Level of evidence for efficacy	Comments
Psychotherapy	Cognitive and cognitive behavioural	Borderline personality disorder	Ib	Improvement noted in a single rigorous trial
Psychotherapy	Dialectical behavioural therapy	Borderline personality disorder	Ia	Better retention rate, decrease in suicidal thoughts, self-destructive and other parasuicidal acts
Psychotherapy	Various cognitive forms	Antisocial personality disorder	III	No effect on outcome though lowered recidivism
Psychotherapy	Various cognitive forms	Avoidant personality disorder	Ia	Behavioural gains are attained but overall impact on social functioning is questionable
Day hospital	Psychodynamic orientation	Mixed personality disorders	IIb	Improvement in a number of symptoms with decreased need for inpatient hospitalization, but questionable impact on overall social functioning
Pharmacotherapy	Low-dose risperidone	Schizotypal personality disorder	Ib	Assumption can be made that low doses of other atypical as well as typical antipsychotics would probably be effective depending upon any individual's ability to tolerate side effects

Pharmacotherapy	SSRI – fluoxetine	Borderline personality disorder	Ia	Decrease in anger independent of mood. Impact on other symptoms is controversial
Pharmacotherapy	SSRI – fluvoxamine	Borderline personality disorder	Ib	Decrease in rapid mood shifts but no change in anger or impulsivity
Pharmacotherapy	SSRIs and other antidepressants (fluoxetine, venlafaxine, sertraline)	Borderline personality disorder	III	Decreases in various symptoms of BPD
Pharmacotherapy	Atypical antipsychotic – clozapine	Borderline personality disorder	III	Studies confounded by Axis I or Axis II comorbid disorders. Improvement shown across a number of symptoms and behaviours
Pharmacotherapy	Atypical antipsychotic – olanzapine	Borderline personality disorder	Ib	Reduced various symptoms of BPD
Pharmacotherapy	Atypical antipsychotics – aripiprazole	Borderline personality disorder	Ib	A double-blind placebo-controlled study found decreased anxiety, depression, anger, and global ratings of psychopathology
Pharmacotherapy	Mood stabilizers – divalproex sodium	Borderline personality disorder	Ib	Decrease in aggression and overall psychopathology. Methodological limitations and diagnostic comorbidities make results difficult to interpret

Table 35.1 (cont.)

Treatment	Form of treatment	Psychiatric disorder/target audience	Level of evidence for efficacy	Comments
Pharmacotherapy	Mood stabilizers – lamotrigine	Borderline personality disorder	III	Case reports. Improvement in impulsive behaviours
Pharmacotherapy	Mood stabilizers – topiramate	Borderline personality disorder	Ib	Decrease in mood lability, aggression, anxiety, interpersonal problems
Pharmacotherapy	Omega-3 fatty acids	Borderline personality disorder	Ib	Improvement in aggression and depression

Most studies examining treatment of ASPD are within prisons and are of limited generalizability. D'Silva et al. (2004) reviewed 24 studies specifically related to psychopaths; only three were of a design appropriate to determine the benefits of treatment.

Psychosocial interventions

A NICE review of the literature (National Collaborating Centre for Mental Health, 2009b) concludes that people with ASPD, including those with substance misuse, should be offered, in community and mental health services, group-based cognitive and behavioural interventions, to address problems of impulsivity, interpersonal difficulties, and antisocial behaviour. For those with an offending behaviour history who are in community and institutional care, programmes focusing on reducing offending and other antisocial behaviour may be useful. Davidson and Tyrer (1996) in a small and methodologically limited CBT study found some positive outcomes. Most studies outside the penal system investigate patients comorbid for substance misuse and ASPD rather than address primary outcomes for the personality disorder.

Avoidant personality disorder

There has been some research on treatment of avoidant personality disorder (AvPD) but no adequate research on the other Cluster C disorders. Patients with AvPD show a pervasive pattern of social inhibition, feelings of inadequacy, and hypersensitivity to negative evaluation. The disorder appears on the boundary between Axis I and Axis II because of overlap with generalized social phobia (GSP). Most studies suggest that patients with GSP with and without AvPD exhibit equivalent levels of change independent of pretreatment severity (Herpertz et al., 2007).

One RCT of CBT versus psychodynamic therapy in AvPD (Emmelkamp et al., 2006) found CBT superior. While other studies report patients making substantial gains, many patients still demonstrate low levels of social functioning. Treatment gains appear to be maintained up to 1 year post-treatment.

Conclusions

There are now a few RCTs but little evidence to suggest specificity of any treatment. Perhaps the milieu of treatment protocols, often a well-constructed, well-structured, and coherent interpersonal endeavour, impacts success of these treatments as much as the interventions. Pharmacological treatment remains adjunctive with only moderate results in the best of outcomes.

Interventions discussed in this chapter are summarized in Table 35.1.

36

Other treatments for persistent disturbances of behaviour

Based on "Other treatments for persistent disturbances of behaviour" by Peter Tyrer and Stephen Tyrer in Effective Treatments in Psychiatry, Cambridge University Press, 2008

Introduction

Persistent behavioural problems are linked to personality disorders but are not always a consequence of them and so they are discussed in this separate chapter. Sometimes these may be considered to be part of a personality disorder that is almost unrecognized by both therapist and patient. There is a tendency for all therapists to be shy of diagnosing personality disorder in case the label is used pejoratively as a reason for not continuing treatment and so even in populations in which personality difficulties and disorders are highly prevalent only a minority of staff will consider using this diagnosis (Bowden-Jones et al., 2004; Newton-Howes et al., 2008).

In this way personality and behavioural disorders differ from most other mental disorders and can be postulated more as diatheses that make a person vulnerable to mental health and behavioural problems rather than being judged as disorders *per se* (Tyrer, 2007). Treating these conditions requires a subtlety of touch not usually necessary with other conditions. Because of the difficulties it is more common in clinical practice to treat abnormal behaviours rather than a specific diagnosis.

Aggressive challenging behaviour

There are a group of disorders within those with intellectual disability that are not yet formal diagnoses (although provision is likely to be made for them in the revisions of ICD and DSM). These are recognized clearly and often constitute the most persistent behavioural problems that need intervention. These behaviours include inappropriate social behaviour, disinhibition, physical aggression, other forms of aggressive, oppositional and threatening behaviour, wandering, sexually inappropriate behaviour, self-injury, and persistent demanding behaviour.

As there are many causes of these behaviours it is valuable, if time permits, to determine what has precipitated them. By careful observation of the subject concerned over a period of time, ideally 24–48 hours, it is possible to assess the relationship between the antecedent conditions and the manifestations of the behaviour (O'Neill et al., 1997).

"Challenging behaviour" is the term that is used to describe behaviour of this type. It does not have a simple equivalent in general adult psychiatry but is recognized in the behavioural problems of older people, particularly when cognitive function is impaired (see Chapter 2). In intellectual disability challenging behaviour is often quite different from the aggressive behaviour seen, for example, in antisocial personality disorder.

Some 10–15% of patients with intellectual disability in contact with services exhibit such behaviour (Emerson et al., 2001) with increasing proportions accompanying greater severity of disability.

Treatments for this condition include drug treatments (mainly antipsychotic drugs), general management strategies (of which person-centred planning is the most common), and a range of psychological treatments with wide variation in their degree of evaluation. There are very few randomized controlled trials in this subject.

Anger management

Two trials of psychological interventions have been carried out with people with learning disabilities living in secure settings (Taylor et al., 2002) and in the community (Willner et al., 2002). These studies both randomized subjects to either a waiting list control group or to a group treated over 12 or 9 weeks, respectively, using a package based on the methods introduced by Novaco (1976) and Black et al. that included both self-management and cognitive techniques. The offenders study (Taylor et al., 2002) reported significant improvements in anger control in the treated group, as assessed by participants' self-reports. Staff ratings of participants' anger tended to move in a similar direction, but the effect was not statistically significant; however, staff rated participants' behaviour on the ward as significantly improved post-treatment and at 1-month follow-up. In the community study (Willner et al., 2002), the treated group improved significantly and these gains were maintained at 3-month follow-up. A large definitive trial of this approach is currently under way in the UK.

Behaviour therapy

Standard behavioural techniques based on operant conditioning were once extremely common in those treated in institutions for those with learning disability, including common behavioural approaches such as "time out" (removal of the subject to an environment lacking the possibility of social reinforcement), seclusion (Rangecroft et al., 1997), overcorrection, and physical restraint. Alternative conditioning techniques involving positive reinforcement following the general principles of contingency management used more commonly now for drug misuse (Petry, 2006), differential reinforcement of other behaviour (DRO), and differential reinforcement of incompatible behaviour (DRI) are now used more frequently. A meta-analysis carried out of all studies between 1976 and 1987 found serious methodological deficiencies (Scotti et al., 1991). Consequently the authors concluded that "the results largely failed to support several widespread assumptions regarding precepts of clinical practice".

A form of DRO has been proposed recently which is termed functional communication (Fisher et al., 2005). This term refers to an approach to help alter inappropriate behaviour by encouraging the individual to communicate his or her wishes in an acceptable way with appropriate reward. This is carried out by reinforcing all efforts by the person undergoing scrutiny to indicate his or her feelings in a non-challenging way. Some studies have shown encouraging effects (Peck Peterson et al., 2005).

Cognitive behavioural therapy

Although cognitive behavioural therapy has been adapted for intellectual disability it has no real evidence supporting it as no controlled trials have been carried out.

Person-centred planning

Person-centred planning has been introduced to learning disability in an attempt to give greater power to those who have this condition, by a combination of promoting increased choice, listening more to their needs and wishes, building relationships, and promoting better support systems (Browder et al., 1997). It makes sound sense but has not been evaluated formally despite its widespread use.

Nidotherapy

Nidotherapy is a "collaborative treatment involving the systematic assessment and modification of the environment to minimize the impact of any form of mental disorder on the individual or on society" (Tyrer et al., 2003b). The notion of improving the adaptation of people to suitable environments rather than trying to change them to be different transfers the emphasis on change in the person to change in the environment. Although environmental changes have always been part of interventions in psychiatry these have not previously been incorporated systematically into a formal treatment strategy.

Nidotherapy can be considered for three forms of mental illness: (a) those in whom no gains in terms of the core features of the disorder can ever be expected (e.g. profound learning disability), (b) people in whom some improvement has been made following direct treatment but this has come to a halt and no further improvement has taken place (e.g. chronic depression, including dysthymia), and (c) those for whom treatment may or may not be helpful but this is immaterial as the patient refuses treatment.

The full process of treatment in nidotherapy is described elsewhere (Tyrer, 2009), but generally involves a single therapist (nidotherapist) working closely with the patient to get a full environmental analysis of physical, social, and personal environments and then collaboratively constructing a set of planned changes, with time scales, to achieve a better fit between the patient and the environment.

Only one randomized controlled trial has been carried out with nidotherapy (Ranger et al., 2009). Fifty-two patients with a severe mental illness and comorbid personality disorder (with 70% having substance misuse disorders also) were randomized to nidotherapy plus standard care from an assertive outreach team or standard care alone. The primary outcome of days in hospital over 1 year showed a gain for nidotherapy, which was greatest for those with the substance misuse group (Tyrer et al.,

2011). Nidotherapy has also been tested in an open trial in those with antisocial personality disturbance leading to a corresponding reduction in aggression, but in the absence of a control group this finding is of limited value, although a qualitative study has indicated both its assets and deficiencies (Spencer et al., 2010).

Psychopharmacological treatments

Drug treatment has been used for many years to treat those with learning disability who show behavioural problems and is usually, if not always appropriately, the first choice of management.

Antipsychotic drugs

The extent of use of antipsychotic drugs in learning disability is enormous. In a systematic review Brylewski & Duggan (2004) found over 500 citations to this treatment but only nine randomized controlled trials could be included in the analyses, and could not conclude if these drugs had any real value. However, some of these trials, even the less satisfactory ones, are worth looking at more closely, and there is some recent evidence from new randomized trials that could revise this verdict.

Van den Borre et al. (1993) carried out a (complicated) crossover trial involving the administration of risperidone (4–12 mg daily) or placebo to existing medication for 3 weeks followed by placebo washout for 1 week and then another 3 weeks' treatment using the alternative crossover medication. Thirty-seven patients were recruited and 30 finished the study. The results suggested a positive effect with risperidone but were completely compromised by differing results in the crossover arms, a common problem when there are carry-over effects from one treatment to another.

Buitelaar et al. (2001) also examined the efficacy of risperidone in a 6-week double-blind, randomized, parallel-group design in the treatment of aggression in 38 hospitalized adolescents with mild, borderline intellectual disability and dull normal intelligence. Risperidone, at a mean dose of less than 3 mg, was associated with significant improvement in severity of illness and behaviour disturbance. Gagiano et al. (2005) compared risperidone (1–4 mg daily, mean 1.45 mg) and placebo in 77 patients with intellectual disability (including 18% with borderline intelligence in the risperidone group) over a 4-week period in a combined randomized trial, with outcome determined primarily by the Aberrant Behaviour Checklist (ABC).

Patients on risperidone improved by 22% more than those allocated to placebo (p < 0.04) but those on placebo improved by 31%, showing the extent of non-specific factors in the treatment of aggressive challenging behaviour.

Very recently, a discontinuation study with zuclopenthixol (Haessler et al., 2007) showed possible benefit of the drug, as following successful treatment, withdrawal of the active drug was followed by a worse outcome in those randomized to placebo compared with zuclopenthixol. However, it would be a mistake to assume that a discontinuation study in itself shows evidence of efficacy for reasons which are spelt out more clearly in Chapter 19.

Mood stabilizers

Two randomized trials (Tyrer et al., 1984; Craft et al., 1987) have been carried out with lithium in the treatment of aggressive challenging behaviour in learning disability. Tyrer et al. (1984) treated 25 inpatient adults with learning disability and persistent aggressive behaviour in a double-blind crossover trial lasting 5 months comparing the effects of lithium with placebo on aspects of aggressive behaviour. All patients were receiving neuroleptic and/or anticonvulsant drugs which were continued during the trial. Seventeen of the patients showed greater improvement with the lithium phase of treatment compared to placebo. Craft et al. (1987) in a parallel group trial lasting 4 months involving 42 mentally handicapped patients compared aggression in patients randomized to lithium and placebo. In the lithium-treated group, 73% of patients showed a reduction in aggression during treatment and somewhat better scores than placebo. Although neither of these studies used an accepted scale, no instrument was available at the time and this was not a major problem in design. The results persuaded the Committee on Safety of Medicines to license lithium for the treatment of aggression in this population. Despite this, the drug is not widely employed in practice.

Topiramate, an anti-epileptic drug, has also shown promise, but only in open trials (Janowsky et al., 2003). Other anticonvulsants, including carbamazepine and sodium valproate, have also been used but the evidence base for benefit is meagre.

Selective serotonin reuptake inhibitors

Although selective serotonin reuptake inhibitors (SSRIs) have been used repeatedly for the treatment of

Table 36.1 Evidence base for treatments of persistent behavioural problems

Treatment	Form of treatment	Psychiatric disorder	Level of evidence for efficacy	Comments
Functional Communication Training (a form of DRO)	Individual treatment	Behavioural disturbance in moderate or severe intellectual disability	IIb	Evidence from one meta-analysis of single case studies only
Anger management	Group	Challenging behaviour	Ib	Some small evidence of efficacy with maintenance of effects
Cognitive behavioural therapy	Individual	Aggressive challenging behaviour	III	No good comparative studies
Nidotherapy	Individual	Comorbid personality disorder and severe mental illness	Ib	Reduced bed usage with nidotherapy
Person-centred planning	Individual	Learning disability in general	III	No adequate controlled studies
Antipsychotic drugs	Risperidone (1-4 mg)	Aggressive challenging behaviour	Ia	The best evidence to date with positive results from industry-funded trials but not from one independent one (NACHBID) (Tyrer et al., 2008)
Lithium	Standard dosage for correct blood levels	Aggressive challenging behaviour	Ib	Reduction in aggressive behaviour with lithium reasonably well demonstrated
Topiramate	200 mg daily	Aggressive challenging behaviour	III	Case studies only

aggressive challenging behaviour there have been no adequate trials of effectiveness and the evidence is circumstantial or based on simple open-label studies (e.g. Janowsky et al., 2005).

Summary

In the absence of a good evidence base it is comfortable to adopt the Hippocratic precept of "Primum non nocere" in treating behavioural problems in those with learning disability. However, the recent work on encouraging choice in functional communication training, which is supported by a meta-analysis, suggests a way forward in those with less profound intellectual disability. Drugs, particularly antipsychotic drugs, should be used sparingly and certainly not routinely, and only after psychological (or environmental) methods of treatment have failed (Oliver-Africano et al., 2009). This last recommendation follows a recent randomized trial carried out in the UK and Australia, NACHBID (Neuroleptics in Aggressive CHallenging Behaviour in Intellectual Disability) which showed that haloperidol and risperidone were less cost-effective than placebo in the treatment of aggressive challenging behavior in intellectual disability in a parallel design trial (Tyrer et al., 2008; Romeo et al., 2009). This suggests that antipsychotic drugs should not be used in the routine management of this condition and opens the door to further studies of psychological treatments whose evaluation is still in its infancy (Table 36.1).

It is hoped that this advice can become less delphic in the future. One randomized trial carried out in the UK and Australia, NACHBID (Neuroleptics in Aggressive Challenging Behaviour in Intellectual Disability), has recently been completed and as this compares haloperidol, risperidone, and placebo in a parallel-design trial the results will be of considerable interest. However, the relatively small numbers of controlled treatment studies carried out in the past 5 years (less than in the 1980s) gives a misty view of the future.

Acknowledgement

We thank Freya Tyrer for her help in the preparation of this chapter.

Sexual and gender identity disorders

37

Sexual therapies

Based on "Effectiveness of treatments of sexual disorders" by Michael King in Effective Treatments in Psychiatry, Cambridge University Press, 2008

Introduction

The so-called sexual liberation in Western countries in the 1960s threw off decades of conservative public morality in which it was barely possible to talk about sexual matters. The early seeds had appeared immediately after World War II when Alfred Kinsey and his colleagues shocked America with their pioneering (but flawed) studies of usual sexual behaviour (Kinsey et al., 1948). In the 1950s and 60s William Masters, a gynaecologist and Virginia Johnson, a psychologist, developed instruments to measure human sexual response and began a project that included direct laboratory observation and measurement of hundreds of men and women while they

were having intercourse or masturbating. Sexual therapy expanded rapidly after the publication of Masters and Johnson's book *Human Sexual Inadequacy* (Masters and Johnson, 1970). They advocated a short, intensive therapy, combining sexual education with a mainly behavioural intervention aimed at reducing anxiety about sexual performance and increasing mutually pleasurable sexual arousal. Masters and Johnson claimed that only 20% of couples failed to respond.

Although the medical view of sex met increasing and well considered criticism (e.g. Illich, 1975), it took off at an even greater pace after the British physiologist, Giles Brindley, stepped onto the platform at the American

Urological Association meeting in 1983 and displayed his own phentolamine-induced erection (Marks, 2003). The introduction of oral treatments has been the most recent advance in treatment of erectile dysfunction but it is fast becoming a routine treatment in the hands of primary care physicians (Meuleman, 2003).

Classification of sexual dysfunction

Sexual problems that are not due primarily to physical disorders can be divided into difficulties of desire, arousal, orgasm, and pain. The first three terms arose from the early work of Masters and Johnson who were radical in their observational, laboratory-based approach to the study of usual sexual function.

Desire is conceptualized as a wish to engage in sexual activity and the occurrence of sexual fantasies. Arousal or excitement is the temporary, immediate feeling of sexual excitement together with the bodily changes that accompany it, such as erection or vaginal lubrication. Orgasm is the peak of sexual pleasure which is accompanied by genital and perineal muscle contractions, contraction of anal sphincters, and (usually) ejaculation in the man. Resolution is the final phase of penile detumnescence, restoration of vaginal volume

to normal, and physical and mental relaxation. A refractory phase in men follows when it is difficult or impossible to achieve an erection, lasting between 10 minutes and 48 hours depending on age and physical health.

Until the pharmaceutical industry entered the fray, the classification of sexual problems in men was relatively uncontroversial beyond the realms of philosophical debate. Now there is widespread concern that industry-funded epidemiological studies report inflated prevalences of sexual disorders and that drug companies will fail to regard many symptoms "as aspects of normal sexuality but as the symptoms of medical conditions that are widespread and treatable with pills" (Moynihan & Mintzes, 2010, p. 4). The word *dysfunction* implies a state of *dis-ease* that requires treatment. Some consider that women's sexual function is completely different to men's, in that it is responsive rather than spontaneous and more dependent on emotional closeness with her partner (Basson et al., 2001).

Male sexual dysfunction

Erectile disorder

As for most diagnoses, deciding whether a problem exists requires a degree of subjectivity. The simplest definition is an inability to initiate or sustain a penile erection (hard enough for penetrative sex) until orgasm. Its prevalence is 7–9% (Laumann et al., 1999; Nazareth et al., 2003).

Drug treatments

The earliest successful drug treatments for erectile dysfunction in men were injectables such as *alprostadil* or prostaglandin E. Prostaglandin E remains a useful alternative for men who do not respond to *sildenafil*, particularly after radical prostatectomy. Other injectables are *phentolamine*, an alpha-blocker, and *papaverine*, a non-specific phosphodiesterase inhibitor. Rates of success in a head-to-head comparison of *alprostadil, papaverine-phentolamine* combination, and *papaverine* alone were 72%, 61%, and 31%, respectively (Porst, 1989). They are largely reserved for men who fail on oral phosphodiesterase-5 inhibitors and men after radical prostatectomy.

The first licensed oral drug for erectile dysfunction, the phosphodiesterase-5 inhibitor *sildenafil*, revolutionized treatment of men with erectile difficulties and has become the first line of treatment. It prolongs smooth muscle relaxation and facilitates erection. Adverse effects include headache, flushing of the skin (particularly of the face and neck), stomach upsets and nasal stuffiness. However in randomized, controlled studies, only 1% of men stop taking the drug because of adverse effects

(Goldstein et al., 1998). Although initial trial reports indicated efficacy rates of 80% to 90%, success in clinical practice is closer to 50% (Morgentaler, 1999). A meta-analysis of trials involving over 2200 men indicated that *sildenafil* led to a higher percentage of successful intercourse attempts (57% to 21%; weighted mean difference 33.7%, CI 29.2, 38.2) than placebo and a greater percentage of men experiencing at least one intercourse success during treatment (83% versus 45%; relative benefit increase 1.8, CI 1.7, 1.9) (Fink et al., 2002). Efficacy is less in diabetes and after radical prostatectomy. Nitrate drugs must not be taken with *sildenafil* as they may lead to profound and life-threatening hypotension. *Tadalafil* is a second phosphodiesterase-5 inhibitor with a half-life at least twice that of *sildenafil*, has similar results to sildenafil, and was effective for up to 36 hours after dosing, a much longer window of effect than for *sildenafil* (Carson et al., 2004).

Unfortunately, there is already evidence that the drug has a street value and can be misused by men with normal sexual function. Where performance anxiety is very high, however, *sildenafil* can reduce tension enough to re-establish a sense of relaxation, help the man to focus on his anxious cognitions, and eventually return to normal sexual function (Schover and Leiblum, 1994). *Apomorphine* is a sublingual medication that acts centrally on dopamine systems to promote erection. Two placebo-controlled, randomized trials involving a total of just over 800 men have indicated modest success in terms of proportion of successful attempts at intercourse (Dula et al., 2001; von Keitz et al., 2002). A third trial involved 43 men in a comparison of *apomorphine* with *sildenafil* in which *apomorphine* behaved little differently from placebo in the principal *sildenafil* trials (Perimentis et al., 2004). Its action on dopamine means that it may also increase sexual drive.

Yohimbine is an indole alkaloid that has a moderate effect on erectile dysfunction at doses of 15 to 30 mg daily. In a meta-analysis *yohimbine* was found superior to placebo in the treatment of erectile dysfunction (odds ratio 3.85, 95% CI 6.67–2.22) with rare but reversible adverse reactions (Ernst & Pittler, 1998), but a subsequent review was more conservative in its conclusion (Tam et al., 2001).

Psychological treatments

There have been no well-conducted clinical trials of psychoanalytical treatment of sexual dysfunction. Traditional sexual therapy using a Masters and Johnson approach has also little controlled trial evidence to back it up. Anxiety was allegedly a cause of poor performance but is only a problem in people who are *already* dysfunctional (van den Hout & Barlow, 2000). Extreme anxiety, for example in soldiers on the battlefield, may induce erection and even ejaculation in the absence of sexual feelings (Bancroft, 1989).

Helen Kaplan in the 1970s advocated using brief analytical methods if a behavioural approach failed (Kaplan, 1974), and today most sex therapists take a pragmatic approach in which they combine several approaches – psychological and biomedical. Cognitive and behavioural approaches lack careful appraisal in large, multicentre trials and brief versions of the approach appear to add no benefit when examined as an adjunct to biological treatments such as intracavernosal *alprostadil* (Van der Windt et al., 2002).

Pelvic floor muscle (or Kegel) exercises have been shown to be effective in a small randomized trial involving men aged 20 and over with erectile dysfunction of at least 6 months' duration (Dorey et al., 2004).

Orgasmic disorders in men

Premature ejaculation

Prevalence estimates for premature ejaculation vary widely, between 4% and 30% (Laumann et al., 1999; Nazareth et al., 2003). Medical treatments for this problem have been described since *clomipramine* was first reported to retard orgasm in up to 80% of men and women who took it (Monteiro et al., 1987). The best randomized trial evidence supports the efficacy of most selective serotonin reuptake inhibitors (SSRIs) (except *fluvoxamine*) with little difference between *sertraline*, *fluoxetine*, and *paroxetine* in delaying ejaculation (Waldinger et al., 2001).

Topical anaesthetics have long been used by men with premature ejaculation. A small randomized trial has recently shown a clear advantage of a *lidocaine–prilocaine* solution over placebo with a 5- to 6-fold increase in intravaginal ejaculatory latency time (Busato & Galindo et al., 2004). However one-third of participants dropped out of the trial.

Despite no meta-analysis being available, the American Urological Association has just issued guidelines for the pharmacological management of premature ejaculation (Montague et al., 2004) in which they recommend *paroxetine*, *sertraline* and *clomipramine* in continuous or intermittent dosage. Despite lack of evidence of safe, long-term efficacy, they also suggest that a topical anaesthetic applied to the penis combined with use of a condom may be useful.

Retarded ejaculation and anorgasmia

Delayed or retarded ejaculation is a less common, but particularly troubling problem in men with prevalence rates of almost 3% in the UK (Nazareth et al., 2003) and under 2%

in the USA (Laumann et al., 1999). Evidence for effective pharmacological treatment is poor.

Psychological and behavioural treatments for orgasmic disorders

Like psychological treatments for sexual dysfunction, those for ejaculatory disorders have a long history. There is no evidence that psychoanalysis is effective in this condition. Behavioural techniques developed by Masters and Johnson and their colleagues include the squeeze technique and subsequently the stop-start technique taken up particularly by Kaplan (1974) is one where the man close to orgasm stops moving or actually withdraws his penis, but no good evidence of their value exists.

A meta-analysis of bibliotherapy (written material) for a range of sexual disorders, mainly orgasmic function, reported a sample size adjusted effect size of 0.5 (van Lankveld, 1998). Bibliotherapy is an intervention in which written material plays a central role and a description of a particular treatment method is typically its focus. This may show that simple advice and education is as effective as anything else in these disorders.

Female sexual dysfunction

Female sexual dysfunction has a complex mix of biological, psychological, and interpersonal determinants and that appears to be age related. Unfortunately, our knowledge of the physiology of the female sexual response has lagged far behind that of the male. It is generally accepted that the clitoris is central to sexual arousal in women (Caruso et al., 2004). However, the physical aspects of sexual arousal, lubrication, and orgasm are not strongly correlated with sexual distress.

Drugs such as tricyclic antidepressants and SSRIs that inhibit sexual function in men cause similar dysfunction, such as retarded orgasm, in women (Monteiro et al., 1987). It also seems likely that androgens are primarily responsible for sexual drive in women (Shifren, 2004).

Hypoactive sexual desire in women

Lack of sexual desire in women is commonly reported in epidemiological studies. Depending on the narrowness of definition, prevalence rates range between 17% in the UK (Nazareth et al., 2003) and 30% in the USA (Laumann et al., 1999). There are strong associations between low sexual drive and anxiety, depression and discord with spouse or partner, and with use of psychotropic medication. It is also common in the 8 months after childbirth.

When a woman lacks sexual drive, it is well worth asking "who is complaining?" It has been suggested that the disorder definition should include persistent lack or deficiency of indicators of sexual desire and that this lack leads to personal distress (King et al., 2007). Thus women who lack desire in certain situations such as marital conflict would not qualify. Similarly, an imbalance between the woman's desire and that of her partner (given similar age and health) would not necessarily be a sign of disorder (Basson, 2001).

Drug treatments

Although *sildenafil* has been considered as a treatment for low sexual desire in women, female arousal disorder has been its main focus, even though it is largely ineffective in this condition. Testosterone therapy in women with low sexual drive appears to have beneficial effects in women who have undergone oophorectomy and hysterectomy, although placebo response is high (Shifren et al., 2000). *Tibolone*, a synthetic steroid that has oestrogenic, progestagenic, and androgenic activity, is used to treat menopausal symptoms and may have a place in enhancing sexual function in postmenopausal women.

Psychological approaches

Adopting the Masters and Johnson Model of sex therapy for women has

Table 37.1 Effectiveness of treatments for sexual disorders

Treatment	Form of treatment	Psychiatric disorder	Level of evidence for efficacy	Comments
Phosphodiesterase-5 inhibitors	Sildenafil (tab)	Erectile dysfunction	Ia	Large effect size, with lower success rates after radical prostatectomy. Contraindicated with nitrates
Phosphodiesterase-5 inhibitors	Tadalafil (tab)	Erectile dysfunction	Ia	Longer duration of action (36 hours) and twice half-life of sildenafil
Phosphodiesterase-5 inhibitors	Vardenafil (tab)	Erectile dysfunction	Ib	Likely to be similar to sildenafil
Dopaminergic drugs	Apomorphine (sublingual)	Erectile dysfunction	Ib	Conflicting results from clinical trials. Probably not as effective as phosphodiesterase-5 inhibitors
Alpha$_2$-adrenoceptor antagonist	Yohimbine (tab)	Erectile dysfunction	Ia	Of some value, but not as effective as other drugs for this condition
Prostaglandins	Alprostadil (intracavernosal injection)	Erectile dysfunction	Ia	Second-line treatment in view of form of treatment and risk of priapism
Behavioural approaches	Masters & Johnson techniques	Erectile dysfunction	III	Widely used but little tested
Cognitive behavioural therapy	Standard treatment to reduce dysfunctional thinking	Erectile dysfunction	III	Little formal evaluation

Table 37.1 (cont.)

Treatment	Form of treatment	Psychiatric disorder	Level of evidence for efficacy	Comments
Couples sexual therapy	Combined with counselling or physical treatment (e.g. vacuum erectile device)	Erectile dysfunction	IIa	One study supports joint physical/couple counselling approach
Pelvic floor muscle exercises	–	Erectile dysfunction	Ib	One trial showed positive results when biofeedback incorporated
Selective serotonin reuptake inhibitors (SSRIs)	Sertraline, fluoxetine	Premature ejaculation	Ia	Good evidence
Topical anaesthetics	Lidocaine-prilocaine	Premature ejaculation	Ib	Some evidence of effectiveness
Alpha-adrenergic antagonists	Pseudoephedrine, ephedrine	Retarded ejaculation/anorgasmia	III	No good evidence of efficacy
Pause-squeeze technique	Linked to Masters & Johnson	Retarded ejaculation/anorgasmia	IIa	Some slight evidence of value
Penile vibrators	–	Retarded ejaculation/anorgasmia	III	Probably effective to some extent but not tested formally

Treatment		Indication	Level	Efficacy
Bibliotherapy	Written material only	Disorders of sexual function generally	Ia	Small but consistent level of efficacy
Hormone therapy	Testosterone	Hypoactive sexual drive (women)	III	Possible benefit
Hormone therapy	Oestrogen replacement/tibolone	Hypoactive sexual drive (women)	III	Little evaluation to date
Phosphodiesterase-5 inhibitors	Sildenafil (tab)	Poor sexual arousal (women)	Ia	Little evidence of value
Dopaminergic drugs	Apomorphine (sustained release tab)	Poor sexual arousal (women)	Ib	On trial showed benefit
Dilator therapy		Vaginismus	Ia	No documented evidence of benefit

received fierce criticism in recent years because it is perceived as equating male and female sexuality. However, advocates of the joint approach contend that such therapy has placed men and women on an equal footing and encourages the view that pleasure in love making is also a female prerogative.

Sexual arousal disorder in women

Lack of arousal in women is complex and probably over-reported. Drug treatments such as *sildenafil* and *phentolamine* do not help generally and Pfizer has not pursued a licence for *sildenafil* in women. Another drug that has received some attention in women complaining of low arousal is *apomorphine*, and a sustained release dose of *apomorphine* in women with arousal disorders *and* low sexual drive has been shown to improve orgasm, sexual enjoyment, and satisfaction in one small placebo-controlled trial (Caruso et al., 2004).

Vaginismus

In this disorder, involuntary vaginal and adductor muscles of the thighs make penetration difficult or impossible. It most commonly presents as primary in young women embarking on their first sexual relationships or secondary following sexual assault or similar trauma. There are no available drug treatments for vaginismus. Over and above non-specific sexual therapy about which little can be added here, behavioural interventions, mainly dilator therapy, have figured commonly in the management of this condition. A recent Cochrane Review has considered all randomized, controlled trials published up to 2002, where treatment for vaginismus was compared to another treatment, either placebo, treatment as usual, or a wait-list control (McGuire & Hawton, 2003). Only two trials were identified and neither showed effectiveness for any particular type of intervention.

Conclusions

Erectile dysfunction and premature ejaculation have good evidence supporting drug treatment but for other disorders the findings are much less clear (Table 37.1) and intelligent reading is a useful precursor for prospective patients before they seek therapy.

38

Disorders of gender identity

Based on "Disorders of gender identity" by James Barrett in Effective Treatments in
Psychiatry, Cambridge University Press, 2008

Introduction

Disorders of gender identity are rare
but constant. The incidence of transsexualism is very roughly 1 in 60 000
males and 1 in every 100 000 females
(Landen et al., 1996). These disorders
did not come to the attention of psychiatric services until the early 1950s,
after the first recognition and description of gender identity problems by
Dr. Harry Benjamin, who together
with other practitioners, formed an
association named the Harry
Benjamin Gender Dysphoria
Association. Initially, problems with
gender identity were thought to represent severe mental illness, but subsequent studies have supported the
view that transsexualism was usually

an isolated diagnosis and not part of
any general psychopathological
disorder.

Currently, but this is unlikely to
remain the same in ICD-11, disorders
of gender identity are classified as
disorders of adult personality and
behaviour in the 10th revision of
the International Classification of
Diseases (ICD-10), and comprise
transsexualism (F64.0), dual role
transvestism (F64.1), gender identity
disorder of childhood (F64.2), other
gender identity disorders (F64.8), and
gender identity disorder, unspecified
(64.9). Transsexualism is described in
ICD-10 as a desire to live and be
accepted as a member of the opposite
sex, usually accompanied by a sense
of discomfort with one's anatomical

325

sex. For the diagnosis to be made transsexual identity should have been present for at least 2 years, and must not be a symptom of another mental disorder, such as schizophrenia, or associated with any intersex, genetic, or sex chromosome abnormality.

Transsexualism is the diagnosis for which most treatment evidence is available. There is little research into dual role transvestism, nor much into related disorders such as dysmorphophobia, autogynephilia, or gynandromorphophilia (Blanchard, 1993). These differential diagnoses may require different management to transsexualism (for example, Blanchard, 1993).

It is now thought possible for transsexualism to be coincidental with another mental illness and yet not caused by it. Successful treatment of a disorder of gender identity in the presence of another psychiatric illness is common and is probably an example of true comorbidity (i.e. two separate illnesses existing in the same person at the same time).

Treatment

Most early approaches to the management of transsexualism involved either an individual patient's case being reported or else publication of a very small series, which could never have amounted to a satisfactory level of evidence. What emerged from these reports was that individual psychotherapy did not act significantly to change the disorder of gender identity although it did help with other aspects of daily living. The failure of psychotherapy alone in these isolated patients led to it never being extensively employed. Instead, surgical approaches to change bodily form closely to resemble that of the opposite sex took the place of psychological treatment. Some psychoanalysts feel that the near abandonment of psychoanalytical approaches was premature, and that such approaches are more possible as psychoanalysis has developed. Others, including Lothstein (1981), reported good success with a mixed psychotherapeutic and surgical approach noting that of 50 gender dysphoric patients, 70% had adjusted to non-surgical solutions, 20% were receiving treatment, and 10% had received gender reassignment surgery and psychotherapy.

Initially, surgical approaches were also reported individually or in small numbers. This meant that benefit could not be statistically proven, although the case reports were in the main positive, with only occasional negative reports (Van Putten & Fawzy, 1976), so such treatment continued.

The qualification criteria and timing of surgical intervention have always been contentious. Often, people with disorders of gender identity have pressed for fewer hurdles and earlier intervention. Before the formation of the Harry Benjamin International Gender Dysphoria Association, it had been possible for individuals with sufficient financial resources to obtain gender reassignment surgery essentially upon request. Outcomes were highly variable, with some said to have been exceedingly poor. The Harry Benjamin International Gender Dysphoria Association set an arbitrary, but not capricious, minimum period for qualification for gender reassignment surgery of at least a year, despite case reports such as that of Levine & Shumaker (1983) suggesting this might be too short a period. This year had to be spent living wholly in the new gender role, with demonstrable psychological and social success.

This period was arrived at because it was felt to be the greatest increase from the previous "surgery on demand" position that surgeons and their patients would be prepared to accept. This period became known as the "real life test", and was subsequently renamed the "real life experience". It became incorporated into a set of "Minimum Standards of Care" formulated by the Harry Benjamin Gender Dysphoria Association. These standards are periodically revised, the changes at each revision reflecting the ever-changing dynamic between empirical changes in clinical practice, new research evidence, local legal imperatives, and patient and political pressures.

Mate-Kole et al. (1988) found that patients who were on a waiting list for surgery showed lower neurotic scores on the Crown–Crisp Experiential Index (a measure of symptoms and personality status), while postoperative transsexuals obtained scores lower than either of the other groups. This suggests that a social change of gender role with hormone treatment is itself helpful, as is subsequent gender reassignment surgery, a finding reiterated by Blanchard et al. (1983), who found a statistically significant negative correlation between depression and social feminization and between tension and social feminization.

In general terms, under the Harry Benjamin Gender Dysphoria Association Standards of Care, both male and female patients are required to change gender role prior to a doctor initiating hormone treatment. Such treatment, when it occurs, is with cross-sex hormones. There is debate about any need for antiandrogen or progestrogenic therapy in male patients, but agreement that high-dose oestrogen therapy is indicated. The treatment seems to be acceptably safe (Van Kesteren et al., 1997), the major risk being that of thromboembolic disease. Female patients require treatment with androgens, either by implant or by intramuscular injection. Oral treatment may be associated with a raised rate of hepatocellular carcinoma. It is thus ethically and legally challenging to use oral agents.

Children and adolescents with gender identity disorders pose particular problems. Instinctive caution has led to surgery and hormones being delayed, although all the evidence is that with carefully selected patients early surgical intervention carries a good outcome (Cohen-Kettenis et al., 2008). There is a trend towards postponing puberty by means of gonadotropin releasing hormone analogues and introducing cross-sex hormone treatment when the child is old enough to give valid consent. There is the suggestion that for males earlier age of onset of transsexualism was associated with better outcome (Tsoi, 1993), which may reflect 'core' transsexualism. The question is rendered more problematic by studies such as that of Davenport (1986), who followed up 10 feminine boys, of whom only one became transsexual, and four heterosexual. He concluded that childhood gender dysphoria appears to be a necessary but not sufficient factor in a transsexual outcome.

Those patients who show improved psychological, social, sexual, and occupational functioning in their new gender role for a period of at least a year are considered appropriate candidates for gender reassignment surgery. Such surgery has been subject to most investigation, since as treated patient numbers grew, it became possible to assess psychological and social outcomes properly after gender reassignment surgery, and to relate these outcomes to some features of the patients' presenting histories.

Regrettably, though many studies show good outcome, most make no greater comment on the selection process for surgery candidature than to delineate what is often little more than a demographic description of the selected group. The process of psychological assessment leading to subsequent selection seems rarely described in any depth at all. The timing of surgery was addressed by Mate-Kole et al. (1991) in a rare randomized controlled study, which established that once patients had been approved for surgery, those fast-tracked showed better psychological function than those who joined a standard waiting list.

The functional results of gender reassignment surgery have been assessed in sexual terms by Green (1998). Rehman et al. (1999) noted general satisfaction was expressed over the quality of cosmetic (normal appearing genitalia) and functional (ability to perceive orgasm) aspects. Lief and Hubschman (1993) found orgiastic capacity after gender reassignment surgery declined in male patients and increased in female ones. Despite the decrease in orgasm in the males, satisfaction with sex and general satisfaction with the results of surgery were high in both. Blanchard & Steiner (1990) suggested that in purely mechanical terms modest vaginal depth could be compensated for by a change of sexual technique.

There seem to have been good outcomes in settings as disparate as Serbia (Rakic et al., 1996) and Holland (Kuiper & Cohen-Kettenis, 1988) and the strong suggestion from several studies that the technical success of surgery and a subsequent legal recognition of a change of sex is associated with a good psychological and social outcome (Tsoi et al., 1995). Indeed, in one study technical surgical outcome accounted for nearly all the variation in postoperative psychopathology (Ross & Need, 1989). This is reiterated by Stein et al. (1990) who reported good outcomes in a group of 10 patients, but noted that none reported being discovered as having had a prior operation by their sexual partner, suggesting technically good results in the group. Much worse psychological outcomes were reported by Lindemalm et al. (1986) but in the 13 patients studied surgical outcome was disappointing, and only one-third of the patients where a vaginal construction was carried out had a functioning vagina,

again supporting a connection with surgical outcomes.

It seems increasingly clear that psychological support is needed after surgery (Rehman et al., 1999) to optimize outcomes since social stressors may persist despite treatment, particularly if the patient has children. In connection with the welfare of children, Green (1978) found there to be no evidence that a change of parental gender role has any effect on the sexual development of children. Despite this, many patients have experienced impaired access to their children on the grounds of their change of gender role.

Landen et al. (1998) showed in a regression analysis that regrets about gender reassignment surgery were associated with poor family and friend support, a lack of an earlier history of childhood gender identity disorder, and a lack of attraction to the same biological sex. This was reiterated in another study by Blanchard et al. (1989) which found attraction to the opposite biological sex was associated with a poorer outcome. Another study by Bodlund & Kullgren (1996) showed personality disorder and Axis II diagnoses to be associated with a worse outcome, and that female patients tend generally to fare better than male. Another study found no preoperative variables could predict good adjustments for female transsexuals (Tsoi, 1993).

Table 38.1 Effectiveness of treatments for gender identity

Treatment	Form of treatment	Psychiatric disorder/target audience	Level of evidence for efficacy	Comments
Psychosocial	Psychotherapy	Gender identity disorder/ transsexualism	IV	Did not change the gender identity disorder but perhaps helped with aspects of daily living
Somatic	Gender reassignment surgery	Transsexualism	III	Better psychosocial adjustment (better scores on items of neurosis) than those on a waiting list and those in no treatment, though those on a waiting list did better than those not in any type of programme. Postoperative psychopathology may be most related to level of satisfaction with the surgery
Somatic	Hormonal treatment	Transsexualism	III	Those who were treated with hormones and were living as the opposite gender had better scores on measures of neurosis than those not in treatment but less than those who received actual surgery

Lindemalm et al. (1987) found traumatic loss of both parents in infancy to be associated with poor outcome and an overprotective mother and a distant father with good. Contrary to other reports, high sexual activity and bisexual experience was associated with fair sexual adjustment and with non-repentance after sex change. Completed military service, a history of typically masculine, hard jobs, and a comparatively late (more than 30 years of age) first request for surgery, were found to be negative prognostic factors in sex-reassignment evaluations, and it was thought that both too much and too little ambivalence may suggest a poor prognosis.

Much less studied have been transsexual people who did not have gender reassignment surgery. Kockott and Fahrner (1987) found that those with an unaltered wish for surgery, but who had not had gender reassignment surgery, did not differ substantially from transsexuals who had had surgery. By contrast, the "hesitating" patients were noticeably older, more often married, more often had children of their own, their partnerships were of long duration, and exclusively with partners of the opposite biological sex. These characteristics had been seen when the diagnosis was first made and were thought to be prognostic for this sub-group. Transsexual people who relinquished their wish for surgery did not differ substantially from transsexuals

with an unaltered wish for surgery. Their reasons for relinquishing the wish for surgery could not clearly be established. It was concluded that it was hesitating patients who required particular scrutiny.

Genital surgery for female patients is a very much more technically challenging procedure and much less studied and reported. Patients' functional demands are high (Hage et al., 1993) and surgical results often fail to match them. Despite this one study found that phalloplasty does not appear to be a critical factor in orgasm or in sexual satisfaction, concluding that it is possible to change one's body image and sexual identity and be sexually satisfied despite inadequate sexual functioning (Lief and Hubschman, 1993). It is strongly suspected that much greater psychological benefit to female patients is conferred by a bilateral mastectomy than by phalloplasty.

In summary we can conclude that transsexualism is not indicative of serious psychopathology and that in carefully selected patients, with psychological support, a change of social gender role does much to improve the psychological state of the patient and (if the improvement can be sustained for at least a year), gender reassignment surgery will probably further improve it.

Interventions discussed in this chapter are summarized in Table 38.1.

Child psychiatry

39

Psychological treatments for children and adolescents

Based on "Psychological treatments for children and adolescents" by Brian W. Jacobs, Stefanie A. Hlastala, and Elizabeth McCauley in Effective Treatments in Psychiatry, Cambridge University Press, 2008

Introduction

Psychological treatments in child and adolescent psychiatry must take into account the complexity of biological development, environmental impact as children grow, and legal frameworks designed to protect their welfare. With this in mind, adult treatments have been adapted and novel treatments developed appropriate to children and their situations.

Children live in intricate, dependent contexts. Environmental disturbance can result in psychiatric distress and disorder; experiences can exacerbate disorders even when the root

cause is predominantly biological. The emotional, cognitive, and moral environments to which children are exposed are crucial for healthy development and failures in early emotional care can result in long-lasting biological changes in brain function (Heim et al., 2001). With age, children encounter increasingly complex social networks mixing with other children in school. These networks provide opportunities but also exposure to peer relationship complications. Puberty and adolescence present increasing opportunities for adult-like decisions though lack of experience and continuing emotional and physical development makes

335

youth more vulnerable to difficulties while allowing greater flexibility in personality development. Children and adolescent treatments take these networks and developmental factors into account.

Confidentiality, consent, legislation, and psychological treatments

Confidentiality and consent issues are complex for children. Parents may know a lot about their children's behaviour and actions but probably know less about their children's thoughts and feelings than they think they do. Adolescence often brings demands for more independence. Therapists recognize that a child's right to confidentiality at the lower ends of childhood and adolescence is limited since parents are most likely their protectors. To protect from harm, parents need to be informed. Confidentiality is more complex with adolescents. If not respected, the adolescent may refuse to see the mental health professional, but if unthinkingly preserved, lives may be placed at risk.

In the UK, young people over the age of 16 are now treated as adults with regards to consent issues; if they have the capacity, as defined by The Mental Capacity Act 2005, they are able to make decisions about treatment on their own behalf. Below that age, the test is one of whether they understand the decision they are making and its implications for the future. A parent can agree to mental health treatment of a younger child in hospital against their wishes provided the parent is seen as acting in the child's interest and the decision is one that it is reasonable to ask the parent to take. Otherwise the law has to be invoked by the doctor.

In the USA, informed consent and confidentiality in children and adolescents are subject to specific federal and state laws. Age of consent can vary significantly from state to state. In Washington State (Seattle), children age 13 and older can consent to care without parental consent and can refuse care despite their parents' consent. Age of consent is often 16 and older in other states. Exceptions to confidentiality include harm to self, to others, or in situations where the child is being harmed by someone else. The clinician is required to act in the minor's best interest. Whether or not to disclose information revealed by an adolescent is complicated. For example, non-life-threatening self-harm may be held in confidence to address in treatment. Additional laws that vary by state apply to substance use and misuse to protect youths' choices to keep this information confidential.

General issues concerning psychological treatments

More than 1500 empirical studies examining the effects of "traditional" (mainly psychodynamic) child psychotherapy suggest that clinically guided care found in usual practice is not effective treatment (Weiss et al., 1999; Weisz et al., 2004). Comprehensive care systems with case management and a menu of mental health services increase treatment access and improve client satisfaction, but show little evidence of benefit (Salzer et al., 1999; Kazdin, 2000). Meta-analyses of research-based treatments reveal better psychotherapy outcome for the average child aged 4–18 than 76% of control group children with an effect size similar to that found in adults (0.71 to 0.79) (Casey & Berman, 1985; Weisz et al., 1987; 1995; Kazdin et al., 1990). This treatment effect often disappears in ordinary clinical settings, and the question of effective versus efficacious treatment arises. Carefully controlled research treatment trials focus on efficacious treatment, but what are effective treatments in clinical settings?

- Behavioural treatments appear more effective than non-behavioural treatments (Casey & Berman, 1985; Weisz et al., 1987; 1995), but for specific disorders and/or populations non-behavioural therapies have shown efficacy (e.g. interpersonal therapy for depressed adolescents (Mufson et al., 1999)).

- Children at higher cognitive developmental levels appear to benefit from more complex interventions than children at lower cognitive developmental levels (Shirk, 2001), though studies specifically examining the relationship between age and psychotherapy have mixed outcomes (Weisz et al., 1987; Dush et al., 1989; Durlak et al., 1991; Weiss et al., 1999).

- The therapeutic alliance appears to influence psychotherapy outcome in youth. Children whose parents have a better relationship with the therapist fare better (Kazdin & Wassel, 1999).

Specific psychological approaches

Behaviour therapy

Behaviour therapy (BT), applicable across diagnoses, uses a problem-solving approach. But it is understood that behaviours carry meanings for the actor and for those around them and require attention to help understand them. Behavioural approaches are used in learning difficulties, autism spectrum disorders, ADHD, and externalizing behaviour disorders, as well as with intensely anxious children and those with OCD. BT has been applied in classroom settings and to promote positive playground social interactions (Dolan et al., 1993). As children become older, more cognitive elements are introduced.

Cognitive behavioural therapy

Cognitive behavioural therapy (CBT) can be applied to a wide range of child and adolescent disorders. Good evidence exists for treatment of anxiety and mild depressive disorders with less good evidence for moderate and severe depression (Compton et al., 2004). Age, gender, and cognitive ability modify the techniques used with children and families. Cognitions are often embedded in feelings though children are thought to have a limited repertoire for emotion recognition while young contributing to limited and distorted cognitions around social interactions. Designing CBT interventions for particular disorders takes these factors into account, modifying it for the particular child's needs. The stronger behavioural focus of CBT designed for children gives way to increasing cognitive components during adolescence (Graham, 1998; Kendall, 2000).

Delivery of CBT to children and adolescents in the context of internalizing disorders employs certain principles. Children rarely seek treatment by themselves and may resent being brought for help. A working alliance needs to be established. Education about CBT's methods is useful for adolescents so that they can become independent in their treatment, improving chances of treatment success. For younger children, family involvement in goal setting and in helping the child improve socialization is essential. These considerations reduce the therapy dropout rate. Often parents are made anxious by their child's difficulties and a family anxiety management component can improve outcome (Barrett et al., 1996a; Brent et al., 1998). Family members can deliver CBT to their younger children (Barrett et al., 1996a). Family discord, poor cohesion, and a lack of external support contribute to poorer outcome (Birmaher et al., 2000; Brent et al., 1998).

Family and systemic therapy

Family and systemic therapy, an important child treatment approach because children develop in family contexts and are affected by familial behaviours and beliefs, has some empirical research support. Family therapies that incorporate BT techniques assume greater prominence with younger children; those linked more to the family belief systems or discussion of relationship qualities become more useful in later childhood and adolescence. Typically a behavioural family therapy model will be employed with children with oppositional defiant disorder. In anorexia nervosa, a style combining elements of a structural family therapy with a non-blaming examination of family belief systems, is used (Seifer et al., 1992).

Not all adolescent problems respond well to an approach focusing on improved understanding of family beliefs. That approach appears ineffective in delinquency, but a primarily behavioural approach involving some negotiation with the adolescent does have an evidence base. Underorganized families do better with more structured, directive approaches; families that are relatively wellfunctioning benefit from more narrative/social constructionist approaches (Hampson & Beavers, 1996).

The research literature for family therapy remains small. Most outcome research is slanted towards behaviourally based interventions. Yet many of the ideas of family therapy are incorporated into child and adolescent mental health practice so that systemic approaches are embedded even in non-family therapy psychotherapy. Involving parents directly in family therapy or in a parallel cognitive style of therapy easily integrated with the child's therapy has been shown to be effective.

Parent training

Parent and family skills training has growing evidence for its efficacy. The programmes concentrate on working with the parents of preschool and middle childhood children with adaptations for parents of adolescents. The goals are improvement of the relationship between the parents and target child through age-appropriate shared activities, learning to give specific praise to the child and to establish behavioural reward programmes. Methods include non-aggressive techniques for limiting unwanted behaviours while emphasizing and reinforcing wanted behaviours rather than those they wish to extinguish (Bank et al., 1991).

Elements of parenting programmes that increase efficacy:

- therapist's ability to establish good relationships with families;
- a structured, active, and focused approach;
- avoiding confrontation by offering support, asking questions, and engaging the parents in discussion;
- using dialogue to help parents and families discover what they should work on and how to reach their goals;
- employing manualized programmes with rigorous training,

standardized delivery, and supervision;

- providing a sufficient dose of the programme (for most families, 10–18 sessions produces significant, clinically important change) though in some cases higher doses (frequency and length of programme) are necessary.

Parent skills training techniques are important with oppositional defiant disorder and obsessive compulsive disorder. Adaptations have been used with children who have ADHD.

Individual psychodynamic therapy

Psychodynamic approaches to the treatment of children and adolescents have a long history. Drive theory has been replaced by object relations theory and attachment theory, theoretical frameworks that can more easily be empirically tested. Working with parents to enable them to support the child's therapy is essential (Kennedy, 2004). Child psychotherapists frequently provide consultation to other professionals working in a variety of settings with distressed children.

Interpersonal therapy (IPT)

Adapted for use with adolescents, individual interpersonal therapy for depression is designed as a once weekly therapy for 12 weeks (Mufson et al., 1999).

Experiential therapies

The evidence base for experiential therapies in child and adolescent mental health is extremely limited. Nonetheless, music therapy, art therapy, dance and movement therapies, and drama therapy are used for children and adolescents in conditions ranging from autism to severe eating disorders. Some children seem better able to explore their feelings and their interactions through these media than through talking therapies.

Group therapy

Group therapies, surprisingly limited in their application, can be effective interventions (Kazdin et al., 1990). Group content must be adapted to the patients' developmental stage and may have restricted age ranges because of developmental issues. Some groups are designed to try to address specific issues such as sexual abuse. Strategies for psychodynamic and other non-directive relationship-based group therapies have become more similar over time with a clearer focus on current interactions being common.

Table 39.1 Effectiveness of psychological treatments for children and adolescents

Treatment	Form of treatment	Psychiatric disorder/target audience	Level of evidence for efficacy	Comments
Clinically guided individual psychotherapy	Psychodynamic and other clinically guided psychotherapies	Child psychiatric disorders in general	Ia, II	Variable evidence with better results in research settings that may not be generalizable
Clinically (research) structured individual psychotherapy	Often CBT but other manualized treatments	Child psychiatric disorders in general	IIa	More evidence that behavioural treatments may be more effective for some disorders than psychodynamic, but definitive studies have yet to be conducted
Family therapy	From psychodynamic and systems through behavioural and cognitive behavioural	Child psychiatric disorders in general	IIIa	Most empirical research has been done on behavioural therapy which can lead to the (false) impression that this is the only type of family therapy that is effective

Table 39.1 (cont.)

Treatment	Form of treatment	Psychiatric disorder/target audience	Level of evidence for efficacy	Comments
Parent and family skills training	Essentially psychoeducational approaches	Child psychiatric disorders in general	IIb	Appears to be particularly useful in externalizing disorders
Group therapy	Psychodynamic and non-directive	Child psychiatric disorders in general	IV	Probably useful in older children and adolescents. Widely used but probably without sufficient empirical support
Group therapy	Social skills and problem solving (psychoeducational and directive)	Child psychiatric disorders in general	III	Slightly more evidence base than for non-directive groups but still empirical support is quite thin

Social skills groups and problem-solving skills training

Social skills training is used in a variety of situations with children including oppositional defiant disorder, conduct disorder, anger management, and ADHD. It has been applied to child sexual abuse, drug abuse, anxiety disorder, depression, and separation and divorce. Many use social skills training in group settings but others, particularly when focusing on externalizing disorders in older children, utilize individual therapy.

Interventions discussed in this chapter are summarized in Table 39.1.

40

Drugs and other physical treatments

Based on "Drugs and other physical treatments" by Brian W. Jacobs, Jennifer A. Varley, and Jon McClellan in Effective Treatments in Psychiatry, Cambridge University Press, 2008

General issues in paediatric psychopharmacology

In the USA, an estimated 6% of young people under the age of 20 years receive prescriptions for psychotropic medication with a two- to three-fold increase over the past 15 years, particularly among adolescents. Prescribing rates now closely approximate adult populations (Zito et al., 2000; 2003). In the early 1990s, there was a three-fold increase in stimulant usage for preschoolers (Zito et al., 2000). In the UK, though medication is used less and has been studied less, there has also been a sharp increase in prescribing over the past decade. Clark (2004) found that 73% of drug prescriptions were accounted for by eight drugs (methylphenidate, methylphenidate/placebo trial, paroxetine, fluoxetine, risperidone, imipramine, dexamphetamine, and melatonin), and there is concern about this increase in prescribing, especially in the prescribing of psychostimulants (Wong et al., 2003).

Ethics and psychotropic drug prescribing

There have been increasing concerns about the lack of evidence for the safety and efficacy of medicines prescribed for children and adolescents. As evidence increases, the balance between the risks and benefits of medications can become clearer (Jureidini et al., 2004). In the USA, there is an FDA "black box" warning specifically advising clinicians of the increased risk of suicidality in children and adolescents with the use of SSRIs. In the UK, advice from the Committee on the Safety of Medicines resulted in dramatic restrictions in the use of these medications for depression in people under the age of 18 (Department of Health, 2003b). Research exploring whether this restriction will reduce the rate of completed or attempted suicide in depressed adolescents suggests that there has been an increase in the suicide rate. Data from the USA (2003–2004) as well as from the Netherlands (2003–2005) suggest that while there was about a 20% decrease in the rate of SSRI prescriptions in both countries, the suicide rate increased by 14% in the USA and by almost 50% in the Netherlands in patients up to the age of 19 (Macey et al., 2005; Gibbons et al., 2007).

Biological development and drug metabolism and distribution

Brain

The rapid development of the brain prenatally and in the early years has major implications for all aspects of child and adolescent treatment and certainly for psychopharmacological treatment (Carrey et al., 2002). Overdevelopment of neurons and synapses with subsequent pruning occurs in early childhood and then again later in early adolescence (Insel, 1995). Monoamine-secreting neurons have been shown in animal models to play an important time-specific role in orientating the arrival of other axons into the cortex (Zecevic & Verney, 1995). These neurotransmitters are detectable by week 5 of human gestation. Serotonin levels in the postnatal cortex of mice are approximately twice those seen in adult mice (Hohman et al., 1988). In children aged 3 months to 3 years there are high levels of monoamine neurotransmitters that decline after age 5 years (Whitaker-Azmitia et al., 1996). We are only beginning to understand the complex development of the brain. This suggests caution in the administration of psychotropic medication to children since psychotropic drugs impact neurotransmitter concentrations.

Physical and hormonal development

Children grow continuously but with a marked growth spurt in early to mid-adolescence accompanied by a changing metabolism with some enzyme systems becoming less prominent whilst others become more prominent. As the child grows up, these changes can impact pharmacological handling of medication and potential drug interactions. Further, hormonal changes of puberty, first evident in children of 6 years, affect young people's psychological development, their self view, and the disorders to which they are vulnerable.

Drug distribution and metabolism

Children's bodies handle drugs differently from adults (Vinks & Walson, 2003). Depending on their age and pubertal status, they have lower ratios of adipose tissue to water compared to adults (Morselli et al., 1980; Kearns & Reed, 1989) that can markedly affect drug distribution as well as the accumulation of fat-solvent medicines and their metabolites. Body fat is greatest during the first year, falling until puberty when it rises again (Milsap & Szefler, 1986). But rather than expecting to see a higher plasma concentration for the lipophilic neuroleptics and antidepressants in proportion to the dose administered when compared to adults, the reverse is usually true because of higher drug metabolism and clearance rates in these younger people.

Drug protein binding also differs between children of different ages (Grandison & Boudinot, 2000), and protein binding differentially affects the bioavailability of medication. Serum albumin concentrations do not change markedly from early childhood so that this will not be a major factor for binding sites for acidic drugs. Protein binding is affected by diseases that reduce the protein levels. For example, sodium valproate (used as an anti-epileptic and also as a mood stabilizer) can saturate the protein at therapeutic levels producing sudden toxicity as bioavailability increases.

Relative to their size children have a greater hepatic metabolic capacity with kidneys more efficient than those of adults in eliminating drugs. Thus given sufficient hydration, children dispose of lithium more rapidly than adults.

There is poor information on the absorption of medication by children. Parents often administer drugs in ways unplanned in their formulation, e.g. crushing tablets, dissolving medications in soft drinks, etc. The effects of these modifications on the absorption and stability of medicines is largely unknown. Drug concentrations often peak earlier in children than in adults because of a more rapid clearance of the drug by children (Vinks & Walson, 2003). The apparent reduced volume of distribution for drugs in children also reduces the half-life of drugs given to children relative to adults. This can be important in drugs with a

Table 40.1 Effectiveness of drugs and other physical treatments

Treatment	Form of treatment	Psychiatric disorder/ target audience	Level of evidence for efficacy	Comments
Psychopharmacology	SSRIs	Depression and anxiety	Ia–IIb	Improvement over placebo in both depressive and anxiety disorders. Greater efficacy in depression. Fluoxetine is the SSRI with the most supporting evidence. OCD is the anxiety disorder most responsive to SSRIs
Psychopharmacology	Antipsychotics	Autism	Ib	Improvement in stereotypes, withdrawal, irritability, temper outburst. Risperidone just approved for autism in USA
Psychopharmacology	Antipsychotics	Schizophrenia	Ib	Superior to placebo. Clozapine may be very effective but side effects even more prominent here
Psychopharmacology	Antipsychotics	Tourette's	Ia	Superior to placebo. Reduces tics and outbursts
Psychopharmacology	Antipsychotics	Conduct disorder	IIb	Studies lack good methodology
Psychopharmacology	Lithium	Bipolar disorder	IIb	Improvement in mood
Psychopharmacology	Mood stabilizers	Disruptive/explosive behaviours	III	Open studies. Other methodological problems
Somatic therapy	ECT	Mood disorders	III	No real comparison studies done. Very small numbers

narrow therapeutic dose range and result in a need for more frequent administration than in older adolescents or adults. An example is provided by imipramine which has a half-life of 11–42 hours in children aged 5–12 whilst in adolescents aged 13–16, its half-life increases to 14–89 hours.

Physical therapies

ECT

Child and adolescent psychiatrists have generally been antagonistic to the use of ECT in the UK and elsewhere. In the USA, there has been some use of ECT in adolescents, and guidelines are available though in actuality there are few good data-driven indicators as to when to offer ECT to adolescents (Ghazziuddin et al., 2004a). Use as a treatment for adolescents seems to be growing in Australia and New Zealand (Walter & Rey, 2003). Taieb et al. (2000) found that adolescents who had had ECT for a severe mood disorder were generally positive about the treatment particularly after a lack of responsiveness to medication made it easier for the parents to agree to this treatment. In the midst of these differences of opinion we must consider the risk of the error of omission, i.e. not giving an effective treatment because of a fear of the risks when there is not much evidence for such risks (Rudnick, 2001).

Interventions discussed in this chapter are summarized in Table 40.1.

41

Educational interventions and alternative treatments

Based on "Educational interventions and alternative treatments" by Brian W. Jacobs, Michael Storck, Ann Vander Stoep, and Wendy Weber in Effective Treatments in Psychiatry, Cambridge University Press, 2008

Interventions in schools

Various interventions have been developed to help manage young people's psychological difficulties in schools. Examples include, but are not limited to:

- To consult or train, e.g. to the teacher to help better manage the child in class.
- To deal with school-wide issues such as bullying.
- To deliver and present early intervention programmes designed to inhibit escalation of difficulties into clinical problems. These programmes may be applied to small groups of children or as a universal programme to classes of children.
- To develop tactics and strategies to help with psychological difficulties in children and staff after traumatic episodes or disasters.

An advantage of intervening in a school setting is that one can gain more regular access to the child once appropriate consent has been obtained. Making a whole school or whole class intervention avoids identification of the target child/children. This approach aims to enhance the understanding and capacity of other children and teachers to help children with particular difficulties by improving the social problem-solving skills of all class members.

Providing parent skills programmes in school settings can be a non-stigmatizing way of reaching parents of vulnerable children. The concern is that the parents who are prepared to attend such programmes will only be the anxious parents of those who do not need the help though in practice little evidence supports this concern.

Teacher training

Teacher training may be purely educational about particular disorders, e.g. autism, epilepsy, ADHD, etc., or may aim to achieve change in classroom management or intervene specifically in classroom discipline. These are often clinic programmes adapted to the classroom or other settings.

Small group therapy in school settings

There are anger management programmes developed to deliver to small groups of pupils in school settings (Nelson III & Finch, 2000). CBT for secondary school youngsters at high risk for depression have been successfully delivered; results suggest reductions in subsequent affective disorders by almost half (Clarke et al., 1995).

Assisting selected children to improve their social skills through specific school programmes has not produced durable changes in the number of friends of the child, although it was possible to improve the child's social network (Oden & Asher, 1977; Gresham & Nagle, 1980). Using a parent-requested parent-assisted social skills training for parents of children aged 7–12 showed promising early results for boys with poor social skills (Frankel et al., 1996).

Bullying interventions and whole school positive behaviour programmes

McCarthy and Carr (2002) review whole school strategies to prevent bullying. Bloomquist and Schnell (2002) review school-wide interventions designed to promote positive behaviour in children with aggressive and conduct problems. Olweus et al.'s (2000) work in Norway has been seminal in this field.

Successful programmes pay attention to system responses to ensure correct procedures will be consistently followed throughout the school and to foster a positive atmosphere in the school within a positive school climate (Bloomquist & Schnell, 2002). They do their best to create a positive school climate. They define behavioural expectations clearly and support positive behaviour while providing consistent and effective responses to problem behaviours with a clear and predictable hierarchy of responses. There are strategies that are applied at a whole school level for classrooms and at the individual level (McCarthy & Carr, 2002). At an individual level, incidents are discussed with the bully, victim, and their parents as soon as they are discovered. Sanctions are applied jointly with parents, but if an incident cannot be resolved, the bully and not the victim changes class. Victims receive assertiveness training. Bully courts may be used in which peers hear both sides of the story.

Whole class interventions as prevention/early intervention

Theoretically, a whole class intervention enables change in the high-risk target children while producing more highly skilled social behaviour in the children around the target child, with the goal of insulating the particular child against his or her particular vulnerability. Since children quickly decide on the social acceptability of their peers, opinions can be difficult to change even with improvement in the target child's behaviour (Hymel et al., 1990). Whole class interventions can be beneficial for children vulnerable to developing behavioural difficulties.

Webster-Stratton & Reid (2004) have adapted their clinical social skills and social problem-solving skills programme, intended to protect children vulnerable to developing oppositional defiant disorder and conduct disorder, for use as a universal classroom intervention. Webster-Stratton et al. (2008) showed medium to large effect sizes on both teacher behaviour in improved discipline style and on child behaviour and management with very large effect sizes for the most behaviourally disturbed children. The class teacher co-presents this programme, the Dinosaur School, together with a trained Dinosaur School interventionist as a twice weekly lesson during the school. The programme uses puppets about the same size as a 5-year-old child to help the children learn classroom rules, recognize emotions, and engage in social problem-solving scenarios such as how to join games, share, pay compliments, etc., that children with behavioural difficulties typically fail with compared with their peers. There are many opportunities during classes to practise skills being learnt. Between lessons the teacher uses every opportunity to remind the children about the concepts and helps students apply them. The programme is captivating for children and has the advantage that the whole cohort of children in the class are given the same language and tools for social negotiation and conflict management.

The vulnerable child is then, hopefully, in a "super-skilled" classroom environment during the year and, if the class stays together, in the future.

Reid and colleagues (Eddy et al., 2003) have developed a programme for grade 2–5 children with similar principles although with a different presentation style. This programme provided some protection against arrest and alcohol use subsequently in middle school.

Multisystemic therapy

Child mental health services have traditionally engaged families for quite prolonged periods of a year or more but many of the most vulnerable families would drop out of treatments early. Satterfield et al. (1981) found that a variety of different approaches were often required over a 2-year period for children with ADHD to produce lasting change, illustrating the complexity of these cases.

Up to 80% of offending adolescents who are involved in the criminal justice system have psychiatric disorders. Recognizing that psychiatric disorders may reduce the likelihood of successful rehabilitation, the juvenile justice system and UK government have supported the development of evidence-based interventions to reduce criminal recidivism and improve reintegration to home, school, and community.

Multisystemic therapy (MST) (Henggeler et al., 1998) aims to empower parents with the skills and resources needed to successfully deter adolescents from engaging in criminal activities. During the 3–5 month intervention, MST therapists work with families, schools, and communities to reorganize behavioural contingencies to reinforce protective factors and lessen risk factors within all systems in which the adolescent operates. The effectiveness of MST in controlled clinical trials with impoverished inner-city juvenile offenders and adolescent sexual offenders was supported with a more than 50% decrease in arrests than would be expected with usual service conditions and individual therapy (Henggeler et al., 1992; Borduin et al., 1995). MST has been disseminated widely and currently supports licensed sites in 7 countries and 28 states in the USA. Developing similar systems in the UK has been hampered by a chronic lack of resources in child and adolescent mental health services (CAMHS).

Results of intensive home-based treatments are variable. Some programmes have produced reduced symptomatology and improved quality of life (Burns et al., 1996) whilst others have had less encouraging results (Bickman, 1996). Case management with high quality of the individual components of treatment available within it appears essential (Henggeler et al., 1998).

Treatment foster care

Treatment foster care and multisystemic therapy are described as exemplary service modalities offered to children with psychiatric disorders within the child welfare and juvenile justice systems. More than half a million US children presently live in foster homes. The majority of these children have psychiatric illness (Clausen et al., 1998) that can compromise their likelihood of stability in foster care placement. Implemented within child welfare systems since the 1980s, therapeutic (or treatment) foster care (TFC) combines the normalizing influence of family-based foster care with specialized treatment interventions. The goal is to create a structured therapeutic environment within the context of a nurturant family and neighborhood (Chamberlain, 1990).

TFC is one of the most widely used forms of out-of-home placement for children with severe emotional and behavioural disorders and is considered to be the least restrictive form of residential care. Core elements of the TFC model include: pre-service training; augmented financial support for foster parents; a mental health therapist or case manager assigned to assist treatment foster parents; weekly support and training meetings with other TFC parents; 24-hour, 7-day a week on call access; and respite services. Studies have shown that youth who participate in TFC experience better post-discharge adjustment and stability compared to youth served in congregate care facilities (Clarke et al., 1995; Chamberlain & Reid, 1998). Family-Centred Intensive Case Management (FCICM), an innovative variation on TFC, involves similar specialized training, with intensive professional and peer support, and respite care provided to the child's biological or adoptive family. There is mixed evidence from trials thus far.

The family preservation services (FPS) model keeps the young person at home with parents but includes very intensive home-based and community interventions (Chamberlain & Rosicky, 1995). The programme takes place over 2–4 months and requires many hours of professional time each week. It has a mixed outcome. One RCT determined that children who remain at home with their own family while receiving these supports experience the same or better outcomes than children placed in the homes of professional parents (Evans et al., 1998).

Inpatient treatment

There is a radically different model of using inpatient services in the USA

Table 41.1 Effectiveness of educational and educative interventions

Treatment	Form of treatment	Psychiatric disorder/target audience	Level of evidence for efficacy	Comments
Small group therapy in schools	Psychoeducation	School children to prevent depression	Ib	Found reduction in subsequent incidence of affective disorders
Social skills training in schools	Designed course	School children	III	Preliminary evidence of improvement in social skills of boys
Bullying and whole school positive behaviour programmes	Designed programmes	Schools where bullying is a problem	IV	Though practised widely, no real controlled studies found
Whole school prevention programmes	Designed programme	School population	IV	May provide some protection against arrest and alcohol use in middle school
Multisystemic therapy	Designed programme	General psychiatric disorders of childhood and adolescence	IIa	A decrease in arrest rates
Foster care treatment	Intensive designed treatment	General psychiatric disorders of childhood and adolescence	IIb	Better post-discharge stability
Inpatient treatment	Various programmes	Severe and dangerous behaviour	III	Evidence suggests that longer lengths of stay may be valuable especially in reducing the need for intensive specialty services post discharge

and the UK. In recent USA practice, admissions are limited to a few days in length. Inpatient admissions funded through health insurance in the USA were reduced in length from 14.4 days in 1997 to 11.5 days in 2000. Admissions that previously treated crisis conditions and situations now focus on triaging cases for treatment elsewhere. Admissions are increasingly restricted to very high risk cases of danger, often to others. This state of affairs has raised concern over the past few years.

In the UK, admissions are usually substantially longer with an average of 117 days in a recent study (Green et al., 2007). The admission is used as treatment in its own right. A recent US outcome study showed some change by discharge but the change was lost 1 month later (Dickerson Mayes et al., 2001), whilst the UK study of four adolescent and four children's units with longer admissions produced change that lasted a year post discharge (Green et al., 2007). Longer lengths of stay were associated with a better outcome at 1 year follow-up post discharge.

Jacobs and colleagues (Jacobs et al., 2009) suggest that inpatient child and adolescent psychiatry in the UK is an effective treatment for severe, complex cases. The treatment reduces severity from needing highly specialized services to that of cases more typically seen in community mental health services. The study was not controlled with random allocation because such a design would currently be unethical with these very severe cases but it has a number of internal features that suggest that the improvements seen are not just due to the passage of time.

Complementary and alternative medicine

The evidence base for the use of complementary medicines in children and adolescents is poor. This does not deter desperate parents. Complementary medicines are more frequently used in the USA (36%) than the UK (10%). A survey of parents in the Washington DC area found that 21% of parents had used CAM treatment for their children (Ottolini et al., 2001). In families where the child has a chronic mental health condition such as ADHD, the percent of families utilizing CAM treatments is even higher. The variance is most likely due to the definitions of CAM used in each of the surveys. While the Internet provides a plethora of testimonials of cures associated with CAM treatments, the scientific research on CAM therapies is limited. Well-controlled trials conducted in paediatric populations are particularly scarce.

Interventions discussed in this chapter are summarized in Table 41.1.

42

Attachment insecurity and attachment disorder

Based on "Attachment insecurity and attachment disorder" by Jonathan Green, Ming Wai Wan, and Michelle DeKlyen in Effective Treatments in Psychiatry, Cambridge University Press, 2008

Introduction

Attachment refers to the affectional bond or relationship of a child to a caregiver. Its quality is known to be strongly associated with social development and mental health. Research on normative patterns of infant attachment finds that "attachment insecurity" (including "disorganization") is a psychosocial risk factor, best conceptualized as a developmental risk variable within multiaxial classification (Green & Goldwyn, 2002).

Two relatively uncommon forms of developmental disturbance associated with severe disruption or absence of early attachment relationships are recognized as Axis 1 clinical disorders in both DSM and ICD systems. ICD-10 describes two separate syndromes: (1) "disinhibited attachment disorder", characterized by indiscriminate sociability and associated particularly with absence of early attachment relationships (as in institutional care); and (2) "inhibited" or "reactive" attachment disorder (RAD), typically associated with disrupted attachment, neglect, or maltreatment. DSM-IV defines "reactive attachment disorder" with two subtypes closely paralleling the separate disorders in ICD-10. The generic term "attachment disorder" is used to apply to both syndromes here.

Research into attachment security/insecurity and attachment disorder suggests that they be thought of as occurring on a spectrum. Green (2003) has suggested that attachment disorder in later childhood may be better characterized as an independent social impairment syndrome and will be considered separately here.

Interventions for attachment insecurity

Characteristics of the attachment relationship are inferred from either the behaviour of the child within the relationship, particularly on reunion after separation, or from the child's mental representation of the relationship. Determinants of child attachments have been found in both caregiver behaviour (responsiveness or sensitivity) and caregiver attachment representation. Intervention strategies have largely addressed one of these caregiver aspects, either as primary prevention in high-risk groups or as intervention in children with attachment insecurity. No interventions are officially endorsed or widely used.

Behaviourally based interventions focused on increasing caregiver sensitivity

Carefully tailored behavioural interventions that are brief, use personalized feedback on interaction (often videotaped), and encourage parenting sensitivity and responsiveness are most effective for the short term. In an RCT of three sessions with parents of irritable infants aged 6–9 months from low socioeconomic status (SES) families (known to be at risk of developing insecure attachment), infant security significantly increased and attachment disorganization decreased at 1 year, compared to controls (van den Boom, 1994; 1995).

Another brief intervention with biological and adoptive parents of infants including video feedback targeting sensitive parenting accompanied by written materials has increased attachment security (Juffer et al., 1997) and reduced attachment disorganization (Juffer et al., 2005) for some children. Written materials alone were not effective. Sensitivity-focused techniques combined with enhancing motor skills and coordination in low birth weight infants were effective in improving attachment security (Sajaniemi et al., 2001). Other interventions involving other high-risk groups (Murray et al., 2003) have not found significant effects on attachment despite increasing parents' sensitivity. Maternal sensitivity is easier to influence than infant attachment behaviour.

Psychodynamic or representation-focused interventions

One US RCT of intensive psychodynamic mother–infant psychotherapy work with high-risk mothers and their infants increased attachment security and reduced attachment disorganization compared with controls; so did a psychoeducational intervention (Cicchetti et al., 2006). Another study found improved empathy in parenting but no significant alteration in child attachment behaviours (Lieberman et al., 1991). An RCT of parent psychotherapy with depressed mothers and their toddlers (mean age 20 months) showed a positive effect on security at 36 months (Cicchetti et al., 1999).

Three European studies used interventions focused on changing parent's own underlying cognitions ("representations") in relation to attachment relationships; either alone (Murray et al., 2003) or in conjunction with behavioural techniques (Klein Velderman et al., 2006). Positive effects were found for maternal mood (Cooper et al., 2003) and sensitivity but not for child attachment status. It was suggested that mothers with a "preoccupied" attachment representation may

differentially benefit from such a representation-focused intervention. No evidence currently exists to either confirm or refute this hypothesis.

Psychosocial support and counselling for caregivers

Psychosocial support and counselling for caregivers is probably the most widely used intervention involving relatively non-specific support over the prenatal period or first 2 years. Three RCTs (2 US, 1 UK) show the benefits of such programmes on general maternal functioning and sensitivity in high social adversity situations but no associated effect on infant attachment (Barnard et al., 1988; Beckwith, 1988; Murray et al., 2003). In contrast, two US studies showed no effect on maternal sensitivity but some increase in infant security over controls (Lyons-Ruth et al., 1990; Jacobson & Frye, 1991).

Attachment-focused group interventions for parents

A 20-week group intervention for high-risk insecure parent–child dyads utilizes videotaped feedback, parent education, and psychotherapy to shift caregivers' views of and interactions with their children. Pre-post studies indicate an increase in secure attachments (Hoffman et al., 2006).

Placement with foster parents

While this is arguably the most radical intervention, foster parenting is widely used in high-risk situations. Dozier et al. (2001) studied 50 children from very adverse environments (typically associated with risk for attachment disorganization) who had early alternate care placement (mean 7.7 months). After several months (mean 9.2 months) attachment pattern distribution was similar to low-risk birth families, suggesting the consequences of the early risk had been avoided by alternate care. Stams et al. (2001) studied 146 internationally early-adopted infants at 7 years follow-up compared to birth siblings from the same family. Outcome for adopted children was similar to birth children. Attachment security was related to adoptive mothers' sensitivity and led to better social and cognitive development.

Children in foster care typically exhibit poor social emotional outcomes. Initial evidence from a 10-week home visiting programme (Dozier et al., 2007) designed to support and educate foster parents so that they will provide more nurturing and appropriate care indicates higher post-treatment rates for secure attachment as well as more normal cortisol patterns compared to controls (Dozier et al., 2006).

Summary

A variety of programmes have been developed to alter insecure attachment. European studies have tended to focus on specific high-risk groups (inter-racial adoptive families, extremely low birth weight infants, infants whose mothers have post-natal depression) whereas many American studies involved disadvantaged families whose risk factors are broader, multiple, and complex. European interventions have tended to be brief and focused while many US studies have been of multifaceted psychosocial interventions and psychotherapy. Comparisons between intervention approaches are hampered by the diversity of interventions and heterogeneity of samples and outcome measures. There have been limited replication studies.

A meta-analysis of interventions for enhancing maternal sensitivity and infant attachment (Bakermans-Kranenburg et al., 2003) found an overall positive but small effect size ($d = 0.20$) on attachment security. Evidence to date suggests that interventions with best effect specifically targeted caregiver sensitivity and behaviour. There is some evidence from the USA to support psychodynamically oriented approaches. Early placement in alternate care may have a positive impact on attachment outcomes, particularly if accompanied by well-designed supportive intervention. No interventions are recommended in official national guidelines.

Treatment choice should be guided by its congruence with attachment theory, the clarity of its objectives (e.g. focus on developing caregiver sensitivity or changing internal working models of attachment), and appropriateness to the population (e.g. biological versus foster parents, multi-risk versus well-functioning families).

Interventions for attachment disorders

No intervention for attachment disorder has been endorsed in national guidelines. There is broad consensus that research has been insufficient to recommend any specific treatment. Placement in a foster or adoptive home may be the most common intervention.

Provision of "normal" caregiving as a non-specific intervention

Romanian children in a "standard" orphanage were compared with others in a small unit designed to provide more consistent caregiving and a group of never-institutionalized toddlers. Inhibited and indiscriminate behaviours were less evident among children raised in the environments with fewer and more consistent caregivers. Two or more years after placement the developmental status of many of these Romanian orphans had improved (Rutter, 1998; O'Connor et al., 1999); they were more likely to be securely attached but some were still indiscriminately sociable (O'Connor et al., 1999; Rutter & Sonuga-Barke, 2010). Similar findings have been reported by Zeanah et al. (2002). Many adoptees in a Canadian sample became securely attached several months after adoption, but indiscriminate sociability had not diminished. Indiscriminate sociability, associated with length of time in an institution, appears particularly intransigent but not necessarily associated with attachment security. Parallel findings have been made in UK children in care after early maltreatment (Minnis et al., 2009).

Psychoeducational intervention with caregivers

Short-term treatment based on the TEACCH programme, originally developed for autistic children, resulted in improved social, language, and behavioural development in young children with attachment disorder following maternal depression and neglect (Mukaddes et al., 2004). TEACCH focuses on supporting

Table 42.1 Effectiveness of intervention approaches to attachment in security and attachment disorder

Treatment	Form of treatment	Psychiatric disorder/ target audience	Level of evidence for efficacy	Comments
Parental sensitivity training	Various short-term interventions	Parents of children at risk of attachment insecurity	Ia	Maternal sensitivity to the infant is increased but the question remains as to whether this actually improves infant attachment
Psychodynamic or representation-focused interventions	Psychodynamic	Parents of children at risk of attachment insecurity	Ia	Maternal sensitivity to the infant is increased but the question remains as to whether this actually improves infant attachment
Psychosocial support and counselling for caregivers	Non-specific supportive therapy	Parents of children at risk of attachment insecurity	Ib	Existing data are equivocal but suggest some benefits for the parents
Attachment focused groups for parents	Short-term group for parents using psychotherapy and parent education	Parents of children at risk of attachment insecurity	IV	Increase in secure attachments
Placement with selected foster parents	Outplacement from family home to foster home	Children at risk of attachment insecurity	III	Outcome appears to be positive and can reduce or eliminate risk of future disturbed attachment patterns

Table 42.1 (cont.)

Treatment	Form of treatment	Psychiatric disorder/ target audience	Level of evidence for efficacy	Comments
Normal caregiving in alternate situations (i.e. adoption)	Adoption	Children with attachment disorder	III	Attachment became more secure, children improved developmental status, but indiscriminate social behaviour persisted
Psychoeducation for caregivers	TEACCH Programme	Children with attachment disorder	III	Improved attachment and behavioural (social and language) adjustment

Note: Contraindicated treatment: so-called "holding therapy" techniques present potentially serious risks to children and are contraindicated (see text).

parents by teaching them to cope with aggression, to enhance language, and to improve self-care skills while practising child-directed play.

"Attachment therapy" or "holding therapy"

"Holding therapy" and other similar so-called "attachment therapies" involve intrusive, coercive, and sustained restraint of the child. They have been widely criticized for inconsistency with attachment theory, lack of efficacy research, and potentially harmful effects. Such interventions have been in use for some years but only one, non-randomized outcome study has been published; it was marred by serious methodological shortcomings, and neither its definition of disorder nor its outcome measures (aggression and delinquency) are specific to attachment disorder. The American Psychiatric Association (2002) specifies that these coercive therapies are contraindicated and potentially dangerous (child deaths have been reported). It is a serious concern that, despite this, the techniques remain in use by some practitioners and parents in the USA and UK.

Summary

Placement of children with attachment disorders in adoptive homes often results in improved functioning, but social and attentional symptoms may linger. Effective treatments are likely to include components to: (1) build a nurturant, secure parent–child relationship, (2) address behaviour problems, (3) remedy skill deficits (e.g. language, emotional regulation, and social skills), and (4) support caregivers.

All interventions should address other problems these children may exhibit, such as behaviour problems, language and cognitive delays, attention deficits, poor social skills, and post-traumatic stress. Programmes that teach foster parents to manage difficult behaviours are particularly promising. Studies in the USA and Europe have shown much convergence in this area.

Interventions discussed in this chapter are summarized in Table 42.1.

43

Feeding and sleeping disorders in infancy and early childhood

Based on "Feeding and sleeping disorders in infancy and early childhood" by Heather Carmichael Olson, Nancy C. Winters, Sally L. Davidson Ward, and Matthew Hodes in Effective Treatments in Psychiatry, Cambridge University Press, 2008

Treatment of feeding disorders

Background

Feeding disorders imply a relationship context (Chatoor, 2002) and can have medical and behavioural components. Feeding disorders are distinguished from failure to thrive (FTT). FTT is defined as either: (1) not maintaining expected rate of weight gain over time (weight < 5% on a standardized growth grid); or (2) deviation downward by two major centiles for at least 1 month in duration. FTT is an *outcome* of any condition resulting in growth impairment and is *not* a diagnosis. The DSM-IV-TR diagnostic term "feeding disorder of infancy and early childhood" requires both feeding refusal and growth impairment. The ICD-10 definition is broader, including: Criterion A, "persistent failure to eat adequately, or persistent rumination or regurgitation of food"; Criterion B, "the child fails to gain weight, loses weight, or exhibits some other significant health problem over at least 1 month". The broader construct, "feeding problems NOS," may include behaviourally driven food refusal or disordered eating not necessarily adversely affecting growth or physical health.

Feeding disturbances are common in children (Reau et al., 1996). In one large UK study, parents reported about 10% of 3-year-olds had "faddy eating" and 16% with poor appetite, symptoms that cluster and show continuity with other behavioural problems. Severe feeding problems that interfere with growth have a prevalence of 1–5% in infants and as high as 80% among children with developmental delays.

Aetiologies of feeding disturbances are not well understood but thought to be multifactorial. Proposed feeding disorder subtypes range from those with presumed underlying organic/ medical aetiology to those thought of as primarily behavioural. Given their multifactorial nature and the transactional process of child development, multidisciplinary treatment (teams including a paediatrician, speech or occupational therapist, nutritionist, and mental health professional) is common (Black et al., 1995; Winters, 2003). Specific interventions can be primarily medical (i.e. tube feeding to correct malnutrition) or can address behavioural, developmental, or relational aspects of feeding refusal (Chatoor, 2002). Recent literature explores treatment for feeding difficulties in special populations (Kodak & Piazza, 2008).

Treatment approaches by category of feeding disturbance

Feeding disorder of infancy or early childhood (infant feeding disorder of non-organic origin)

Treatment of children with primarily organic/medical explanations for food refusal that require appropriate medical interventions are not discussed here. But some cases of food refusal can be viewed as conditioned responses from prior experiences of irritation or trauma to the oropharynx or oesophagus or following an episode of choking (e.g. "post-traumatic feeding disorders") (Benoit & Coolbear, 1998). Other feeding disturbances are influenced by medical factors (e.g. developmental delay due to neurological impairment; chronic health conditions).

The evidence base for feeding disorder interventions is complicated by diversity in study samples, heterogeneity of disorders, changing classification systems, lack of subtype clarity, age-specific treatment, and limited data (Bryant-Waugh et al., 2010; Winters, 2003). No national treatment guidelines exist. A summary of recommended, valuable or common treatments is given below:

- Hospitalization: for severe malnutrition, when no response to outpatient treatment, and where abuse/ neglect is suspected. Benefits: direct feeding observations, multiple specialty assessments, treatment initiation (Maggioni & Lifschitz, 1995; Linscheid & Murphy, 1999).

- Medical interventions: invasive interventions such as enteral feeding. Used primarily for behaviourally based feeding disorders to correct significant malnutrition when other interventions are unsuccessful.

- Dietary manipulation: for nutritional repletion and "catch-up" growth including structuring mealtimes, changing diet (Maggioni & Lifschitz, 1995), manipulating hunger. Accompanied by parent education.

- Speech or occupational therapy: addresses mechanics of eating and/or dealing with sensory problems (Winters, 2003).

- Parent–child interaction intervention: parent education to establish regular mealtimes/seating, age-appropriate food choices/utensils, self-feeding when appropriate, minimize environmental distractions, employing reinforcement, increasing reciprocal feeding interactions (Linscheid & Murphy, 1999).

- Behaviour modification: widely used by behavioural specialists accompanied by parent training (Mueller et al., 2003). Interventions: manipulate reinforcement contingencies, apply extinction strategies to eliminate feeding avoidance (e.g. Casey et al., 2009).

- Addressing parental psychiatric disorder or symptoms re abnormal eating attitudes and patterns (e.g. McCann et al., 1994).

- Treatments by expert opinion: (a) medication to enhance appetite; (b) individual specialized interventions (e.g. Chatoor, 2003).

Treatment trials show mixed results and limited success and must be applied to appropriate populations.

- Community-based/home health visits have been less effective.

- Clinic-based team interventions show weight gain benefit.

- Well-designed randomized and quasi-randomized controlled trials involving combinations of psycho-educational and behavioural components reveal some efficacy for most, but not all, groups studied.

- Outpatient and intensive inpatient behaviour modification show efficacy in selected situations (often with very severe feeding disorders).

- Long-term enteral feeding (naso-gastric or gastrostomy), often used for children with medical compromise or resistance to other interventions, can result in resistance to oral feeding or food aversion; use for shortest period possible and continue oral feeding throughout.

- Parent–child interventions, often applied to younger children, show promise.

Feeding difficulties and/or mismanagement (feeding problem not otherwise specified)

This may include food refusal not significantly impairing growth, refusal of food types (e.g. solids or liquids), or very difficult, picky, or slow feeding behaviour (e.g. Reau et al., 1996). These issues have medium predictive power to later eating problems in retrospective studies (Kotler et al., 2001), but unclear predictive power in longitudinal prospective studies (Jacobi et al., 2004). There are no national guidelines.

Child and family distress is the first consideration. Intervention type depends on distress level. Expert opinion supports a phased multiple-component approach. Parent education alone may be adequate. Nutritional and medical evaluation is important. If no medical abnormality (such as swallowing problems) exists, treatment will be occupational or sensorimotor therapies using systematic desensitization and gradual exposure to increasing textures and dietary manipulation as needed. Direct individualized behavioural approaches can be efficacious (with improvements beyond those seen with parent education), though their use with less severe feeding problems is controversial because parent–child control issues may arise, undermining the child's natural motivation to eat (Kerwin, 1999). Invasive medical interventions are generally not appropriate.

Pica

Pica, often described as treatment-resistant, is a persistence of developmentally inappropriate eating of non-nutritive substances that is not a culturally sanctioned practice for more than 1 month. Pica includes eating a wide variety of substances, can result in medical risks including those associated with lead poisoning, and is often considered self-injurious or automatically reinforced behaviour. It may occur in association with developmental disabilities (e.g. Arbiter & Black, 1991; Nchito et al., 2004), or underlying disease. Little is known about associated psychopathology. Pica is less prevalent in adolescence than childhood, but may occur in adults during pregnancy or associated with iron deficiency anaemia. More commonly, pica and vitamin deficiencies co-occur in the context of poverty, neglect, and poor parental supervision (Linscheid & Murphy, 1999).

No national guidelines exist. Evaluation includes assessment of medical issues, home environment and family functioning, cognitive and psychiatric status, and a careful description and functional analysis of the ingesting behaviour (Casey et al.,

2009). Recommended treatment has multiple components: proper supervision of young children, removing access to noxious substances, parental education re adequate/balanced diets, and provision of appropriate developmental stimulation. Decision-making algorithms have been developed for ethical and quality of life concerns (LeBlanc et al., 1997). Behavioural treatments include some combination of differential reinforcement, discrimination training, extinction, and punishment, though data show mixed success. Supplementation with iron, vitamins, and minerals is needed in nutritional deficiency, but an RCT of pica associated with iron deficiency in 406 African children with geophagy ("eating earth") found no benefit for iron over multimicronutrient supplementation or placebo (Nchito et al., 2004).

Rumination disorder

Rumination, voluntarily bringing already-ingested food back into the mouth and then ejecting or rechewing and swallowing, often occurs in infants and individuals with intellectual disability through adolescence. Prevalence ranges from "rare" to 10% (e.g. Linscheid & Murphy, 1999). Major concerns are weight loss and negative effects on social interaction. Ruling out an organic cause is important. Rumination is often complicated by comorbid medical or psychiatric conditions that may require treatment. Early recognition is essential; delayed diagnosis is associated with morbidity. Parent education to optimize home conditions and parent–child interaction is recommended in less severe situations. Behavioural treatments are most commonly used in rumination with more severe consequences (Chial et al., 2003). There are no national guidelines.

Treatment of sleep disorders

Practice parameters and a literature review were published in 2006 by the American Academy of Sleep Medicine for treatment of bedtime problems and night waking (behavioural insomnias), addressing young children without developmental disabilities or comorbid medical or psychiatric conditions (Mindell et al., 2006; Morgenthaler et al., 2006). An evidence-based book on this subject has recently been published (Mindell & Owens, 2010). The practice parameters state that, in general, behavioural interventions are effective and are recommended for treatment of bedtime problems and night waking. Unmodified extinction and extinction of undesired behaviour with parental presence appear effective but have limited parental acceptance. With decreasing levels of evidence, the following are considered effective and are recommended: parent education/prevention; graduated extinction; delayed bedtime with removal from bed/positive bedtime routines; and use of scheduled awakenings. Evidence is insufficient to recommend any single therapy or combination or multifaceted interventions.

Experts believe a preventative approach to infant sleeping difficulties is important. Establishing healthy sleep habits supported routinely through parent education either before or shortly after birth re normal infant sleep and the vital role of sleep hygiene include: (a) keeping bedtime routines brief, pleasant, predictable, calming; (b) avoiding vigorous mental or physical activity the hour before bedtime; (c) avoiding bedtime hunger but scheduling mealtime more than an hour before bedtime; (d) avoiding foods, beverages, and, if possible, medications containing alcohol or caffeine; (e) helping infants and young children learn to fall asleep alone without parent intervention; (f) keeping sleeping environment cool, dark, quiet; (g) using bed or crib exclusively for sleeping; (h) eliminating television or electronic games from bedroom; (i) avoiding excessive fluid intake before bedtime and during night; (j) observing a regular wake time; and (k) encouraging age-appropriate naps only.

Behavioural insomnia of childhood: sleep onset association type

Sleep onset association disorder occurs when infants and toddlers habitually fall asleep in one environment (parent's arms or bed) and then, after normal arousal, find themselves in an unfamiliar sleep environment, such as their crib, and are unable to return to sleep until the sleep-promoting environment is restored ("night waking"). Typical parental response often reinforces this behaviour. Parent education about their role in the sleep disorder comes first and may be sufficient in itself. Clinically, graduated extinction is the most commonly applied treatment (Ferber & Kryger, 1995), and parents must be committed to its success. Treatment involves conditioning the child to initiate nighttime sleep using positive bedtime routines and return to sleep following spontaneous arousals in the desired sleeping environment. Infants gradually learn sleep initiation on their own, usually in less than 1 week, though in toddlers more time may be needed (Ferber & Kryger, 1995). Graduated extinction is associated with improved sleep and improved family well-being (Eckerberg, 2002).

Behavioural insomnia of childhood: limit-setting type

The limit-setting type of childhood sleep disorder ("bedtime problems") is characterized by inadequate parent enforcement of bedtimes resulting in child refusal to go to bed or stalling techniques often not problematic until children become ambulatory. This can persist through adolescence. Once sleep is initiated, there are no abnormalities of sleep architecture or arousal. Certain parenting styles can be associated with this disorder.

In clinical practice, parent education emphasizes consistency and supportive firmness without anger (Ferber & Kryger, 1995; Mindell & Owens, 2010) with age-appropriate bedtime rituals using strictly followed routines. Parent education may sometimes be sufficient (Eckerberg, 2002). Child sleep time may be temporarily adjusted. Valid fears the child has associated with sleep must be acknowledged and dispelled; this may require the parent to spend more time in the child's room at sleep onset. Limit-setting sleep disorder may occur in the context of a wider parenting disorder, a chaotic household, or with marital discord, so underlying issues should be addressed before determining the child has a sleep disorder. Sedating medications are not indicated.

Sleep terrors

Sleep terrors (previously called "night terrors"), with onset generally between ages 2 and 4, are abrupt events that represent an incomplete arousal from non-rapid eye movement sleep accompanied by autonomic activation. Episodes usually occur during the first half of the night, last several minutes, and terminate with sudden return to deep sleep. The child does not remember the event. Sleep terrors typically peak at 5–7 years, usually with spontaneous resolution before adolescence.

No national guidelines exist. Therapy begins with reassuring parents about the benign nature of sleep terrors. Parent education and implementation of good sleep hygiene and a safe sleep environment are often sufficient. The child should not be aroused from sleep, as this can induce confusion and prolong the episode (e.g. Anders & Eiben, 1997). Scheduled awakening just before the expected time of night terrors can be helpful. Medication may be appropriate only when terrors are severe, persistent, and there is safety risk; then referral to a sleep specialist is recommended in these cases. Treatable disorders that disrupt sleep (sleep apnoea, reflux disease, nocturnal seizures), should be ruled out prior to starting pharmacotherapy. Both

Table 43.1 Feeding disorders

Treatment	Form of treatment	Psychiatric disorder/target audience	Level of evidence for efficacy	Comments
Multidisciplinary approach	Designed programme involving both clinic and home interventions	Feeding disorders	Ia	Growth status improved, and improved cognitive status with home intervention in some studies
Multidisciplinary approach	Often individually designed intervention	Pica	IV	Many of the studies come from single case or case series analyses
Multidisciplinary approach	Both home and clinic interventions to increase stimulation and attention	Rumination	IV	Many of the studies come from single case or case series analyses; recommended for less severe cases
Behavioural intervention	Designed clinic programme	Feeding disorders	Ia	More weight gain with behavioural interventions; nutritional counselling may or may not add to effectiveness
Behavioural intervention	Reinforcement, discrimination training, extinction, and punishment	Pica	III	Improvement found in pica behaviour but difficult to generalize because many studies are single case studies with specific individualized behavioural intervention

Table 43.1 (cont.)

Treatment	Form of treatment	Psychiatric disorder/target audience	Level of evidence for efficacy	Comments
Behavioural intervention	Various behavioural methods; for older children, habit reversal	Rumination	III	Behavioural treatments used for more severe cases, and can include aversive conditioning
Parent-focused or parent–child focused	Designed programmes such as play-focused or psychoeducation	Feeding disorders	III	Improved parent (and sometimes child) behaviour and child weight gain
Nutritional supplementation	Zinc and/or iron supplementation	Pica	III	Effective for pica associated with deficiencies but not as a general treatment for all situations of pica

Table 43.2 Sleep(ing) disorders

Treatment	Form of treatment	Psychiatric disorder/ target audience	Level of evidence for efficacy	Comments
Behavioural approaches	Primarily but not limited to graduated extinction	Sleeping onset disorders	Ia	Quite successful and in young infants, results are often obtained within a week
Behavioural approaches	Primarily but not limited to graduated extinction	Limit-setting disorders	Ib	Quite successful
Behavioural approaches	Positive bedtime routine	Limit-setting disorders	Ib	No more successful than graduated extinction but greater marital satisfaction
Psychopharmacology	Benzodiazepines, tricyclic antidepressants	Sleep terrors	III	Probably effective, but should be used only for the most severe cases and medical illnesses need to be ruled out
Parent education	Specific educational programme	Sleeping onset disorders	III	Improvement in sleep and sleep patterns
Scheduled awakening	Probable change to sleep architecture	Sleep terrors	III	Reports indicate success

benzodiazepines and tricyclic anti-depressants have been used.

Summary

Eating: While there is no consensus or guidelines, there are multiple available therapies. Behavioural approaches with a multidisciplinary team have the largest evidence base. The child's relationship context plays a role in feeding dynamics.

Sleep: Parents need to establish healthy sleep habits early in life as part of routine health care. Most sleep disorders can be prevented with good parenting practices or with simple behavioural measures. Interventions discussed in this chapter are summarized in Tables 43.1 and 43.2.

44

Autism spectrum disorders

Based on "Evaluating interventions for children with autism and intellectual disabilities" by Patricia Howlin and Hower Kwon in Effective Treatments in Psychiatry, Cambridge University Press, 2008

Introduction

Autism spectrum disorders (ASDs) are a complex and heterogeneous group of conditions that affect around 1% of the population and have a pervasive effect on functioning from infancy through to adult life. When first described in the 1940s autism was considered a psychiatric disorder of psychogenic origin. However, over time the cognitive, social, and communication deficits underlying ASD became more widely recognized, leading to much greater awareness of the role of communication deficits in contributing to many of the "challenging behaviours" frequently associated with the disorder (Howlin &

Rutter, 1987). Research has also demonstrated the importance of early intervention, the need for individually based treatments, structured education, and the involvement of parents in therapy. Nevertheless, the evidence base for many treatments for children with ASD remains weak.

"Miracle cures"

"Miracle cures" include numerous dietary and vitamin treatments, endocrine and other injections, physical therapies (including "facilitated communication" and "holding therapy"), sensory therapies (including sensory integration, auditory integration, and music therapy), and "psychoeducational" therapies, such as the Son-Rise programmes (see Howlin, 2010). Despite the dramatic claims made for many of these therapies (and their high cost), evidence for their effectiveness is generally lacking.

Pharmacological interventions

The use of psychotropic medication for young children with autism varies greatly from country to country. US practitioners have generally been more willing than their counterparts in the UK to use psychotropic medications in children with autism. Even when psychotropic medications are used, they have been reserved largely to treat specific problems such as hyperactivity, self-injurious behaviour, depression, and irritability, with the hope that improving these behaviours will allow these patients to become more amenable to benefits from educational and other therapeutic approaches.

The antipsychotic agents have been the best-studied class of medications in treating symptoms associated with autism. Two large, multisite, randomized, double-blind trials, one performed in the USA (Research Units on Paediatric Psychopharmacology, RUPP) and one in Canada, found risperidone to be effective in treating irritability, aggression, and repetitive behaviour in children with autism (McCracken, 2002; Shea et al., 2004). In the RUPP study, improvements in behaviour and adaptive skills appeared to persist for 6 to 8 months following the start of treatment with risperidone (Williams et al., 2006). Moreover, therapy combining risperidone and parent training was found to be superior to risperidone alone in reducing tantrums, self-injury, and aggression (Aman et al., 2009). Combination therapy also allowed for lower doses of the medication to be used. In October 2006, risperidone became the first drug to receive approval by the US FDA for treatment of symptoms related to autism: irritability, aggression, self-injury, and tantrums. Aripiprazole was shown in two large randomized, placebo-controlled trials to reduce behaviours such as tantrums, aggression, and self-injurious behaviour (Owen et al., 2009; Marcus et al., 2009). Other atypical antipsychotics such as olanzapine, ziprasidone, and quetiapine have support in smaller studies.

Though SSRIs have been used to address various problem behaviours in autism, there are few RCTs to rigorously examine their effectiveness. A distinction should be drawn between the use of SSRIs for psychiatric symptoms commonly seen in children affected by autism, such as anxiety and depression, versus their use to address the core symptoms of autism. Whereas the use of SSRIs to treat associated psychiatric symptoms in children with autism is widespread and potentially effective (Kolevzon et al., 2006), results of studies examining their use for core autistic symptoms have been mixed. A large, multisite, placebo-controlled, randomized trial examining citalopram found no improvement in repetitive behaviour in children and adolescents with autism (King et al., 2009). Citalopram was more likely to cause adverse reactions, including increased energy, impulsivity, hyperactivity, and stereotypies.

Fluoxetine was found to be more effective than placebo in treating repetitive behaviours in childhood autism (Hollander et al., 2005). In a study involving adults with autism, fluvoxamine had clinically significant effects on repetitive thoughts and behaviour, aggression, and impaired social relatedness (McDougle et al., 1996). Clomipramine, a non-SSRI antidepressant, has been shown in a double-blind crossover study to be significantly superior to desipramine and placebo in reducing stereotypies and compulsive and ritualized behaviours (Gordon et al., 1993), though serious side effects, including tachycardia, QT prolongation, seizures, and tremor, were noted.

Guanfacine and clonidine are alpha$_2$ adrenergic agonists with potential benefits for symptoms of hyperactivity, impulsivity, and tics. Retrospective studies have shown benefit for a variety of symptoms in children with autism. A small randomized prospective study of guanfacine in children with autism and other developmental disorders showed improvement with guanfacine in hyperactivity (Handen et al., 2008). Stimulants have shown some effectiveness in managing symptoms associated with ADHD, although concerns exist about side effects in children with autism (Hazell, 2006).

Psychoeducational programmes

There are very many and varied psychoeducational programmes for children with ASD. The TEACCH programme (Teaching and Education of Autistic and Related Communication Handicapped Children; Schopler, 1997) which emphasizes individually based teaching, the need for structure, and the use of visual cues is amongst the most widely used but many other educational models exist (see National Research Council, 2001 for review). There is also a range of programmes that focus on the encouragement of play and pleasurable interactions between preschool children with autism and their parents or peers (e.g. the Developmental Intervention Model, the Waldon Program, the Hanen Approach, and the Early Bird Project). Other interventions focus specifically on the social-communication and developmental impairments in autism. These include the Preschool Autism Communication therapy (PACT; Green et al., 2010) which focuses on the early social-communication interaction between mothers and children; the developmentally based Early Start Denver Model (ESDM, Dawson et al., 2010); programmes to develop joint attention and symbolic play (Kasari et al., 2008); the Picture Exchange Communication System (PECS; Bondy & Frost, 1996); and Social Stories (Gray, 1995). However, many of these interventions lack a sound evidence base and few are supported by independent or randomized controlled trials. The exceptions are recent RCTs of PECS (Yoder & Stone, 2006; Howlin et al., 2007), PACT (Green et al., 2010), joint attention/symbolic play (Kasari et al., 2006), and the Denver Model (Dawson et al., 2010). These trials indicate that while the effects of treatment are positive and significant, the impact tends to be on skills that are specifically targeted by the intervention. Generalization to other areas is limited, and core autism symptoms often show relatively little change (Green et al., 2010).

Pre-school intensive behavioural programmes

Among the most widely publicised of these is the Early Intensive Behavioural Intervention (EIBI; Lovaas, 2002), which employs a highly prescriptive, applied behavioural analysis (ABA) approach. Children are expected, beginning at age 2, to spend at least 40 hours a week for 2 years or more in therapy which is supervised by experienced behavioural consultants. Although most trials of EIBI have reported significant improvements in the treatment group (with IQ gains of up to 30 points) the extent of change is variable and progress in other areas of development is often more limited. Moreover, recent systematic reviews/meta-analyses (e.g. Howlin et al., 2009; Reichow & Wolery, 2009; Seida et al., 2009; Virtué-Ortega, 2010) conclude that in all EIBI studies there are children who fail to improve, and others who regress during the course of intervention. This has led to attempts to identify the characteristics of the children who do and do not respond to early intensive intervention.

Interventions for older children

Most of the best evaluated interventions for autism spectrum disorders have been conducted with children aged 6 years or younger. However, mental health difficulties, particularly anxiety and depression, affect many children with ASD as they move into adolescence. Cognitive behaviour strategies are being increasingly used with this group although there are only a few positive RCTs reported, mainly for anxiety disorders, anger management, and social difficulties (see review by Howlin et al., 2009).

Understanding the research-based evidence for effective approaches to intervention

Recent reviews highlight the limited quality of much intervention research, and the failure of any one treatment to demonstrate superiority over all others. There are concerns, too, that interventions proven to work in highly controlled experimental settings (efficacy trials) may prove less effective in real-life settings.

It is also apparent that other factors, such as degree of parental involvement, integration of multicomponent approaches and, to some extent, duration of therapy (there is no evidence of the enduring effects of short-term interventions), are all crucial in determining treatment effectiveness.

Finally, it is important to recognize that autism spectrum disorders persist throughout life. The types of intervention needed in early childhood (which focus mainly on behaviour and communication) may be very different from those required in adolescence or adulthood (when social, emotional, and mental health problems may be of more concern). Thus, there is a need for provision that can both monitor and meet individual's changing needs over the years.

- There is a range of approaches that – although not resulting in "cures" for autism – can result in improvements in many areas, including communication, social functioning, and behavioural difficulties. However, no single intervention approach has been demonstrated to be effective for all children, or across the life span.

- Successful interventions should build on approaches that have a strong evidence base, but should also be adapted to meet the needs of individual children and their families, and take into account the individual's cognitive level, severity of autistic symptomatology, and overall developmental level.

- Intensive behavioural interventions are among the most widely evaluated, but although some children do show significant gains from such programmes this is not the case for all. Other children may respond better to interventions

Table 44.1 Effectiveness of treatments for autism and intellectual disabilities in children

Treatment	Form of treatment	Psychiatric disorder/target audience	Level of evidence for efficacy	Comments
Psychopharmacology	Antipsychotics	Autism and developmentally disabled	1b	Reduction of temper tantrums, aggression, some stereotypies, and self-injurious behaviour
Psychopharmacology	Antidepressants (SSRIs)	Autism and developmentally disabled	1b	Improvement of repetitive thoughts and behaviours, aggression, and social relatedness
Psychopharmacology	Antidepressants (TCAs)	Autism and developmentally disabled	IIb	Clomipramine reduced stereotypies and compulsive and ritualized behaviours but substantial side effects
Educational programmes	Multiple models of structured educational interventions	Autism and developmentally disabled	IIa	Empirical validation remains weak. Predictable structure and a heavy emphasis on visual cues appear to be most helpful
Behavioural programmes	Multiple models including EIBI	Preschool children with autism and developmental disorders	IIa	These are probably effective, but data are needed as to the specificity of the effectiveness and what programmes or what elements of which programmes are effective. It appears that programmes that concentrate on social-communication skills can improve social functioning and interactions

that focus on communication and early parent–child interaction.

- Programmes that combine a developmental, naturalistic approach to intervention, together with behavioural strategies and the involvement of parents, are likely to have an optimal impact.

- A focus on structure, predictability and consistency, with an emphasis on visual rather than verbal cues is most likely to provide children with ASD with the environment they need to minimize confusion and distress, to enhance learning, and reduce stereotyped or disruptive behaviours.

- Family-centred treatment approaches appear to ensure more effective generalization and maintenance of skills. The development of management strategies that can be implemented consistently and in ways that do not demand extensive sacrifice in terms of time, money, or other

aspects of family life, seems to offer benefits for all involved.

Conclusions

There are no miracle cures for ASD and although systematic reviews generally conclude that early educational/behavioural programmes are a good option for children with ASD there remains little evidence in support of any one specific methodology or intensity of treatment. Certain pharmacological treatments seem to be effective but further research is required. There is little or no scientific evidence in support of most other treatments. There are general approaches to intervention, based on psychological and developmental research, but to be effective these must be adapted in order to take account of individual differences and needs.

Interventions discussed in this chapter are summarized in Table 44.1.

45

ADHD and hyperkinetic disorder

Based on "ADHD and hyperkinetic disorder" by Paramala J. Santosh, Amy Henry, and Christopher K. Varley in Effective Treatments in Psychiatry, Cambridge University Press, 2008

Introduction

Attention deficit hyperactivity disorder (ADHD) or hyperkinetic disorder (HKD) are worldwide common childhood conditions found across cultures (Biederman et al., 1991; Rohde et al., 2001). ADHD, a DSM disorder, is characterized by impulsiveness, hyperactivity, and/or inattention to a degree beyond what is expected in the normal continuum in developmentally similar children. HKD, a narrower ICD-10 diagnosis, requiring the presence of inattention, impulsivity as well as hyperactivity, is a subgroup of ADHD. The aetiology of ADHD is unknown but thought to be multifactorial with some genetic components.

In HKD symptoms occur before the age of 6 (age 7 for ADHD) and be present in more than one setting (in ADHD as well). Its prevalence is about 1.5% (3–5% for ADHD) in school-age populations. With HKD, the presence of another disorder, such as anxiety, is an exclusion criterion, but ADHD is commonly associated with comorbid conditions, such as oppositional defiant disorder, conduct disorder, anxiety disorders, depressive disorders, pervasive developmental disorders, tic disorders, and learning disorders (Biederman et al., 1991). ADHD has subtypes: primarily inattentive, primarily hyperactive-impulsive, or combined type. In the UK, where ICD-10 is usually employed,

ADHD is used by both clinicians and families.

ADHD affects more males than females (roughly 3:1) and is associated with a variety of functional impairments in academic, family, and social functioning (Wellset al., 2000). ADHD prevalence appears to be rising in the USA for unknown reasons. Significant controversy surrounds the frequency of diagnosing ADHD and prescribing of medication. While ADHD is recognized in many cultures, there are substantial differences between countries in percentage of youth prescribed medication for it. All treatments suffer from failure to maintain improvement after discontinuing treatment and failure to generalize to settings where treatment has not been active. Situations where symptoms cause most impairment should be treatment targets.

Pharmacotherapy

Medication is usually necessary for treating HKD and is considered for ADHD especially if psychological treatments have not managed symptoms well. Young people with greater hyperactivity, inattention, and clumsiness without comorbidities improve more completely. Patients without hyperactivity (ADD) may benefit from lower stimulant doses. If hyperactivity is present in only one situation, then that situation should be identified and stresses reduced as first-line management. With school-specific problems, learning disabilities should be professionally assessed with adjustment of educational techniques and expectations prior to antihyperactivity treatments. If behaviour is confined to home, the possibility of adverse parenting influences needs consideration and parent training approaches contemplated.

First-line agents: stimulants

Pharmacotherapy with psychostimulants (methylphenidate, dexamphetamine, and others) are first-line treatments. More is known about stimulant use in this age group than about any other psychotropic medication. Onset of action is rapid, dosage easy to titrate, and positive response frequently predicted from a single dose. Modern formulations achieve specialized medication effects (e.g. longer duration of action). There is little evidence for superiority of one stimulant preparation over another.

Meta-analyses supported by published clinical guidelines supply the evidence base for methylphenidate for the short term and periods of up to 3 years (National Institute for Health and Clinical Excellence, 2000; AACAP Official Action, 2002; Taylor et al., 2004). Pemoline, associated with increased risk of liver toxicity/

failure, has been removed from the US market.

Stimulant medications have been found effective against ADHD symptoms in more than 100 trials across settings (effect size ~ 0.8): fewer disruptive behaviours, more sustained classroom attention and task persistence, improved on-task home behaviours, and increased attentiveness during sporting activities (Carlson et al., 1992; Pelham et al., 1991; Richters et al., 1995; Schachter et al., 2001). Positive effects are found for secondary impairments: academic performance, peer relationships, family interactions, compliance with instructions, and self-esteem (Barkley & Cunningham, 1979; Whalen et al., 1990), and for comorbid externalizing symptoms, including verbal and physical aggression, covert antisocial behaviour, and oppositional behaviour (Klein et al., 1997). Families where ADHD children have a positive stimulant response appear more amenable to psychosocial interventions (Schachar et al., 1997).

Methylphenidate was superior to placebo in 6/8 short-term RCTs in 241 preschoolers (AACAP Official Action, 2002). Eight RCTs of stimulants in 214 ADHD adolescents found statistically significant improvement (Smith et al., 2000). Longer-term studies demonstrate continued effectiveness over 12–24 months (MTA Cooperative Group, 1999; AACAP Official Action, 2002). Only variable benefits are found in young adults previously treated with psychostimulants.

Stimulants are contraindicated in schizophrenia, hyperthyroidism, cardiac arrhythmias, angina pectoris, glaucoma, or a history of hypersensitivity to drug and are used with caution in youth with hypertension, depression, tics (or family history of Tourette's syndrome), pervasive developmental disorders, severe mental retardation, or a substance use history.

Adverse effects of stimulant medications are generally mild: irritability, headaches, abdominal pain, and loss of appetite. Mild appetite suppression is almost universal. Rebound effects are increased excitability, activity, talkativeness, irritability, and insomnia beginning 4–15 hours after a dose. Decreased sleep is frequent though it is important to distinguish insomnia as an unwanted drug effect from insomnia that may be due to medication effects subsiding. In general there are no adverse cardiovascular effects of stimulants. In the USA, there is a warning of possible cardiac side effects particularly where known cardiovascular illnesses are present. There is little evidence that stimulants produce a clinically significant decrease in the seizure threshold (Crumrine et al., 1987), and little evidence of addiction resulting from prescribing stimulants. Long-acting preparations seem less likely to be diverted or abused.

Children on stimulants need pulse and BP monitored at each increase and every 6 months, and weight and height measured on a growth chart at least every 6 months.

Second-line agents: non-stimulant medication

Non-stimulant drugs without abuse potential are available.

Atomoxetine

Atomoxetine, a selective norepinephrine reuptake inhibitor, is the first non-stimulant drug FDA approved for ADHD with four RCTs in children and adolescents demonstrating effectiveness, with sustained effects in subsets for at least 2 years (Michelson et al., 2002; Spencer et al., 2002). Atomoxetine is significantly more effective than placebo and does not differ significantly from, or is non-inferior to, immediate-release methylphenidate; however, it is significantly less effective than the extended-release methylphenidate formulation OROS® methylphenidate and extended-release mixed amphetamine salts (Garnok-Jones and Keating, 2010). Primary side effects: GI upset, decreased appetite, fatigue, dizziness, and mild increases in pulse and systolic blood pressure. Atomoxetine can be dosed either once or twice daily and is considered quite safe. It may be used with comorbid tics and anxiety/depression. Parents need to know that symptoms take about 6 weeks to improve (unlike stimulants). Rare, but serious, hepatic side effects have been reported.

Bupropion

Bupropion is a common second-line ADHD treatment. In three RCTs, bupropion demonstrated significant decreases in ADHD symptoms. Adverse effects are generally mild: sedation, nausea, decreased appetite, dizziness. A serious side effect is that bupropion lowers seizure threshold and is contraindicated in patients with known seizure disorder, eating disorder, or at substantial risk for seizures for other reasons. Though not FDA approved for any paediatric indication, bupropion is a relatively attractive second-line treatment for those who are not at significant risk for seizures (Conners et al., 1996).

Tricyclic antidepressants (TCAs)

Thought not FDA approved, RCTs of TCAs in children and adolescents demonstrate efficacy. Desipramine and imipramine have been most studied. A robust response was found in 12/18 controlled trials; a moderate response in 5/12 (Spencer et al., 1996). Drawbacks include potential cardiotoxicity, especially in pre-pubertal children, danger of accidental or intentional overdose, sedation, anticholinergic side effects, lowered seizure threshold, and possibly declining efficacy over time. Medication administration needs supervision. Pills should be placed in a safe place. Cardiac monitoring is essential at baseline and throughout treatment. While TCAs may have a role in ADHD, other agents offer a better benefit-to-risk profile.

Alpha-agonists

A meta-analysis of 10 studies of clonidine and guanfacine, centrally acting alpha$_2$-adrenergic agonists, found positive effects in paediatric ADHD (moderate effect size of 0.58). Side effects included sedation, hypotension, tachycardia, dizziness, and rash from the transdermal clonidine patch. Pulse and blood pressure need monitoring for bradycardia and hypotension. When discontinuing clonidine, the dose should be tapered to avoid rebound hypertension.

Extended-release guanfacine (Intuniv), a novel long-acting, once-daily formulation of guanfacine, has been approved by the FDA for ADHD in 6- to 17-year-old children and adolescents (Connor and Rubin, 2010). In doses of 1 to 4 mg/day, guanfacine extended-release (GXR) significantly improves the symptoms of ADHD compared with placebo. Because of different pharmacokinetics, GXR is not substitutable on a mg-for-mg basis with immediate-release guanfacine. Although GXR does not demonstrate clinically significant ECG changes, mild slowing of the heart rate and some lowering of systolic and diastolic BP does occur and requires vital sign monitoring during treatment. Children with a clinically significant cardiovascular history should not be prescribed GXR. Guanfacine has been shown to help both tics and ADHD symptoms in children with ADHD and tic disorders.

Other pharmacological interventions

Antipsychotics

In 8/12 controlled trials of antipsychotics in 242 children antipsychotics had moderate or robust effectiveness (Spencer et al., 1996) though no more than 50% of ADHD patients improve with antipsychotics. Antipsychotics can cause serious adverse effects and should be reserved for extreme treatment of refractory cases.

Carbamazepine

A meta-analysis of carbamazepine in three RCTs involving 53 patients found that 71% of carbamezapine-treated subjects showed significant improvement versus 26% on placebo (effect size of 1.01) (Silva et al., 1996). Because of significant potential haematological and hepatic side effects, carbamazepine is generally reserved for those whose ADHD has not responded to standard treatments and who have a comorbid seizure disorder or significant brain damage.

Combination of a stimulant and non-stimulant

The most common combination currently used for ADHD is a stimulant and clonidine. The safety or efficacy of this combination is unknown. Combinations of imipramine and methylphenidate have been associated with confusion, affective lability, marked aggression, and severe agitation. This combination can increase plasma levels of imipramine; monitoring blood levels may be necessary.

Developmental trajectory and medication response

- **Pre-schoolers**: Behavioural interventions first. Stimulants are probably less effective and produce greater side effects.
- **School-going children**: Medication superior to behavioural interventions.
- **Adolescence**: Non-compliance and risk of misuse are problems. Diversions to peers is more common than abuse by the patient. Options are extended-release stimulant preparations or atomoxetine.
- **Adults**: Since adult ADHD often presents differently from childhood ADHD, it is important to consider the differential diagnoses.

Both stimulants and atomoxetine are effective but effect size is marginally lower than in children.

Pharmacological management of HKD in Europe

The importance of treating hyperactivity is established. A variety of different clinical approaches exist within Europe. In some countries, notably Britain and France, there has been public hostility to psychotropic medication use even though guidelines recommend them (Taylor et al., 2004). Controversy surrounds the extent to which a narrower definition of HKD or a broader definition of ADHD should guide clinical practice. HKD appears more stimulant and less behavioural intervention responsive than ADHD.

Psychosocial interventions

Behaviour therapy (BT) and cognitive behavioural therapy (CBT)

BT is commonly used to address both primary symptoms and associated functional impairments of ADHD with the goal of preventing and discouraging maladaptive behaviours while rewarding and eliciting positive behaviours. BT has been shown to improve the classroom behaviour in the short-term relative to control settings (Carlson et al., 1992), but positive effects are rarely sustained after discontinuation. Effects do not appear to generalize. BT is generally not as effective as stimulant medication (Carlson et al., 1992). CBT has had mixed results and does not appear to offer benefits beyond the behavioural component alone.

Neurofeedback

Neurofeedback (NF) may help to improve attentional and self-management capabilities in children with attention deficit/hyperactivity disorder (ADHD). In a randomized controlled trial, NF training was found to be superior to a computerized attention skills training (AST) on behavioural improvement, with moderate effect size, and treatment effects continued at 6-month follow-up (Gevensleben et al., 2010). The drawbacks were that large numbers of sessions (at least 36 sessions) were needed, treatment effects were limited, and may not be as cost-effective as medication.

Social skills training

Social skills training to address the social skill deficits commonly associated with ADHD typically utilizes cognitive and behavioural strategies and social learning theory. Limited data exist.

Parent training

Parent training offers psychoeducation and training in learning theory principles to parents of ADHD children to promote the child's positive and minimize negative behaviour. Controlled studies reveal improved functioning in both ADHD children and their parents: improved compliance, more rapid task completion, decreased symptom ratings by parents, and decreased parental stress with improved parental self-esteem (Anastopoulos et al., 1993).

Family therapy

Structural family therapy focuses on altering common maladaptive patterns of family communication and functioning. While family therapy is often provided to ADHD families, there are limited efficacy data.

Combined treatments

Multimodal treatment, medications combined with behaviour therapy and/or parent training, is very common with ADHD. Little data exists to show advantages over medication alone (Klein et al., 1997), though children in combined treatments required 20% less medication (MTA, 1999).

Table 45.1 Effectiveness of treatments for ADHD and hyperkinetic disorder

Treatment	Form of treatment	Psychiatric disorder/ target audience	Level of evidence for efficacy	Comments
Psychopharmacology	Stimulants: methylphenidate, amphetamine salts	ADHD, HKD	Ia	Multiple trials support their use as effective in not only core symptoms of ADHD (increased attention, decreased disruptive behaviours across many settings) but also in some secondary symptoms (academic performance, peer and family interactions). They appear to work across age groups and not only with children. Most studies have been short term
Psychopharmacology	Non-stimulant: atomoxetine	ADHD, HKD	Ia	Found to be significantly more effective in parent and teacher ratings for core symptoms of ADHD than placebo
Psychopharmacology	Non-stimulant: tricyclic antidepressants	ADHD, HKD	Ia	Moderate effectiveness especially with respect to behavioural symptoms. Stimulants overall are more effective
Psychopharmacology	Non-stimulant: bupropion	ADHD, HKD	Ib	Appears to be an effective second-line treatment

Table 45.1 (cont.)

Treatment	Form of treatment	Psychiatric disorder/ target audience	Level of evidence for efficacy	Comments
Psychopharmacology	Non-stimulant: clonidine	ADHD, HKD	Ib	Effect size of 0.58 (moderately effective treatment)
Psychopharmacology	Non-stimulant: guanfacine	ADHD, HKD	Ib	Studied with children with ADHD and ADHD with tics. Improvement in both groups
Psychopharmacology	Non-stimulant: antipsychotics	ADHD, HKD	IIa	Are effective in about 50% of the cases but because of side effects, should only be used in the most treatment-resistant cases
Psychopharmacology	Non-stimulant: carbamazepine	ADHD, HKD	IIa	Are effective in about three-quarters of the cases but because of side effects, should only be used in the most treatment-resistant cases
Psychosocial intervention	Behaviour therapy	ADHD, HKD	IIa	Appears effective but not as effective as psychopharmacological interventions. Results do not appear to be generalizable from the specific studied behaviour. Results do not sustain themselves after termination of treatment
Psychosocial intervention	Behaviour therapy	ADHD, HKD	IIb	Questions raised as to whether adding a cognitive component adds anything to the effectiveness of the behavioural approach alone

Psychosocial intervention	Neurofeedback	ADHD, HKD	IIb	Appears effective but not as effective as psychopharmacological interventions. The large number of sessions needed, cost, and limited response are drawbacks
Psychosocial intervention	Social skills training	ADHD, HKD	IV	If it works, works best in a group setting
Psychosocial intervention	Parent training	ADHD, HKD	IIa	Improved functioning in both parents and children
Psychosocial intervention	Family therapy	ADHD, HKD	IIb	Appears to decrease negative communication and family conflicts and improves school performance. Effective in about 30%

Duration of treatment

Treatment trial evidence shows continued benefits for up to 36 months. Discontinuation trial evidence suggests that many children can ultimately discontinue medications without symptom recurrence. It is recommended that a discontinuation trial be undertaken every 12 to 18 months. Long-term treatment may be necessary in some people.

Interventions discussed in this chapter are summarized in Table 45.1.

46

Oppositional defiant disorder and conduct disorder

Based on "Oppositional defiant disorder and conduct disorder" by Brent Collett, Stephen Scott, Carol Rockhill, Matthew Spelz, and Jon McClellan in Effective Treatments in Psychiatry, Cambridge University Press, 2008

Introduction

Conduct disorder (CD), characterized by persisting, inappropriate, and severe antisocial behaviour, in ICD-10 is an overarching term that includes oppositional defiant disorder (ODD) as a milder subtype typically found in younger children and CD as a more severe form found in older youths. In DSM-IV, ODD and CD are classified as separate disorders. Because of the overlap between these diagnoses and other forms of antisocial behaviour, the treatment literature often uses the broad term "conduct problems" (CP) rather than focusing on one diagnosis.

Collectively, conduct problems are the most common reasons for psychiatric care referral for boys.

Many influences contribute to CP including genetic and biological vulnerability; difficult temperament; deficits in verbal skills and executive functioning, inattentiveness, overactivity, and impulsiveness; insecure attachment; and a propensity to interpret ambiguous social situations as hostile and to generate aggressive rather than prosocial responses to conflict. Parental factors include irritability and explosiveness; inconsistent, overly rigid and inflexible discipline; inadequate supervision; low warmth and involvement; and limited use of

393

strategies to increase prosocial behaviour. CP is often complicated by poor academic achievement. Within the peer group, CP children are more likely to be rejected by normal peers and may associate with deviant peers.

Most evidence-based treatments for CP are intended for delivery by specialty care providers (e.g. child/adolescent psychiatrists, clinical child psychologists), and many treatments require specialized training and ongoing treatment fidelity monitoring. However, due to limited availability of mental health resources, primary care physicians often play a key role in initial triage and ongoing treatment such as medication management. Most of these interventions are intended for outpatient or community settings. There is little or no evidence that inpatient admissions lead to gains that are maintained. In the US, the American Academy of Child and Adolescent Psychiatry (AACAP, 1997a) has published practice parameters for the treatment of CD, and several excellent reviews of the evidence-based CP treatments have been published (Brestan & Eyberg, 1998; Woolfenden et al., 2002).

Psychological interventions

Several psychological interventions for CP are considered "well established" or "probably efficacious" by evidence-based standards. The appropriateness of these interventions varies by the patient's developmental level, the unique risk factors contributing to the evolution of CP, and comorbidities. For example, parenting skills interventions are very effective with young children though somewhat less so with older children and adolescents (Ruma et al., 1996). More advanced cognitive development may facilitate participation in individual or group therapies.

Engagement in therapy tends to be difficult with dropout rates up to 60%. Practical measures, assisting with transportation, providing childcare, and holding evening sessions or other family suitable times, may facilitate retention.

Parenting skills

Parenting programmes, designed to improve parents' behaviour management skills and parent–child relationship quality, target skills such as promoting play and developing a positive parent–child relationship, using praise and rewards to increase desirable social behaviour, giving clear directions and rules, using consistent and calm consequences for unwanted behaviour, and reorganizing the child's day to prevent problems. Parenting interventions may also address distal factors likely to inhibit change (e.g. parental drug/alcohol abuse, maternal depression, and relational violence between parents). Treatment can be delivered in individual parent–child appointments or in a parenting group. Individual approaches offer the advantages of "in vivo" observation of the parent–child dyad and therapist coaching and feedback. *Living with Children* (Patterson and Gullion, 1968) and *Parent–Child Interaction Therapy* (PCIT; Eyberg, 1988) are two examples of well-validated individual programmes. Group treatment has been shown to be equally effective and offers opportunities for parents to share their experience with others who are struggling with a disruptive child. Two well-known group treatments are the *Incredible Years Program* (IY; Webster-Stratton, 1981) and the *Positive Parenting Program* (Triple-P; Sanders et al., 2000).

Behavioural parent training is the most extensively studied treatment for CP with considerable empirical support for its effectiveness (Weisz et al., 2004). The *Living with Children* and *IY* programmes are both considered "well established" with multiple randomized trials and replications by independent research groups (Scott et al., 2001). There are RCTs showing the effectiveness of *PCIT* and *Triple P* (Sanders et al., 2000) with at least one independent

replication of the PCIT model (Nixon et al., 2003). Behavioural parent training leads to short-term reductions in antisocial behaviour (moderate to large effect sizes of $d = 0.5$ to 0.8). "Normalization" of children's behaviour following treatment is not consistently observed (Reid et al., 2003) though follow-up studies suggest enduring effects at up to 6 years post-treatment (Reid et al., 2003).

Family interventions

A few family treatment approaches have been systematically investigated and validated. Though these programmes are potentially costly to the community and healthcare system, they may result in a net saving when the costs associated with recidivism are considered. Examples include *Functional Family Therapy* (FFT; Alexander & Parsons, 1982), *MultiSystemic Therapy* (MST; Henggeler et al., 1998), and *Multidimensional Treatment Foster Care* (MTFC; Chamberlain, 2003).

These interventions have been well studied by their originators but with few independent replications. *FFT* studies have demonstrated improved family communication and reduced recidivism compared to controls, and youth continue to show lower rates of criminal offence well into early adulthood, positive findings replicated in a Swedish sample. The effectiveness of *MST* has been studied in multiple trials versus "treatment as usual", with evidence of improved family interactions in direct behavioural observations in MST, decreased chance of being placed out of the home, and a lower rate of re-arrests. Depending on the functional domain assessed, effect sizes range from $d = 0.11$ (peer relations) to 0.76 (observed family interactions) (Curtis et al., 2004) with many of these benefits maintained up to 15 years post-treatment (Schaeffer & Borduin, 2005). *MTFC* results in decreased youth behaviour problems and self-reported delinquency, lower runaway and arrest rates, and fewer days of incarceration. For foster parents and the foster care system, *MTFC* results in better behaviour management strategies, retention of foster parents, and fewer disruptions in child placements.

Youth interpersonal skills

Cognitive behavioural therapy (CBT) targets the social-cognitive errors and limited prosocial behavioural repertoires observed in CP children who are mainly of school-age and older, though elements of CBT have been included in treatments for preschoolers. These interventions may be delivered via individual or group formats. Though groups offer several advantages (e.g. opportunities to practise peer interactions), it is worth noting that there is some research documenting iatrogenic effects in adolescents with CP, especially in larger groups and those with inadequate therapist supervision. A lower patient–therapist ratio is therefore recommended for group work. Two of the more popular treatment models for school-age youth and adolescents are Kazdin's *Problem-Solving Skills Training with in vivo Practice* (PSST-P; Kazdin, 1996) and Lochman and Wells's (1996) *Coping Power Program*. Recently, Webster-Stratton et al. (2004) have added a group child social skills training component to their *IY* program. This program, *Dinosaur School*, is intended for preschoolers and early school-age children.

RCTs found that *PSST* resulted in significant decreases in deviant behaviour and increases in prosocial behaviour. Outcomes were maintained at 1-year follow-up. The addition of in vivo practice and a parent training component have both been found to enhance outcomes. Evaluations of the *Coping Power* programme demonstrate reductions in aggression and substance use and improved social competence. Treatment effects were maintained at 1-year follow-up particularly for those who also received parent training components. Both of these programmes are considered "probably efficacious", though replications by independent research groups are needed. In studies by Webster-Stratton et al. (2004), *Dinosaur School* has been found to result in significant decreases in behaviour problems and increased prosocial behaviour; gains that appear maintained after 1 year. There is at least one independent replication of the *IY* programme, including the *Dinosaur School* component.

Psychopharmacology

Though there are no pharmacological interventions presently approved specifically for CP, medications are used relatively frequently and increasingly in the USA (Zito et al., 2000). Primary care physicians are often in the position of managing such medications, and there are concerns about their lack of adequate training in developmental psychopathology. Primary practice often does not allow adequate time for thorough assessment and monitoring. In the UK medication would generally not be supported as good practice because well-replicated trials of effectiveness are limited, particularly for children with CP without ADHD.

The best-studied pharmacological interventions are psychostimulants (e.g. methylphenidate), as used with children with comorbid ADHD and CP. Reduction in hyperactivity/impulsivity will also result in reduced CP (Connor et al., 2002). Other approaches have tended to target reactive aggression/over-arousal, primarily in highly aggressive and psychiatrically hospitalized youth. These include medications targeting affect dysregulation (e.g. buspirone, clonidine), mood stabilizers (e.g. lithium, carbamazepine), and neuroleptics (e.g. risperidone).

There is at least some evidence supporting psychopharmacological intervention for CP though samples are small and/or treatment design limited. These treatments also have greater risk for side effects and effectiveness does not endure after therapy is discontinued. A meta-analytical review of placebo-controlled studies examining effects of stimulants on aggression identified two studies of CP patients with a primary diagnosis of CD with and without comorbid ADHD (Klein et al., 1997; Connor et al., 2002). Both studies showed robust decreases in aggression following treatment (effect sizes of roughly $d = 0.75$ to 1.5) with one study finding that improvements in CD symptoms were independent of ADHD symptom reduction (Klein et al., 1997). Comparable effects were observed in studies examining the effects of stimulants on children with primary ADHD and comorbid CP

Table 46.1 Effectiveness of treatments for oppositional defiant disorder and conduct disorder

Treatment	Form of treatment	Psychiatric disorder/target audience	Level of evidence for efficacy	Comments
Parenting skills	Living with Children	Individual parent training model	Ia	Among the oldest parent-training programmes, used as a model for many of the newer interventions
Parenting skills	Parent–Child Interaction Therapy	Individual parent training model	Ib	Currently being disseminated for use with high-risk groups (e.g. parents with a history of abusing their child)
Parenting skills	Incredible Years	Group parent training model	Ia	Evidence-based teacher training and child social skills groups are also available, making this a desirable choice for multimodal intervention
Parenting skills	Positive Parenting Programme (Triple-P)	Group and individual parent training model	Ib	Unique given inclusion of multiple levels of intervention (i.e. ranging from public service announcements to targeted interventions for higher risk children/families)
Family interventions	Functional Family Therapy	Combined family systems and behavioural interventions	Ib	Data from delinquent juveniles showing long-term reductions in recidivism. Cost-effectiveness data indicate net savings to the community

	Intervention	Description	Level	Comments
Family interventions	Multisystemic Therapy	Community treatment of family. Intensive with support always available	Ia	Adequate implementation requires considerable staff involvement and commitment. Cost-effectiveness data indicate net savings to the community
Family interventions	Multidimensional Treatment Foster Care	Intensive multidimensional care in foster home	Ib	Enduring effects at up to 4 years post-intervention. Cost-effectiveness data indicate net savings to the community relative to regular foster care
Youth Interpersonal Skills	Problem-Solving Skills Training with in vivo Practice	Individual cognitive behavioural training	Ib	Decreases in deviant and increases in prosocial behaviour. Improvements in family and parent functioning have been observed in addition to child behaviour improvements
Youth Interpersonal Skills	Coping Power Programme	Group training especially on interpersonal cues and skills. Can have a parent training component	Ib	Reduced aggression and substance misuse and increased social competence
Youth Interpersonal Skills	Dinosaur School	Group training in interpersonal skills for young children	Ib	Decrease in behavioural problems and improved social behaviour. Can be integrated along with other components from the IY programme
Psychopharmacology	Psychostimulants	Patients with CP	Ia	Decrease in aggression that appears to be independent of/in addition to reduced ADHD symptoms

Table 46.1 (cont.)

Treatment	Form of treatment	Psychiatric disorder/target audience	Level of evidence for efficacy	Comments
Psychopharmacology	Clonidine	Patients with CP	Ib	Reduced oppositional defiant symptoms
Psychopharmacology	Psychostimulants + clonidine	Patients with CP	Ib	Improvement may be better than with either agent alone
Psychopharmacology	Risperidone	Patients with CP	Ib	Significant improvement in behaviour, including those with CP as well as developmental delay

(average effect size: $d = 0.84$ on overt aggression, $d = 0.69$ on covert aggression).

Clonidine has been studied alone and in combination with psychostimulants. A small (N = 8 per treatment group), placebo-controlled study showed that clonidine alone led to reduced ODD symptoms and clonidine plus stimulants resulted in greater improvement than stimulants or clonidine alone. Comparable findings were reported by Hazell and Stuart (2003) in a larger placebo-controlled, randomized trial (stimulants plus placebo versus stimulants plus clonidine). However, the use of polypharmacy treatment also carries the risk of increased side effects.

In a double-blind placebo-controlled study, risperidone has been shown to be efficacious for the treatment of aggressive youth with CD. Studies of the effect of lithium on aggression are inconsistent (also see Chapter 36).

Uncontrolled (open trials) studies have suggested that carbamazepine reduces aggression and explosive behaviour. However, carbamazepine failed to outperform placebo in a more recent, double-blind placebo-controlled study.

Conclusion

Psychological therapies are the mainstay of CP treatment. However, despite this strong evidence base, in both the USA and UK, only a small percentage of youth receive any treatment and even fewer receive empirically supported interventions. Further, the "effectiveness" of these interventions as practised in community settings tends to lag behind documented "efficacy" in controlled trials (Curtis et al., 2004). The next generation of evidence-based treatments for CP will likely include much greater attention to dissemination, including strategies for ongoing training and supervision to ensure treatment fidelity. The ultimate goal is to ensure that children with these disorders have access to high-quality, empirically based care.

Interventions discussed in this chapter are summarized in Table 46.1.

47

Treatment of depressive disorders in children and adolescents

Based on "Treatment of depressive disorders in children and adolescents" by Kelly Schloredt, Rachel Gershenson, Christopher K. Varley, Paul Wilkinson, and Ian Goodyer in Effective Treatments in Psychiatry, Cambridge University Press, 2008

Introduction

In the US, prevalence rates of Dysthymic Disorder (DD) and Major Depressive Disorders (MDD) in children and adolescents range from 0.6% to 8.2% (Lewinsohn et al., 1993). Rates are lower in childhood and increase dramatically during adolescence. One in 20 adolescents suffer from MDD at any time point; 20% have at least one episode by age 18 (Lewinsohn et al., 1993). In a UK national survey (Meltzer et al., 2003), 4% of children had anxiety or depression and about 1% had depression. Childhood depression is often persistent or recurrent, compromises development by interfering with academic and social functioning, and is a primary risk factor for substance use and suicide.

The UK National Institute for Health and Clinical Excellence (National Collaborating Centre for Mental Health, 2005a) guidelines for the treatment of youth depression proposes psychological treatment as the treatment of choice. Antidepressant medication is shunned for mild depression. In moderate to severe depression, fluoxetine is approved but the guideline suggests that it should be used cautiously and only in conjunction with ongoing psychological treatment. US practice parameters suggest a multi-method approach taking into consideration severity of illness, motivation of patient and patient's family, and severity of other psychiatric and/or medical conditions, with treatment provided in the least restrictive safe environment (Birmaher et al., 1998). Empirical US studies support both psychopharmacological and psychosocial interventions for MDD in children and adolescents with some limitations. There are few controlled studies examining treatment for dysthymia. The discussion here centres largely on MDD.

Pharmacotherapy

Psychopharmacological treatment of childhood and adolescent depression is common in the USA (Delate et al., 2004), though not in the UK (MHRA, 2003).

Selective Serotonin reuptate inhibitors (SSRIs)

The first double-blind, placebo-controlled trial of 96 children and adolescents, randomized to either fluoxetine (20 mg) or placebo over 8 weeks, found a 56% fluoxetine response rate compared to 33% with placebo. A second fluoxetine study of 219 youths found a 41% fluoxetine response rate versus 20% with placebo (Emslie et al., 2002). This led to the FDA approving fluoxetine for treatment of major depression in children and adolescents.

Other SSRI studies, however, have been difficult to decipher. Though generally well tolerated, evidence for efficacy is limited. The MHRA (UK) concluded that there were no or minimal benefits and increased side effects (possibly including increased suicidality) for paroxetine, sertraline, citalopram, and venlafaxine (MHRA, 2003). On one hand, there is evidence for SSRI response rates as high as 70% (Emslie et al., 2002; Wagner et al., 2003); on the other hand, clinical significance for some SSRIs is low (Wagner et al., 2004) or the effect over placebo is minimal (Emslie et al., 2002; Wagner et al., 2003; 2004).

SSRIs are the US psychopharmacological treatment of choice with some caution; only fluoxetine is the treatment of choice in the UK. There is a debate concerning the extent of positive reported benefits, the number of unpublished trials showing negative results, and possible mood related side effects that might lead to suicidal thinking and suicide attempts (Whittington et al., 2004). This has led to formal regulatory action. In June 2003, the MHRA declared paroxetine contraindicated for major depression treatment in individuals under age 18. Then the US FDA followed suit. SSRI medications were declared contraindicated by the MHRA for use in depressed youth include venlafaxine, citalopram, escitalopram, sertraline, nefazodone, and mirtazapine, in the belief that the risks of treatment with these agents outweigh benefits. Most studies excluded patients with comorbid conditions, more severe depression, and pre-existing suicidality. There is concern about extrapolating empirical findings to the more severely ill patients seen in clinics, though there may be greater medication–placebo differences in more severe depression. Despite these criticisms, a meta-analysis (Jureidini et al., 2004) of five published RCTs of SSRIs showed a small, but statistically significant, effect size of 0.26 (95% confidence interval 0.13 to 0.40).

An FDA sponsored meta-analysis of all paediatric SSRI studies revealed significantly increased suicidality and self-harm events in those given SSRI compared with placebo (Dubicka et al., 2006), though absolute differences are small (4.8% of children and adolescents given SSRIs versus 3.0% given placebo). Despite push-back from the academics, the FDA issued a "black box" warning regarding an increased risk of suicidal behaviour in antidepressant-treated children and adolescents. This "black box" warning led to significant decreases in the annual number of antidepressant prescriptions written in the USA, reversing a several years' trend of increasing numbers. Coincident with this decrease in antidepressant prescribing has been an increase in the rate of suicide in youth, raising questions of unintended negative consequences. A subsequent meta-analysis with a larger data set of second generation antidepressants in youth concluded that the risk was smaller, with the number needed to harm in depression, 112, in obsessive compulsive disorder (OCD) 200, and 143 in other anxiety disorders (Bridge et al., 2007). In addition there were no completed suicides in the over 4000 youth in antidepressant RCTs.

Practitioners are currently expected to inform their patients and families of possible side effects including suicidality, agitation, and clinical worsening of symptoms and to monitor them closely. The initial results of the TADS (Treatment for Adolescents with Depression Study, 2004) suggested that fluoxetine is more effective than placebo and more effective than CBT alone. Treatment reduced suicidality in all groups.

While some depressed children and adolescents appear to benefit from antidepressants, studies suggest that up to 40% are "non-responders" (Reinecke et al., 1998), highlighting the need for effective psychosocial treatment options. In view of the lack of evidence for other treatments (particularly psychological treatments) in severe depression, and the fact that subjects in treatment studies tend to have less severe depression, it is generally accepted that SSRIs are valuable in treating severe depression.

Tricyclic antidepressants (TCAs)

A Cochrane meta-analysis (Hazell et al., 2009) found 13 RCTs comparing TCAs with placebo in 506 children and adolescents aged 6–18. Results suggested marginal effectiveness in reducing depressive symptoms in depressed adolescents (effect size = −0.47, 95% CI −0.92 to −0.02) but not children (effect size = 0.15, 95% CI −0.34 to 0.64). Significantly higher side effect rates occurred with TCAs.

Other antidepressants

Small uncontrolled case series have shown improvements in depressed adolescents with bupropion, nefazodone, and phenelzine. There is no evidence for the efficacy of mirtazepine.

Somatic treatments

Electroconvulsive therapy (ECT)

The use of ECT in children and adolescents is controversial in the USA and UK. A review of the literature (American Academy of Child and Adolescent Psychiatry, 2004) suggested that ECT may be an effective treatment for adolescents with unipolar and bipolar disorders. Data remain insufficient in assessing its utility in depressed children. ECT is very rarely used in the UK and in the USA for depressed adolescents. Its use tends to be restricted to situations where a very urgent response is needed due to risk of death or in severe, treatment-resistant depression. It is considered best practice to obtain a second opinion before proceeding with ECT.

There have been no randomized ECT trials in adolescents (also see Chapter 20). A systematic review (Walter et al., 1999) of published case reports and case series showed that 33/52 (64%) of adolescents with major depression and 25/35 (71%) adolescents with psychotic depression showed remission or marked improvements after ECT. Publication bias could be present.

Current US practice parameters suggest consideration of ECT with adolescents an appropriate treatment option when adolescents have had two or more failed trials of pharmacotherapy with poor response, or when symptom severity precludes waiting for a response to psychopharmacological treatment (American Academy of Child and Adolescent Psychiatry, 2004). There is a strong need for consent from the adolescent's legal guardian, with a preference to also obtain consent/assent from the adolescent. In addition, there is a need to follow state and institutional guidelines, as well as a need to use techniques with evidence for the greatest efficacy and fewest side effects, and a need for systematic pre- and post-treatment evaluations including symptom and cognitive functioning assessments (American Academy of Child and Adolescent Psychiatry, 2004).

Psychotherapy

While the body of research on psychosocial interventions is growing rapidly, there exist only a small number of controlled studies. The treatment literature covers a variety of psychotherapeutic schools of thought, including psychodynamic therapy and supportive group treatment. Cognitive behavioural therapy (CBT) and interpersonal therapy (IPT) have been more widely studied in controlled trials.

Cognitive behavioural therapy (CBT)

CBT, the most thoroughly researched psychosocial intervention in depressed youth, aims to alter depressogenic behaviours and cognitions through a variety of techniques

including mood monitoring, pleasant events scheduling, and challenging negative automatic thoughts/beliefs. CBT has been delivered to adolescents in both individual and group formats with consistent results. A CBT meta-analysis (Lewinsohn & Clarke, 1999) found a large estimated overall effect size (1.27); 63% of patients across analysed studies made clinically significant improvements by the end of treatment. Other meta-analyses of CBT's effectiveness reached similar conclusions (Reinecke et al., 1998). Improvement rates in children and adolescents with depressive disorders are 54–67% (Brent et al., 1997). Participants in these studies tended to present with less severe symptomatology than those in studies of tricyclic antidepressants. More severe social impairment reduced the efficacy of CBT.

Brent et al. (1997) randomly assigned 107 adolescents with MDD to 12–16 weeks of CBT treatment, systemic behavioural family therapy (SBFT), and non-directive supportive therapy (NST). Short-term outcomes revealed decreased depressive cognitions in the CBT group (Brent et al., 1997; Clarke et al., 1999), but no long-term advantage in rates of remission, recovery, recurrence, and level of functioning (Birmaher et al., 2000). Booster sessions did not reduce the follow-up recurrence rate but did appear to speed the recovery of those still depressed after acute treatment (Clarke et al., 1999).

The Treatment for Adolescents with Depression Study was a large RCT with rigorous methodology, comparing depressed adolescents (about 110 patients per group) on medication alone (fluoxetine), psychotherapy alone (CBT), combined treatment (fluoxetine + CBT), or placebo (Treatment for Adolescents with Depression Study, 2004). Initial results following 12 weeks of treatment revealed response rates of 71% for combined fluoxetine and 'CBT, 63% for fluoxetine alone, 43% for CBT alone, and 31% for placebo. Follow-up data, however, show that these initial treatment differences disappear 36 weeks post-treatment (TADS Team, 2007). More specifically, the effects of CBT only and fluoxetine only treatments converged with those of the combined treatment, and approximately 80% of all participants experienced a significant decline in symptomatology regardless of the type of treatment received. Melvin et al. (2006) compared sertraline, CBT, and combined sertraline and CBT, and demonstrated that CBT was more effective than sertraline. There was no difference between combined and single treatments.

Another RCT of combined treatment, the Treatment of SSRI-Resistant Depression in Adolescents study (TORDIA), randomized 334 adolescents with MDD (12–18 years old) to one of four treatment conditions following an inadequate response to a 2-month SSRI trial (Brent et al., 2008). The four conditions included: (1) switch to a second SSRI (paroxetine, citalopram, or fluoxetine); (2) switch to a second SSRI plus cognitive behavioural therapy (CBT); (3) switch to venlafaxine; or (4) switch to venlafaxine plus CBT. A significantly higher treatment response rate was noted for participants who received either medication with CBT (54.8% response rate) than for participants who received medication alone (40.5% response rate).

Interpersonal therapy (IPT)

In contrast to CBT, interpersonal therapy (IPT) aims to reduce depressive symptoms and increase interpersonal functioning by connecting symptoms to problem areas such as grief, role disputes, role transitions, and interpersonal sensitivities. Originally developed for depressed adult outpatients, IPT has been manualized for adolescents (IPT-A) and applied in both clinic and school settings (Mufson et al., 2004). Initial evaluation of the 12-week treatment suggested positive gains; the majority of adolescents reported fewer depressive symptoms. Improvements in social functioning were maintained

Table 47.1 Effectiveness of treatments for depressive disorders in children and adolescents

Treatment	Form of treatment	Psychiatric disorder/target audience	Level of evidence for efficacy	Comments
Pharmacotherapy	SSRIs	Childhood and adolescent depression	Ia	Only SSRI showing significant improvement in symptoms is fluoxetine. Much controversy about the use of SSRIs in this age group. Other SSRIs and other newer antidepressants have little or negative evidence for effectiveness
Electroconvulsive therapy	(ECT)	Childhood and adolescent depression	III	Recommendation only when depression is so severe that safety or welfare of the patient is at immediate risk
Psychotherapy	Cognitive behavioural	Childhood and adolescent depression	Ia	Meta-analyses reveal effect size from 0.41 to 1.70. Improvement in the range of somewhere between 50% and 70%
Psychotherapy	Interpersonal therapy	Childhood and adolescent depression	Ia	There are RCTs here, but caution should be used because the RCTs have all been conducted by the same group. One study showed both CBT and IPT to be better than waiting list, but CBT and IPT were equally effective
Psychotherapy	Family therapy	Families with and parents with children with childhood and adolescent depression	IV	While it is thought that the family system impacts the depression in childhood and adolescence, little empirical evidence exists to support this viewpoint

at 1-year follow-up (Mufson & Fairbanks, 1996). Findings have been replicated: IPT-A reduces depressive symptoms and improves social functioning and interpersonal problem solving in acutely depressed adolescents. IPT-A appears effective when delivered within a school-based health clinic (Mufson et al., 2004). Both IPT and CBT when compared to each other and to a wait-list control were significantly better than controls with no significant difference in efficacy between them (Rosselló & Bernal, 1999).

Family therapy

Family-based interventions, such as family therapy for the treatment of depressed adolescents (FTDA) and Stress Busters, will likely be an area of increased investigation in years to come and appear to be promising treatments. While family discord can be an important aetiological factor in paediatric depression, randomized controlled trials have not shown family therapy, for the whole family or for the parents, to be any more effective than control treatments (Brent et al., 1997).

Issues to consider about treatment

Regardless of intervention type, psychotherapy or psychopharmacology, approximately 40% of depressed youth are treatment "non-responders" (Reinecke et al., 1998). Of those who "respond" to acute treatment, 1 year relapse rates are significant (Birmaher et al., 2000). We must also consider the natural history of an episode of depression. Current evidence is that the median time to full remission is between 28 and 39 weeks with around 70% of patients recovering by 72 weeks (Goodyer et al., 2003). Many treatments may accelerate time to recovery. Studies that pit interventions directly against each other in RCTs are important.

Interventions discussed in this chapter are summarized in Table 47.1.

48

Treatment of psychoses in children and adolescents

Based on "Treatment of psychoses in children and adolescents" by
Anthony James and Jon McClellan in Effective Treatments in Psychiatry, Cambridge
University Press, 2008

Introduction

The evidence base demonstrating the efficacy of antipsychotic medication in the treatment of early-onset schizophrenia (EOS) is increasing. However, there is a lack of researched-based evidence for psychological treatments, and in this area treatment decisions may need to be based on data extrapolated from adults. Though current evidence suggests that EOS is continuous with the adult form, EOS generally has a more severe course and is less treatment responsive. Progress is also being made in researching treatments for early-onset bipolar disorder (EOBPD); again the early form of bipolar disorder appears more severe and treatment-resistant than the adult form, particularly rapid cycling cases.

Following recent research findings, US (APA, 2009) and UK guidance (National Collaborating Centre for Mental Health, 2010) for adults no longer emphasizes the use of second generation antipsychotics (SGAs) over first generation antipsychotics (FGAs), but do highlight the importance of psychological treatments, family therapy, CBT, psychoeducation, vocational training, as well as support for carers.

Schizophrenia

A Cochrane Review (Kennedy et al., 2007) of treatments for childhood-onset schizophrenia (age of onset <13 years) found improvements with antipsychotic treatment. However, there was little to support the use of one antipsychotic medication over another, with the exception of clozapine over haloperidol. A systematic review and meta-analysis of 15 studies of antipsychotics in children and adolescents (up to the year 2003) showed a 55.7% average response to second generation antipsychotics (SGAs) compared to 72.3% for first generation antipsychotics (FGAs). The effect size of 0.36 in favour of the FGAs was not significant (Armenteros & Davies, 2006). The review was limited by the methodological quality of the studies which included only 2 RCTs of FGA medications, loxapine and haloperidol.

The US multicentre, randomized controlled trial,Treatment of Early-Onset Schizophrenia Spectrum Disorders (TEOSS) (Sikich et al., 2008) involving 119 young people (aged 8–19 years) showed that risperidone and olanzapine (SGAs) were not superior to molindone, an FGA.

Clozapine

Various RCTs have shown clozapine to be more effective than haloperidol (Kumra et al., 1996), olanzapine (Shaw et al., 2006), and high-dose olanzapine (Kumra et al., 2007). Clozapine is effective against both positive and negative symptoms of schizophrenia (Kumra et al., 2007) with improvement evident within the first 6 weeks of treatment. Overall, clozapine appears to be a uniquely beneficial second-line agent for treating children with refractory schizophrenia (Gogtay & Rapoport, 2008), and some argue for its early use in first episode psychosis. Indeed, despite a concerning side effect profile, clozapine is associated with a substantially reduced mortality rate compared to other antipsychotics (Tiihonen et al., 2009).

Bipolar disorder

There is an increasing trend to use antipsychotics in children and adolescents, both in the acute manic phase and as mood stabilizers. A small, double-blind, placebo-controlled study found that quetiapine in combination with divalproex was more effective for the treatment of adolescent bipolar mania than divalproex alone (DelBello et al., 2002), while separately quetiapine appears to act faster than divalproex (DelBello et al., 2006). The evidence base for the use of lithium in youth is limited, but a large open trial showed that lithium in combination with antipsychotic drugs was efficacious in treating mania (Kafantaris et al., 2003). A short-term (3-week), multicentre, double-blind RCT involving outpatient and inpatient adolescents aged 13–17 years with an acute manic or mixed episode showed a significant benefit of olanzapine over placebo in reducing Young Mania Rating Scale scores (effect size 0.84) (Tohen et al., 2007). Risperidone also appears effective in the manic stage of the illness (Haas et al., 2009).

Expert guidelines on the treatment of paediatric bipolar disorder (Kowatch et al., 2005) recommend the use of mood stabilizers and/or SGAs. A combination of mood stabilizers and SGAs is often advocated, though this is controversial. There are also negative RCTs for the use of valproate (Wagner et al., 2009) and oxcarbazepine (Wagner et al., 2006). Thus the role of mood stabilizers in paediatric bipolar disorder remains to be established. The choice of medication also depends on the phase of the illness, presence of psychosis, presence of rapid cycling, risk of side effects, and most importantly patient and family acceptance. SGAs are recommended for treating psychotic symptoms but they also act as mood stabilizers. Premature discontinuation of antipsychotic medication leads to a recurrence of psychotic symptoms in a large percentage of cases (Kafantaris et al., 2004).

Psychopharmacological side effects

The side effect profile of antipsychotics differs according to their receptor blockade potential (for reviews see Correll et al., 2009; Correll, 2008). There are important differences between SGAs and FGAs in terms of metabolic syndromes, with perhaps more similarities than originally thought with respect to extrapyramidal side effects (EPSEs) and hyperprolactinaemia.

Weight gain

Weight gain following the use of SGAs is greater in children and adolescents than adults (Correll et al., 2009). Excessive weight gain is associated with significant medical morbidity and mortality including dyslipidaemia, diabetes mellitus, polycystic ovary syndrome, hypertension, and sleep apnoea. The potential for weight gain is greatest with olanzapine and lowest with aripiprazole and ziprasidone (Correll et al., 2009).

Hyperprolactinaemia

Secretion of prolactin from the pituitary is regulated by tonic dopaminergic inhibition; consequently the majority of antipsychotics elevate prolactin levels. Hyperprolactinaemia can result in amenorrhoea and oligomenorrhoea, erectile dysfunction, decreased libido, hirsutism, and galactorrhoea. Prolactin levels are not closely correlated with these symptoms. Hyperprolactinaemia appears dose dependent, tends to normalize over time, and resolves after antipsychotic discontinuation. The relative potency of antipsychotic drugs to induce hyperprolactinaemia is greatest with risperidone and least with aripiprazole. If the patient develops persistently high prolactin levels, switching to a medication with a lower risk is often helpful. Aripiprazole may actually lower prolactin levels.

Extrapyramidal side effects

Children and adolescents appear more sensitive than adults to extrapyramidal side effects (EPSEs), i.e. parkinsonian side effects and dystonia (Correll, 2008), but perhaps have lower risk of tardive dyskinesia.

Neurological adverse events

Seizures

Children and adolescents taking clozapine may be at higher risk than adults for developing seizures or epileptiform discharges on an EEG.

Sedation/somnolence

Sedation and somnolence are frequent side effects of antipsychotics that are usually dose dependent.

Somnolence appears to reduce with time due to developing tolerance.

Neutropenia and agranulocytosis

There is a risk of neutropenia and agranulocytosis with clozapine treatment; hence the absolute need for regular monitoring.

Cardiac effects

Myocarditis, cardiomyopathy

Clozapine has been associated with a small risk for myocarditis, which occurs early on in treatment. A baseline ECG is necessary and blood pressure and pulse are initially performed daily. Clozapine should be discontinued if either myocarditis or cardiomyopathy develops.

Assessment and monitoring

At baseline and regularly at 3–6 monthly follow-up intervals, weight, blood pressure, and blood tests (full blood count (at baseline only, except clozapine where more regular monitoring is required), liver function tests, fasting lipids, cholesterol, blood sugar, and prolactin) are recommended (Correll, 2008).

Family therapy

Although family therapy is often used with families of adolescents with psychotic disorders, there is only one small trial of family therapy solely in this age group that showed no significant differences between groups in terms of functioning and time spent in hospital, but did show a reduction in overall costs despite the extra input (Rund, 1994). As part of the early intervention programme for psychosis for older adolescents and younger adults, family behavioural therapy with a specific focus on psychoeducation and CBT for relapse prevention, resulted in a significantly lower relapse rate compared to treatment as usual and a significantly longer time to relapse (Gleeson et al., 2009). The number needed to treat was 6 over 7 months. Family therapy also improved the carers' experience and understanding, but it did not reduce overall distress.

For bipolar disorder, adjunctive psychotherapy enhances the symptomatic and functional outcomes over a 2-year period (Miklowitz, 2008), although there is less evidence for early-onset cases. Treatments that emphasize medication adherence and early recognition of mood symptoms such as psychoeducation have stronger effects on mania, whereas treatments that emphasize cognitive and interpersonal coping strategies, e.g. CBT and family therapy, have stronger effects on depression.

Family-focused therapy for adolescents with EOBPD (13–17 years) (FFT-A) involving 21 sessions over 9 months and follow-up at 2 years, showed FFT-A was associated with a faster recovery from depression compared to brief psychoeducation (Miklowitz et al., 2008). High expressed emotion (EE) attitudes among parents are generally associated with an increased likelihood of relapse in EOBPD. This highlights the importance of a family approach with FFT-A, which results in a greater reduction in depressive and manic symptoms in high-EE families (Miklowitz et al., 2008).

CBT

An RCT of CBT versus befriending in older adolescents and young adults with early-onset psychosis found CBT did speed functional recovery initially, but there were no differences in symptomatic recovery, rate of hospitalization or functional recovery over time, with both interventions showing improvements (Jackson et al., 2008). A meta-analysis of cognitive remediation in one adolescent study showed benefits in the domains of cognition, psychosocial functioning, and symptoms, greater if combined with psychosocial rehabilitation (McGurk et al., 2007). There is no evidence of efficacy for social skills training (Pilling et al., 2002a).

Table 48.1 Effectiveness of treatments for psychoses in children and adolescents

Treatment	Form of treatment	Psychiatric disorder/target audience	Level of evidence for efficacy	Comments
Psychopharmacology	Atypical antipsychotics	Youth with schizophrenia	Ia	As effective as typical antipsychotics. Cause more weight gain in youth than adults
Psychopharmacology	Combined antipsychotic and mood stabilizer	Youth with bipolar illness	IIb	There is some, but weak, evidence that youth appear to do better on a combination of an antipsychotic and a mood stabilizer, especially if psychotic features present. But this is controversial with some negative studies for mood stabilizers
Psychopharmacology	Early pharmacological intervention	Psychoses	IIb	Intervention appears to be effective but little evidence that early intervention impacts long-term course and/or ability to remain well after intervention is stopped
Family therapy	Family therapy and other psychoeducational programmes to families	Families of patients with schizophrenia	IIa	Some evidence of family therapy being better than TAU
Psychotherapy	Cognitive behavioural therapy	Schizophrenia	IIa	Few studies specifically for adolescents. CBT may speed initial functional recovery

ECT

ECT is rarely used in adolescents. There are no RCTs, but case series and reports support its use in severe life-threatening psychotic depression or treatment-resistant mania. The response rate for psychotic disorders is 50–60% (Ghaziuddin et al., 2004b). The Practice Parameter of the American Academy of Child and Adolescent Psychiatry recommends ECT for adolescents when there is lack of response to at least two trials of pharmacological treatment or severe symptoms preclude waiting for a response to pharmacological treatment (Ghaziuddin et al., 2004b).

Conclusions

Fortunately, the evidence base for the use of antipsychotics in children and adolescents has increased with a number of RCTs now available; however, the side effect profile is concerning and requires continuous monitoring. Weight gain and metabolic problems associated with SGAs raise important public health concerns, given the widespread use of these medications (Sikich et al., 2008). Caution is further heightened by the finding that generally side effects in children and adolescents appear more severe than in adults. With the notable exception of clozapine, there is no evidence for greater efficacy of one antipsychotic over another in the treatment of psychosis in this age group. Choice may therefore be guided by the side effect profile and the knowledge that switching of antipsychotics is not backed by evidence. Using high doses of antipsychotics does not appear effective (only indirect evidence for high-dose olanzapine; Kumra et al., 2007), and such practice is not recommended. Indeed, dosing should be more conservative in untreated new-onset cases.

Interventions discussed in this chapter are summarized in Table 48.1.

49

Anxiety disorders: Separation anxiety disorder, generalized anxiety disorder, specific phobias, social phobia, panic disorder, post-traumatic stress disorder (PTSD), adjustment disorder, and obsessive compulsive disorder (OCD)

Based on "Anxiety disorders" by Christopher K. Varley, Angeles Diaz-Caneja, and Elena Garralda in Effective Treatments in Psychiatry, Cambridge University Press, 2008

Introduction

Anxiety disorders, often associated with significant functional impairment in multiple domains, are common in childhood, occurring in 3–13% of children and adolescents (Costello & Angold, 1995). Children typically present with more than one anxiety disorder. Comorbidity, primarily with depression, is common. Since anxiety disorders may persist into adulthood, effective treatment is important.

Treatments for anxiety disorders in youth often draw from the adult literature as few controlled studies have been conducted in youth. Recently published RCTs in younger people have limitations (small number of participants, unclear inclusion criteria, comorbidities of other anxiety disorders or depression), and need to be taken cautiously. Pharmacotherapy for anxiety disorders in youth is not generally approved in the UK (except sertraline and fluvoxamine for OCD) and in the USA (except for sertraline, fluvoxamine, fluoxetine, and clomipramine for OCD). Clinicians, however, often use medications based on their clinical expertise or experience, supported a little by RCTs in the scientific literature.

The American Academy of Child and Adolescent Psychiatry (AACAP) published practice guidelines for management of anxiety disorders, PTSD, and OCD (1997b, 1998a, 1998b). The European Society of Child and Adolescent Psychiatry has published guidelines for OCD (Thomsen, 1998). The Royal College of Psychiatrists suggests that psychoeducation about the diagnosis (symptoms, treatment, prognosis) is important before formal treatment. The family is considered important and should be included in any treatment plan (AACAP, 1997, 1998a, 1998b).

This chapter first discusses mixed or non-specified anxiety disorders and then focuses on specific anxiety disorders.

Anxiety disorders in general (includes social anxiety disorder)

Psychotherapy: cognitive behavioural therapy

Many studies do not have defined diagnostic inclusion criteria or included youth with mixed anxiety disorders. Cognitive behavioural therapy (CBT) has proved effective in a number of RCTs or quasi-experimental studies. Participants had generalized anxiety disorder (GAD), separation anxiety disorder, and social phobia. Two RCTs (Kendall et al., 1997) found that a CBT cohort showed clinically significantly reduced anxiety compared to a wait-list control. CBT and CBT plus family anxiety management reduced anxiety compared to a control group; improvements were sustained at 1-year follow-up (Barret et al., 1996b). Combined treatment fared better in the long term.

CBT was also effective with and without parental involvement (Manassis et al., 2002). Children with higher social anxiety may respond better to individual treatment (Manassis et al., 2002).

Psychopharmacology

In two RCTs of SSRIs in children and adolescents with mixed anxiety disorders, an 8-week study found that 76% of those treated with fluvoxamine improved versus 28% on placebo (RUPPS, 2001). In a 12-week RCT, 61% improved on fluoxetine versus 31% on placebo (Birmaher et al., 2003). The first study had an open follow-up phase where participants were divided into three groups and followed for 6 months: (a) continuing with fluvoxamine (96% improved); (b) placebo non-responders switching to fluvoxamine (56% improved); (c) fluvoxamine non-responders switching to fluoxetine (71% improved).

In a small RCT, imipramine was superior to placebo in adolescents with school refusal and anxiety disorders. Data for other antidepressants are limited. Benzodiazepines may be considered in acute anxiety situations, but their effectiveness remains unproved.

Psychotherapy and psychopharmacology

The most important anxiety study to date, CAMS, a multisite RCT funded by the National Institute of Mental Health in the United States, investigated a number of anxiety conditions in youth, separation anxiety disorder, generalized anxiety disorder, and social phobia (Walkup et al., 2008). Treatment consisted of cognitive behavioural therapy, sertraline, or a combination. CBT utilized the "Coping Cat" Model developed by Kendall (Kendall et al., 1997) and was 12 weeks in duration. Sertraline was titrated to a maximum of 200 mg/day. At 12 weeks 81% responded to the combined treatment, 60% to cognitive behavioural therapy, 55% to sertraline, and only 24% to placebo. The mean mg/day dose of sertraline was 131 in combined treatment and 141 on medication alone.

Generalized anxiety disorder (GAD)

Psychotherapy: cognitive behavioural therapy

Behavioural techniques and CBT are recommended as first-line treatment. Where symptoms are severe, medication can be considered. Cognitive therapies include systematic desensitization, exposure and response prevention (ERP), extinction, counter-conditioning, modelling, and operant techniques (Barret et al., 1996b; AACAP, 1997b; Kendall et al., 1997).

Pharmacotherapy

Venlafaxine XR, in an 8-week multicentre RCT, significantly reduced ratings on anxiety scales in doses up to

225 mg/day but side effects included weakness, decreased appetite, pain and somnolence. A 9-week RCT with sertraline in 22 children and adolescents with GAD (Rynn et al., 2001) found significant improvements with sertraline on the Hamilton Anxiety Scale and CGI beginning at week 4. There is no good evidence for TCA use in children. Benzodiazepines may be used cautiously in anticipatory anxiety and panic disorder.

Specific phobia (including school phobia)

Psychotherapy: cognitive behavioural therapy

First-line treatment for social phobia is behavioural and cognitive behavioural treatment, which have been used extensively. Systematic desensitization and exposure and response prevention (ERP) have efficacy. When there are associated complications, individual and/or family psychotherapy and medication should be considered (AACAP, 1997b).

Uncontrolled studies suggest possible efficacy of behavioural management in school. A study comparing three interventions for school phobia (family-based behaviour therapy with in vivo flooding and child returning to school immediately; hospital-based inpatient including milieu, educational and occupational therapy, pharmacological treatment, and liaison with parents and school; home tutoring with psychotherapy for the child and parents) found in vivo exposure superior. Improvement was maintained after a year (Blagg & Yule, 1984). Subjects were not randomly allocated. In an RCT of CBT, educational support therapy, and wait-list control, CBT was effective compared to the control (King et al., 1998) but not superior to educational support therapy. Both treatments reduced anxiety and depression.

Psychopharmacology

One study revealed that imipramine was significantly better than placebo in facilitating school attendance and reducing anxiety symptoms, though other studies did not concur. No studies have compared psychological to pharmacological interventions.

Psychotherapy and psychopharmacology

Medication adjuvant of behavioural or CBT treatment can be considered. An 8-week study comparing CBT plus imipramine to CBT plus placebo in school refusal found medication and CBT significantly more efficacious in improving school attendance and decreasing depression. But at 1-year follow-up, no between-group differences were found in severity of depression or prevalence of anxiety or depressive disorders. Thus, the overall benefit of maintenance treatment remains unclear (Bernstein et al., 2001). Nonetheless, liaison between school, family, and other services emphasizing gradual reintegration into school is essential.

Social phobia (including selective mutism)

CBT (individual or group) and behavioural therapy are recommended first-line treatments. Family interventions should be considered (AACAP, 1997b).

Psychotherapy: cognitive behavioural therapy

Clinic-based treatments: (a) social effectiveness therapy for children addressing social anxiety by combining group social skills sessions and individual exposure sessions was superior to study-skills and test-taking skills (Testbusters) at 6 months follow-up (Beidel et al., 2000); and (b) social skills training, with or without parental involvement, was superior to a wait-list control (Spence et al., 2000). CBT group

therapy for adolescents was beneficial in a preliminary study. A 3-week RCT of CBT versus wait-list for children with social phobia found CBT superior on the majority of child, parent, and interviewer reports of social anxiety symptoms (Gallagher-Heather et al., 2004).

Psychopharmacology

Paroxetine was found beneficial (78% versus 38% with placebo) at a mean dose of 25 mg/day, though paroxetine is not currently recommended in youth. Side effects (typical for SSRIs) include headache, nausea, sedation, and activation. Serotonergic agents (paroxetine, sertraline, and nefazodone) examined in a case series had a positive clinical response and were well tolerated (Mancini et al., 1999). Fluoxetine, in case report series of children with selective mutism, was beneficial for 76% (decreased anxiety, increased speech in social settings). A 12-week RCT of 15 children found improved parent-rated outcome measures with fluoxetine (Black & Uhde, 1994).

Panic disorder

Treatment of panic disorder should be a combination of psychoeducation for the child and family with subsequent CBT. Small time-limited doses of benzodiazepines may be used if symptoms are very severe. SSRIs can be considered.

Post-traumatic stress disorder (includes adjustment disorders)

PTSD treatment should be comprehensive for both the child and parents and include trauma-focused therapy, psychoeducation about PTSD, and address non-PTSD behavioural and emotional difficulties.

Controlled intervention studies have not been done with adjustment disorders. Treatment guidelines generally follow recommendations for PTSD.

Psychotherapy: cognitive behavioural therapy

Seven randomized trials comparing trauma-specific CBT to no treatment or a credible alternative demonstrate the superiority of CBT on at least some outcomes for sexually abused, multiply traumatized, disaster and community violence exposed children (Deblinger, 1999; Cohen et al., 2004). Trauma-focused CBT (TF-CBT) in sexually abused youth leads to improvement. Family involvement did not impact outcome. TF-CBT includes teaching anxiety management skills, correcting maladaptive cognitions, and gradual exposure/desensitization. Most have a parental component. Group CBT for children exposed to a single stressor found that 57% of those who met PTSD criteria at onset did not meet criteria after treatment with 12/14 free of PTSD at 6-month follow-up (March et al., 1998). There was no control group. An RCT of CBT for children with PTSD and depression resulting from exposure to violence found lower scores on PTSD symptoms, depression, and psychosocial dysfunction in the intervention group after 3 months (Stein et al., 2003). Little data supports other psychological interventions.

Psychopharmacology

Psychopharmacological treatments are widely used to treat childhood PTSD (95% on a recent survey), but no empirical research exists. Antidepressants (SSRIs) should be used as adjuvant with psychological interventions if depressive or panic symptoms are present (AACAP, 1998a).

Eye movement desensitization and reprocessing (EMDR)

No controlled studies have evaluated the benefits and risks of EMDR in children and adolescents.

Consensus with PTSD would be that trauma-focused CBT should be used as first-line treatment, with subsequent pharmacotherapy.

Obsessive compulsive disorder

Obsessive compulsive behaviour treatment in youth has the most evidence supporting efficacy. AACAP guidelines (1998a) recommend behavioural therapy or medication initially with similar recommendations in Europe (Thomsen, 1998). A combination of behavioural therapy and medication with SSRIs appears the preferred treatment in severe cases.

Psychotherapy: behaviour therapy and cognitive behavioural therapy

Open trials of CBT involving ERP (exposure and response prevention) reveal efficacy. Manualized group CBT is also efficacious in OCD (Cordioli et al., 2003).

Family participation appears crucial in helping the child to overcome obsessive thoughts and compulsions. Integrated CBT and family treatment (CBFT) appears to improve the child's symptoms and the family's anxiety. It is as effective in reducing youth OCD symptoms as individual treatment (Barret et al., 2004).

Psychopharmacology

Drug treatment should be first line if children are overwhelmed by the symptoms or the family is unable to engage in treatment. Where possible it should be used in combination with ERP (AACAP, 1998b). Antidepressants, SSRIs and clomipramine, are first-line pharmacological options and have shown effectiveness in several randomized control trials, in particular fluoxetine, fluvoxamine, sertraline, paroxetine, and clomipramine.

In the most comprehensive study of OCD, CBT, sertraline, and their combination were studied in 112 patients, ages 7–17. CBT alone ($P = 0.003$), sertraline alone ($P = 0.007$) and combined treatment ($P = 0.001$) were superior to placebo (Paediatric OCD Treatment Study (POTS) Team, 2004). Combined treatment proved superior to CBT alone ($P = 0.008$) or to sertraline alone ($P = 0.006$). The results for clinical remission were as follows: combined treatment, 53.6%; CBT alone, 39.3%; sertraline alone, 21.4%; and placebo, 3.6%. All three active treatments were acceptable and well tolerated with no evidence of treatment-emergent harm to self or others.

A meta-analysis of pharmacotherapy trials in youth OCD found clomipramine superior to SSRIs, but side effects and risk of cardiac

Table 49.1 Effectiveness of treatments for anxiety disorder

Treatment	Form of treatment	Psychiatric disorder/target audience	Level of evidence for efficacy	Comments
Psychotherapy	Cognitive behavioural therapy	Anxiety disorder in general in children and adolescents	Ia	Reduction in anxiety that was maintained at 1-year follow-up. Those receiving CBT plus a family management programme fared even better
Psychotherapy	Cognitive behavioural therapy and techniques	GAD	IV	Recommended as first-line treatment but no real controlled studies
Psychotherapy	Cognitive behavioural therapy and techniques	Specific phobias	IIb	Recommended as first-line treatment and efficacy has been established
Psychotherapy	Cognitive behavioural therapy and techniques	School phobia	III	Behavioural treatment with in vivo flooding better than hospitalization or home schooling plus psychotherapy
Psychotherapy	CBT (individual or group)	Social phobia	IIa	A number of clinic-based studies supports its effectiveness
Psychotherapy	CBT	Panic disorder	IV	Little research but recommended as first-line treatment
Psychotherapy	Trauma-focused CBT	Post-traumatic stress disorder	Ib	Multiple controlled studies plus RCTs to support this intervention

Treatment	Intervention	Disorder	Evidence level	Notes
Psychotherapy	CBT with exposure response prevention (ERP)	Obsessive compulsive disorder	Ib	Found to be effective. CBT with ERP recommended as first-line treatment
Psychopharmacology	Tricyclic antidepressants (TCAs)	Anxiety disorder in general in children and adolescents	Ib	Imipramine improved school refusal and anxiety
Psychopharmacology	SSRIs	Anxiety disorder in general in children and adolescents	Ia	Particularly evidence for fluvoxamine, fluoxetine, and sertraline with somewhere between 50% and 75% responding
Psychopharmacology	SSRIs SNRIs	GAD	Ib	RCTs with venlafaxine, fluoxetine, and fluvoxamine
Psychopharmacology	Tricyclic antidepressants	School phobia	III	Some studies show significant improvement; other studies do not show improvement (imipramine)
Psychopharmacology	SSRIs	Social phobia Selective mutism	Ia	RCTs with fluoxetine primarily but other SSRIs are effective. Paroxetine also found effective but its use in children and adolescents is currently not encouraged
Psychopharmacology	SSRIs	Panic disorder	III	Medications used for panic disorder in adults are not recommended though open studies have revealed that panic disorder symptoms improved with SSRIs in this age grouping

Table 49.1 (cont.)

Treatment	Form of treatment	Psychiatric disorder/target audience	Level of evidence for efficacy	Comments
Psychopharmacology	SSRIs	PTSD	IIa	Controlled trials have been conducted with sertraline and paroxetine. 95% of adolescent psychiatrists have used SSRIs to treat PTSD symptoms in their patients
Psychopharmacology	SSRIs Clomipramine	Obsessive compulsive disorder	Ia	Repeatedly found to be effective. SSRIs recommended over clomipramine due to side effect differences
Psychopharmacology plus psychotherapy	SSRIs plus CBT	Anxiety disorder in general in children and adolescents	Ia	Combined treatment more effective (81%) than CBT (605) or SSRI (55%). All treatment superior to placebo (24%)
Psychopharmacology plus psychotherapy	TCAs plus CBT	School phobias	IIa	Combination was better than CBT alone. But no difference between groups at one year
Psychopharmacology plus psychotherapy	SSRI plus CBT	Obsessive compulsive disorder	Ib	Combined treatment more effective (54%) than the SSRI (sertraline) alone (21%) or CBT alone (395) or placebo alone (4%)

arrhythmias mitigate against it as first-line treatment (Geller et al., 2003).

Summary

- A pooled analysis of all controlled trials of antidepressants in children and adolescents identifies a heightened suicide risk in the treatment of both major depression and anxiety (4% suicide-related behaviours versus 2% on placebo).
- Emphasizing and teaching lifestyle choices such as exercise, peer support groups, and teamwork and effective communication between team members are important.

Interventions discussed in this chapter are summarized in Table 49.1.

50

Treatment of eating disorders in children and adolescents

Based on "Treatment of eating disorders in children and adolescents" by Matthew Hodes, Rose Calderon, Cora Collette Breuner, and Christoper K. Varley in Effective Treatments in Psychiatry, Cambridge University Press, 2008

Introduction

Eating disorders, including anorexia and bulimia nervosa, originate in late childhood and early adolescence. The majority of individuals first diagnosed with eating disorders are less than age 25 years. Age of onset for anorexia nervosa peaks between ages 13 and 15; for bulimia nervosa, between 17 and 25. Prevalence rates for anorexia nervosa are: 0.5–1.0% in females, 0.1% in males; for bulimia nervosa: 1–3% in females, <0.2% in males (Lask & Bryant-Waugh, 2007). The incidence of bulimia nervosa appears to be increasing.

Eating disorders are associated with functional impairment (increased withdrawal from activities and interactions and impairment in academic and work settings) (Lask & Bryant-Waugh, 2007). There is extensive psychiatric comorbidity, anxiety disorders including social phobia and OCD being common, with 50–70% of eating disordered patients having a comorbid depressive disorder (Herpetz-Dahlmann & Remschmidt, 1993; Eisler et al., 2000).

Relatively few controlled treatment studies have been carried out in eating disorders in youngsters. Treatment requires judicious integration of the available evidence base in child and adolescent eating disorders, treatments derived from understanding mechanisms of the disorder, and inferences from adult eating disorder research (Gowers & Bryant-Waugh, 2004). For successful treatment it is unclear whether multiple aspects of the illness must be addressed simultaneously or in sequence or whether, by solely addressing the eating disorder, other comorbid concerns will resolve.

Children and adolescents with eating disorders need to be medically stable before psychotherapy can be utilized. Usually therapists work closely with paediatrics or general medicine, dietetics and mental health providers while employing an eclectic treatment approach that considers the patient's understanding, intellectual ability, and the appropriateness of structured and language-based therapies versus more non-directive and or expressive therapies. All providers should collaborate actively and share a similar philosophy in the understanding and treatment of the disorder.

The initial approach to treatment of child and adolescent eating disorders includes psychoeducation which provides appropriate information about the disorders and effects of unhealthy eating behaviours and weight controlling strategies. Psychoeducation aims to correct any misconceptions about factors that lead to and maintain the illness, reduce resistance to treatment by increasing the adolescents' and parents' awareness of the disorders, and secure engagement and partnership of the young person for behavioural change.

The evidence base for specific interventions for anorexia and bulimia nervosa has been increasing in the first decade of the 21st century. Much of it concerns family-based interventions and CBT (Lock & Fitzpatrick, 2009) which are described here in more detail, but other interventions, while reported as being useful by sufferers, their families and clinicians (Lask and Bryant-Waugh, 2007), lack evidence and are covered only very briefly. The evidence is presented separately for each of the two main eating disorders.

Anorexia nervosa

Psychotherapies and other psychosocial interventions

Family therapy interventions

Considerable work has been carried out on the family therapy of adolescent anorexia nervosa (see reviews in Eisler, 2005 and Lock & Fitzpatrick, 2009). Currently models have converged in agreeing that families with an adolescent with anorexia nervosa have (a) a high level of closeness typically involving the patient and one parent, usually the mother, (b) hidden but ongoing conflict between the parents, and (c) a lack of expressed warmth and emotion recognition in the families. These formulations have produced specific approaches to intervention that include directive elements (as in Minuchin's Structural Family Therapy; Minuchin et al., 1978), reframing, and the avoidance of blame (emphasized in Selvini-Palazzoli's model; Selvini-Palazzoli, 1974).

Tentative conclusions for family therapy effectiveness come from RCTs and suggest: (1) family interventions that have a directive element and focus on parents guiding their offspring to eat more are associated with more rapid improvement than individual psychological treatments and/or no intervention (Russell et al., 1987; Robin et al., 1999); (2) by the end of 12–15 months of treatment, most will make good progress; (3) improvement occurs not only in weight but also in eating attitudes and mood even in the absence of specific therapies targeting these areas; (4) there is significant improvement in family relationships, involving both parents and adolescent, as well as between parents (Eisler et al., 2000); and (5) in families with high conflict, separated family therapy (parents and patient seen separately) shows advantages over conjoint family therapy (Eisler et al., 2000, 2007). Manualized family-based treatments have been described (Lock et al., 2001) and formed the basis for many of the trials mentioned here; they appear effective and applicable in clinical service settings (Loeb et al., 2007). A development from family-based treatments is multifamily therapy groups but the one small RCT published showed this was not superior to conjoint family therapy (Geist et al., 2000).

Cognitive behavioural therapy

Specific techniques of cognitive behavioural therapy include cognitive restructuring to address characteristic eating disordered attitudes about weight and shape and providing extensive psychoeducation (Garner & Vitousek, 1997; Christie, 2007). The challenge in anorexia is the patient's lack of motivation for weight gain. This may be addressed by starting CBT after family-based treatment has resulted in weight gain, typically associated with improved mood, and also motivational techniques (see below). No systematic studies of CBT with adolescents are available.

Body image therapy may be regarded as a variant of CBT. It addresses body image distortion and overemphasis of self-worth being dependent on body image that are hallmarks of eating disorders. Body image therapy, best utilized as an adjunct intervention, is a systematic approach to transforming the young person's relationship with his or her body from a self-defeating struggle to self-acceptance and enjoyment.

Other psychological interventions

Psychodynamic psychotherapy has a long tradition of use in treatment of children and adolescents with eating disorders, but has no evidence supporting its effectiveness. Adolescents provided with the psychodynamic psychotherapy achieved less weight gain and no greater gains in ego functioning than those in family therapy (Robin et al., 1999). Newer psychological treatments include narrative therapy and interpersonal psychotherapy. Motivational interviewing and enhancement are reported to be helpful for teenagers with chronic, entrenched patterns of eating disordered behaviours, especially those who are brought to treatment by parents or under court order rather than by their own desire for change. The initial treatment phase of anorexia is cultivating and sustaining motivation for change (Gowers & Bryant-Waugh, 2004).

Addressing nutritional and physical abnormalities

Nutritional counselling, an important comprehensive treatment component, provides individualized assessment and treatment regarding the physiological aspects of an eating disorder. The nutritionist facilitates the teenagers' and parents' understanding of what he or she needs from a physiological standpoint, teaching how to apply it to normalize food intake, to achieve normal hunger, and satiety signals.

The medical management of an adolescent with moderate to severe anorexia nervosa requires knowledge of the physical presentations and intervention for possible medical complications (Lask & Bryant-Waugh, 2007). The medical complications of anorexia nervosa which may require hospitalization for correction and weight gain include: cardiovascular abnormalities, electrolyte abnormalities, especially those arising from vomiting, and refeeding which may cause hypophosphataemia. Other specific abnormalities include growth retardation, delayed pubertal development and onset of menses, and osteoporosis which may occur in up to 50% of adolescents with anorexia nervosa.

Psychopharmacology

If significant psychiatric symptoms are present, then psychotropic medications may be considered as part of a comprehensive treatment plan, although the primary treatment for anorexia nervosa is eating (Gowers &

Bryant-Waugh, 2004). No controlled trials with children and adolescents exist; evidence is from clinical impressions, multiple single case studies, and inference from adult studies. Antidepressants, mainly fluoxetine, which is the first line drug in child and adolescent depression, is quite widely used when the depression is comorbid with an eating disorder (Gowers et al., 2010). Depression with anorexia nervosa improves with family treatment targeting weight gain and family relationships (Eisler et al., 2000), but for some children and adolescents the depression persists despite weight gain. In this group a trial of fluoxetine may be undertaken (Gowers & Bryant-Waugh, 2004). For high levels of anxiety, particularly at mealtimes, other anxiolytic medications may be tried on a case-by-case basis.

There has been increasing interest in antipsychotic drugs especially olanzapine to help achieve weight gain. Multiple single case studies of children and adolescents with severe anorexia treated with olanzapine suggest clinical improvement, probably by changing the fixed distorted belief systems and taking advantage of the weight gain effect. The beneficial effects of weight gain described in small RCTs of adults with anorexia nervosa (Bissada et al., 2008) have been influential in treatment for the younger patients.

Hospitalization

In addition to the medical indications described above for hospitalization, other indications include loss of more than 30% of ideal body weight, rapid weight loss, psychiatric comorbidity with self-harm risk, and poor progress in outpatient treatment. However evidence suggests admission does not improve the medium-term outcome. A randomized controlled trial of 170 adolescents (mean age 14 years 11 months) showed that inpatient treatment did not result in greater improvement than outpatient treatment, provided over 6 months or at 1 and 2 years after start of treatment (Gowers et al., 2007).

The limited research carried out on inpatient management has resulted in strict and lenient behavioural approaches being replaced by more flexible approaches seeking a greater partnership with patients and their parents (Touyz et al., 1995). Day programmes have been described, and evaluation in open design suggests moderate benefit for participants (Goldstein et al., 2010).

Bulimia nervosa

Family therapy

Family therapy approaches in adolescent bulimia nervosa have been influenced by the model for adolescent anorexia nervosa. The main difference is that the parental task in the first stage of treatment is to prompt the adolescent to eat regular meals thus reducing the starvation and urge to binge (rather than the need to consume greater quantities of food in a day and gain weight). A small open trial of eight adolescents found that during the intervention there was a significant reduction in binge eating, vomiting, and laxative use and an improvement in general outcome (Dodge et al., 1995). This was followed by an RCT with 80 adolescents aged 16 years of family-based intervention compared with supportive psychotherapy that showed the family-based intervention resulted in greater reduction of binge eating and purging, with nearly one-third in this group achieving abstinence (Le Grange et al., 2007).

Cognitive behavioural therapy

Motivation and subsequent engagement of adolescents with CBT may be greater than it is with those with anorexia nervosa because of the greater subjective distress associated with bulimia nervosa. An RCT involving 85 adolescents offered 10 sessions of CBT-guided self-care showed greater improvement than in those receiving family therapy at 6 months amongst older adolescents, but this difference disappeared at 12 months

(Schmidt et al., 2007). Reasons for the more rapid improvement in the CBT group may have been related to age (this group had mean age 17.4 (SD 1.8) years, whereas the family therapy group had mean age 17.9 (SD 1.6) years), and 17% of this group were not living at home with their family. One possibility is that for the older adolescents or young adults, who have more autonomy and many of whom are not living at home, CBT is more effective than family-based treatment, which is more suitable for younger adolescents who are at an earlier life-cycle stage.

Interpersonal therapy (IPT)

IPT, originally developed for use in depression, has been shown to be effective in adults with bulimia nervosa (Fairburn, 1997), but there are no studies of its use with adolescents. Its effectiveness with adult bulimia and benefit in adolescent depression suggest promise.

Psychopharmacology

There is scant evidence available regarding use of antidepressants, mostly SSRIs, for bulimia nervosa in adolescents. One open 8-week trial of fluoxetine along with supportive psychotherapy was associated with reduced binge and purge frequencies (Kotler et al., 2003). Expert advice

Table 50.1 Effectiveness of treatments for eating disorders in children and adolescents

Treatment	Form of treatment	Psychiatric disorder/target audience	Level of evidence for efficacy	Comments
Psychotherapy	Cognitive behavioural therapy	Bulimia nervosa	Ia	CBT-guided self-care showed greater improvement than those receiving family therapy at 6 months amongst older adolescents
Psychotherapy	Interpersonal therapy	Bulimia nervosa	III	No trials on children or adolescents but evidence from adult studies suggests it may be useful in this younger age group as well
Psychotherapy	Motivational interviewing and enhancement	Eating disorders	IV	Work with adolescents and impact of discontinuation of this type of treatment suggests that it could be effective
Family therapy	Various forms of structured and systemic family therapy	Anorexia nervosa	Ia	Weight gain. Better relationships among identified patients and parents. Better relationships between parents
Family therapy	Various forms of structured and systemic family therapy	Bulimia nervosa	Ia	Reduction binge–purge frequency, demonstrated in younger adolescents
Psychopharmacology	SSRIs (especially fluoxetine)	Eating disorders	III	Evidence from studies with adults might apply to adolescents as well. Some studies show worsening with citalopram. A greater body of evidence for treatment success with SSRIs for bulimia nervosa than for anorexia nervosa

| Psychopharmacology | Atypical antipsychotics (especially olanzapine) | Anorexia nervosa | III | May help change fixed ideas about body and weight and may also, because of weight gain side effect, directly contribute to weight gain |
| Hospitalization | Multidisciplinary intervention | Primarily for anorexia nervosa | Ia | May be necessary especially in life-threatening situations. Evidence suggests not associated with medium-term benefit. Evidence suggests no benefit over 1-2 years compared with outpatient management |

is that given the substantial evidence base for fluoxetine as a treatment for bulimia nervosa in adults (Bacaltchuk & Hay, 2003), this would be an appropriate drug for adolescents if adequate progress is not achieved with psychological treatment (Couturier & Lock, 2007).

Practice guidelines for treatment

The American Psychiatric Association's 2000 revision of their 1993 Practice Guidelines for the Treatment of Patients with Eating Disorders (American Psychiatric Association Practice Guidelines, 2000) offers a comprehensive overview and is helpful in orienting practitioners to eating disorders treatment. In the UK, the National Institute of Clinical Excellence has published guidelines on the management of eating disorders (National Collaborating Centre for Mental Health, 2004b) with children and adolescents with anorexia nervosa. The only guideline graded B (based on adequately designed studies without randomization) is that "family intervention that directly addresses the eating disorder should be offered" (National Collaborating Centre for Mental Health, 2004b). For bulimia nervosa, only one paragraph addresses psychological treatments in this younger group: "CBT-BN adapted as needed to suit their age, circumstances and level of development and including the family as appropriate". Other treatments and service recommendations are based on expert committee reports or on extrapolation from adult studies with control or comparison groups.

One survey regarding treatments provided across Europe revealed considerable variation with respect to the availability of inpatient and day services and range of psychological treatments. Psychotropic drugs including SSRIs, antipsychotics, and minor tranquillizers appear to be quite widely used (Gowers et al., 2010).

Interventions discussed in this chapter are summarized in Table 50.1.

Appendix I: Key to effectiveness tables

Ia Evidence from meta-analysis of randomized controlled trials

Ib Evidence from at least one randomized controlled trial

IIa Evidence from at least one controlled study without randomization

IIb Evidence from at least one other type of quasi-experimental study

III Evidence from non-experimental descriptive studies, such as comparative studies, correlation studies, and case–control studies

IV Evidence from expert committee reports or opinion and/or clinical experience of respected authorities

US Agency for Health Care Policy and Research Classification (AHCPR) (US Department of Health and Human

Services, Public Health Service, Agency for Health Care Policy and Research. Acute pain management: operative or medical procedures and trauma. Rockville, MD: Agency for Health Care Policy and Research Publications 1992 – see http://www.ncbi.nlm.nih.gov/books/NBK16501/).

Please move that the level of evidence refers to the strength of the conclusions in the last column of the table, not the level of effectiveness. Thus, for example, on p. 289 the evidence for in-patient, day-patient and out-patient treatment are compared (Table 34.1). As this has been subjected to randomized trial the level of the evidence is Ib, but as this trial showed as differences between the groups there is no evidence that any one is better than any other.

References

AACAP Official Action (2002). Practice parameter for the use of stimulant medications in the treatment of children, adolescents and adults. *Journal of the American Academy of Child and Adolescent Psychiatry*, **41**(2) Suppl., 26S–49S.

Aarsland, D., Larsen, J. P., Cummins, J. L. & Laake, K. (1999). Prevalence and clinical correlates of psychotic symtoms in Parkinson disease: a community-based study. *Archives of Neurology*, **56**, 595–601.

Abramowitz, J. S. (1997). Effectiveness of psychological and pharmacological treatments for obsessive-compulsive disorder: a quantitative review. *Journal of Consulting and Clinical Psychology*, **65**, 44–52.

AD2000 Collaborative Group (2004). Long-term donepezil treatment in 565 patients with Alzheimer's disease (AD2000): randomized double-blind trial. *The Lancet*, **363**, 2105–15.

Agras, W. S., Walsh, B. T., Fairburn, C. G., Wilson, G. T. & Kraemer, H. C. (2000). A multicenter comparison of cognitive-behavioral therapy and interpersonal psychotherapy for bulimia nervosa. *Archives of General Psychiatry*, **57**, 459–66.

Alexander, J. F. & Parsons, B. V. (1982). *Functional Family Therapy*. Monterey, CA: Brooks/Cole.

Alexander, C. N., Robinson, P. & Rainforth, M. (1994). Treating and preventing alcohol, nicotine, and drug abuse through Transcendental Meditation: a review and statistical meta-analysis. *Alcoholism Treatment Quarterly*, **11**, 13–87.

Altshuler, L. L., Bauer, M., Frye, M. A. et al. (2001). Does thyroid supplementation accelerate tricyclic antidepressant response? A review and meta-analysis of the literature. *American Journal of Psychiatry*, **158**(10), 1617–22.

Aman, M. G., McDougle, C. J., Scahill, L. et al. (2009). Medication and parent training in children with pervasive developmental disorders and serious behavior problems: results from a randomized clinical trial. *Journal of the American Academy of Child and Adolescent Psychiatry*, **48**, 1143–54.

American Academy of Child and Adolescent Psychiatry (1997a). Practice parameters for the assessment and treatment of children and adolescents with conduct disorder. *Journal of the American Academy of Child and Adolescent Psychiatry*, **36**, 122S–39S.

American Academy of Child and Adolescent Psychiatry (1997b). Practice parameters for the assessment and treatment of children with anxiety disorders. *Journal of the American Academy of Child and Adolescent Psychiatry*, **36** (Suppl.), S4–S26.

American Academy of Child and Adolescent Psychiatry (1998a). Practice parameters for the assessment and treatment of children and adolescents with posttraumatic stress disorders. *Journal of the American Academy of Child and Adolescent Psychiatry*, **37** (Suppl.), S27–S45.

American Academy of Child and Adolescent Psychiatry (1998b). Practice parameters for the assessment and treatment of children and adolescents with obsessive-compulsive disorders. *Journal of the American Academy of Child and Adolescent Psychiatry*, **37** (Suppl.), S4–S26.

American Academy of Child and Adolescent Psychiatry (2004). Practice parameter for use of electroconvulsive therapy with adolescents. *Journal of the American Academy of Child and Adolescent Psychiatry*, **43**, 1521–39.

American Psychiatric Association (1994). *Diagnostic and Statistical Manual of Mental Disorders*, 4th edn: DSM-IV. Washington, DC: American Psychiatric Association.

American Psychiatric Association (1997). Practice guideline for the treatment of patients with Alzheimer's disease and other dementias of late life. *American Journal of Psychiatry*, **154** (Suppl.), 1–39.

American Psychiatric Association (1998). Practice guideline for the treatment of patients with panic disorder. Work Group on Panic Disorder. American

Psychiatric Association. *American Journal of Psychiatry*, **155** (5 Suppl.), 1–34.

American Psychiatric Association (1999). Practice guideline for the treatment of patients with delirium. *American Journal of Psychiatry*, **156** (May Suppl.), 1–20.

American Psychiatric Association (2000). Practice guideline for the treatment of patients with eating disorders (revision). American Psychiatric Association Work Group on Eating Disorders. *American Journal of Psychiatry*, **157**(1) Suppl., 1–39.

American Psychiatric Association (2002). *Reactive Attachment Disorder: Position Statement.* APA Document No. 200205. Washington, DC: The American Psychiatric Association.

American Psychiatric Association (2006). *Practice Guidelines for the Treatment of Patients with Substance Use Disorders*, 2nd edn. Washington, DC: American Psychiatric Association.

American Psychiatric Association (APA). (2009). *Practice Guideline for the Treatment of Patients with Schizophrenia*, 2nd edn. http://www.guideline.gov/summary/summary.aspx?doc_id=5217 (accessed 22 May, 2010).

American Psychiatric Association Practice Guidelines (2000). Practice guidelines for the treatment of patients with eating disorders (Revision). *Supplement to The American Journal of Psychiatry*, **151**(1), 1–39.

American Society of Addiction Medicine (2001). *ASAM Public Policy Statement.* Retrieved 30 August, 2004, from the American Society of Addiction Medicine website: http://www.asam.org/ppol/treatment.htm

Anastopoulos, A. D., Shelton, T. L, DuPaul, G. J. & Guevremont, D. C. (1993). Parent training for attention-deficit hyperactivity disorder: its impact on parent functioning. *Journal of Abnormal Child Psychology*, **21**, 581–95.

Ancoli-Israel, S., Martin, J. L., Gehrman, P. et al. (2003). Effect of light on agitation in institutionalized patients with severe Alzheimer disease. *American Journal of Geriatric Psychiatry*, **11**, 194–203.

Anders, T. F. & Eiben, L. A. (1997). Pediatric sleep disorders: A review of the past 10 years. *Journal of the American Academy of Child and Adolescent Psychiatry*, **36**, 9–20.

Andersen, A. E. (1999). Using medical information psychotherapeutically. In: P. S. Mehler & A. E. Andersen, eds. *Eating Disorders: A Guide to Medical Care and Complications.* Baltimore: The Johns Hopkins University Press, pp. 192–201.

Andersen, G., Vestergaard, K. & Lauritzen, L. (1994). Effective treatment of post-stroke depression with the selective serotonin reuptake inhibitor citalopram. *Stroke*, **25**, 1099–104.

Anderson, D. (1981). *Perspectives on Treatment: The Minnesota Experience.* Center City, MN: Hazelden.

Anderson, I. M., Delvai, N. A., Ashim, B. et al. (2007). Adjunctive fast repetitive transcranial magnetic stimulation in depression. *British Journal of Psychiatry*, **190**, 533–4.

Anderson, I. M., Nutt, D. J. & Deakin, J. F. (2000). Evidence-based guidelines for treating depressive disorders with antidepressants: a revision of the 1993 British Association for Psychopharmacology guidelines. British Association for Psychopharmacology. *Journal of Psychopharmacology*, **14**, 3–20.

Anderson, P., Chisholm, D. & Fuhr Dipl-Psych, D. C. (2009). Effectiveness and cost-effectiveness of policies and programmes to reduce the harm caused by alcohol. *The Lancet*, **373** (9682), 2234–46.

Andersson, G., Carlbring, P., Holmstrom, A. et al. (2006). Internet-based self-help with therapist feedback and in vivo group exposure for social phobia: a randomized controlled trial. *Journal of Consulting and Clinical Psychology*, **74**, 677–86.

Andersson, G., Waara, J., Jonssonm, U., Malmaeus, F., Carlbreng, P. & Ost, L. G. (2009). Internet-based self-help versus one-session exposure in the treatment of spider phobia in randomized control trial. *Cognitive and Behavioural Therapy*, **39**, 114–20.

Andresen, R., Oades, L. & Caputi, P. (2003). The experience of recovery from schizophrenia: towards an empirically validated stage model. *Australian and New Zealand Journal of Psychiatry*, **37**, 586–94.

Andrews, D. G., O'Connor, P., Mulder, C., McLennan, J., Derham, H., Weigall, S. & Say, S. (1996). Computerised psychoeducation for patients with eating disorders. *Australian and New Zealand Journal of Psychiatry*, **30**, 492–7.

Andrews, G. & Slade, T. (2006). Agoraphobia without a history of panic disorder may be part of the panic disorder syndrome. *Journal of Nervous and Mental Disease*, **190**, 624–30.

Andrews, G., Cuijpers, P., Craske, M. G., McEvoy, P. & Titov, N. (2010). Computer therapy for the anxiety and depressive disorders is effective, acceptable and practical health care: a meta-analysis. *PLoS One*, **5**. pii: e13196.

Anton, R. F., Moak, D. H, Latham, P. et al. (2005). Naltrexone combined with either cognitive behavioral or motivational enhancement therapy for alcohol dependence. *Journal of Clinical Psychopharmacology*, **25**, 349–57.

Anton, R. F., O'Malley, S. O., Ciraulo, D. A. et al. (2006). Combined pharmacotherapies and behavioral interventions for alcohol dependence. The COMBINE study: a randomized controlled trial. *Journal of the American Medical Association*, **295**, 2003–17.

Antonioli, C. & Reveley, M. A. (2005). Randomised controlled trial of animal facilitated therapy with dolphins in the treatment of depression. *British Medical Journal*, **331**, 1231.

Apodaca, T. R. & Miller, W. R. (2003). A meta-analysis of the effectiveness of bibliotherapy for alcohol problems. *Journal of Clinical Psychology*, **59**, 289–304.

Appolinario, J. C., Bacaltchuk, J., Sichieri, R. et al. (2003). A randomized, double-blind, placebo-controlled study of sibutramine in the treatment of binge-eating disorder. *Archives of General Psychiatry*, **60**(11), 1109–16.

Arbiter, E. A. & Black, D. (1991). Pica and iron-deficiency anaemia. *Child: Care, Health and Development*, **17**, 231–34.

Armenteros, J. & Davies, M. (2006). Antipsychotics in early-onset schizophrenia: systematic review and meta-analysis. *European Journal of Child and Adolescent Psychiatry*, **15**, 141–8.

Arnold, L. M., McElroy, S. L., Hudson, J. I., Welge, J. A., Bennett, A. J. & Keck, P. E. (2002). A placebo-controlled, randomized trial of fluoxetine in the treatment of binge-eating disorder. *Journal of Clinical Psychiatry*, **63**(11), 1028–33.

Aschenbrand, S. G., Kendall, P. C., Webb, A., Safford, S. M. & Flannery-Schroeder, E. (2003). Is childhood separation anxiety disorder a predictor of adult panic disorder and agoraphobia? A seven-year longitudinal study. *Journal of the American Academy of Child and Adolescent Psychiatry*, **42**(12), 1478–85.

Ashton, C. H., Rawlins, M. D. & Tyrer, S. P. et al. (1990). A double-blind placebo-controlled study of buspirone in diazepam withdrawal in chronic benzodiazepine users. *British Journal of Psychiatry*, **157**, 232–8.

Asplund, C. A., Aaronson, J. W. & Aaronson, H. E. (2004). 3 Regimens for alcohol withdrawal and detoxification. *Journal Family Practice*, **53**, 545–54.

Atmaca, M., Kuloglu, M., Tezcan, E. et al. (2002). The efficacy of citalopram in the treatment of premature ejaculation: a placebo-controlled study. *International Journal of Impotence Research*, **14**(6), 502–5.

Australian Institute of Health and Welfare (2003). *Alcohol and other drug treatment services in Australia: Findings from the National Minimum Data Set 2001–02*. Vol. 16 Bulletin No. 10, AIHW cat. no. AUS 40. 2003. Canberra: Australian Institute of Health and Welfare.

Avery, D. H., Eder, D. N. & Bolte, M. A. et al. (2001). Dawn simulation and bright light in the treatment of SAD: a controlled study. *Biological Psychiatry*, **50**(3), 205–16.

Babor, T. F. & Grant, M. (1992). *Programme on Substance Abuse. Project on Identification and Management of Alcohol Related Problems. Report on Phase II: A Randomised Controlled Trial of Brief Interventions in Primary Health Care*. Geneva: World Health Organisation.

Babor, T., Carroll, K. M., Christiansen, K. et al. (2004). Brief treatments for cannabis dependence: findings from a randomized multi-site trial. *Journal of Consulting and Clinical Psychology*, **72**, 455–66.

Babyak, M., Blumenthal, J. A. & Herman, S. et al. (2000). Exercise treatment for major depression: maintenance of therapeutic benefit at 10 months. *Psychosomatic Medicine*, **62**(5), 633–8.

Bacaltchuk, J. & Hay, P. (2003). Antidepressants versus placebo for people with bulimia nervosa. *Cochrane Database of Systematic Reviews*, CD003391. Oxford: Update Software Ltd.

Baillargeon, L., Landreville, P., Verreault, R., Beauchemin, J. P., Gregoire, J. P. & Morin, C. M. (2003). Discontinuation of benzodiazepines among older insomniac adults treated with cognitive-behavioural therapy combined with gradual tapering: a randomized trial. *Canadian Medical Association Journal*, **169**, 1015–20.

Baille, A., Mattick, R. P., Hall, W. & Webster, P. (1994). Meta-analytic review of the efficacy of smoking cessation interventions. *Drug and Alcohol Review*, **13**, 157–70.

Baker, A., Boggs, T. G. & Lewin, T. J. (2001). Randomized controlled brief cognitive-behavioural interventions among regular users of amphetamine. *Addiction*, **96**, 1279–87.

Baker, D. G., Diamond, B. I., Gillette, G. et al. (1995). A double-blind, randomized, placebo-controlled, multi-center study of brofaromine in the treatment of post-traumatic stress disorder. *Psychopharmacology (Berl)*, **122**, 386–9.

Bakermans-Kranenburg, M. J., van IJzendoorn, M. H. & Juffer, F. (2003). Less is more: Meta-analysis of sensitivity and attachment interventions in early childhood. *Psychological Bulletin*, **129**, 195–215.

Bakker, A., van Balkom, A. J. & Spinhoven, P. (2002). SSRIs vs. TCAs in the treatment of panic disorder: a meta-analysis. *Acta Psychiatrica Scandinavica*, **106**(3), 163–7.

Baldwin, D. S., Anderson, I. M., Nutt, D. J. et al. (2005). Evidence-based guidelines for the pharmacological treatment of anxiety disorders: recommendations from the British Association for Psychopharmacology. *Journal of Psychopharmacology*, **19**, 567–96.

Baldwin, D. S., Huusom, A. K. & Maehlum, E. (2006). Escitalopram and paroxetine in the treatment of generalised anxiety disorder: randomised, placebo-controlled, doubleblind study. *British Journal of Psychiatry*, **189**, 264–72.

Ballard, C. G., Thomas, A., Fossey, J. et al. (2004). A 3-month, randomized, placebo-controlled, neuroleptic discontinuation study in 100 people with dementia: the neuropsychiatric inventory median cutoff is a predictor of clinical outcome. *Journal of Clinical Psychiatry*, **65**, 114–19.

Ballenger, J. C., Davidson, J. R. T., Lecrubier, Y. et al. (2001). Consensus statement on generalized anxiety disorder from the international consensus group on depression and anxiety. *Journal of Clinical Psychiatry*, **62** (Suppl. 11), 53–8.

Ballesteros, J. & Callado, L. F. (2004). Effectiveness of pindolol plus serotonin uptake inhibitors in depression: a meta-analysis of early and late outcomes from randomized controlled trials. *Journal of Affective Disorders*, **79**(1–3), 137–47.

Bancroft, J. (1989). *Human Sexuality and its Problems*. Edinburgh: Churchill Livingstone, pp. 128–13.

Bank, L., Marlowe, J. H., Reid, J. B., Patterson, G. R & Weinrott, M. R. (1991). A comparative evaluation of parent training interventions for families of chronic delinquents. *Journal of Abnormal Child Psychology*, **19**, 15–33.

Barbaric, N. C., McConaha, C. W., Halmi, K. A. et al. (2004). Use of nutritional supplements to increase the efficacy of fluoxetine in the treatment of anorexia nervosa. *International Journal of Eating Disorders*, **35**(1), 10–15.

Barber, J. G. & Gilbertson, R. (1997). Unilateral interventions for women living with heavy drinkers. *Social Work*, **42**, 69–78.

Barbini, B., Colombo, C., Benedetti, F., Campori, E., Bellodi, L. & Smeraldi, E. (1998). The unipolar-bipolar dichotomy and the response to sleep deprivation. *Psychiatry Research*, **79**(1), 43–50.

Barkley, R. A. & Cunningham, C. E. (1979). The effects of methylphenidate on the mother–child interactions of hyperactive children. *Archives of General Psychiatry*, **36**, 201–8.

Barlow, D. H., Gorman, J. M., Shear, M. K. & Woods, S. W. (2000). Cognitive-behavioral therapy, imipramine, or their combination for panic disorder: a randomized controlled trial. *Journal of the American Medical Association*, **283**(19), 2529-36.

Barnard, K. E., Magyary, D., Sumner, G., Booth, C. L., Mitchell, S. K. & Spieker, S. (1988). Prevention of parenting alterations for women with low social support. *Psychiatry*, **51**, 248-53.

Barnett, S. D., Kramer, M. L., Casat, C. D., Connor, K. M. & Davidson, J. R. (2002). Efficacy of olanzapine in social anxiety disorder: a pilot study. *Journal of Psychopharmacology*, **16**, 365-8.

Barrett, P. M., Dadds, M. R. & Rapee, R. M. (1996a). Family treatment of childhood anxiety: a controlled trial. *Journal of Consulting and Clinical Psychology*, **64**, 333-42.

Barrett, P. M., Dadds, M. R. & Rapee, R. M. (1996b). Family management of childhood anxiety: a controlled trial. *Journal of Consulting and Clinical Psychology*, **65**, 366-80.

Barrett, P., Healy-Farrell, L. & March, J. (2004). Cognitive-behavioural family treatment of childhood obsessive-compulsive disorder: a controlled trial. *Journal of the American Academy of Child and Adolescent Psychiatry*, **43**, 46-62.

Barrows, K. A. & Jacobs, B. P. (2002). Mind-body medicine, an introduction & review of the literature. *Medical Clinics of North America*, **86**, 11-31.

Barsky, A. J. & Ahern, D. K. (2004). Cognitive behavior therapy for hypochondriasis: a randomized controlled trial. *Journal of the American Medical Association*, **291**, 1464-70.

Bashir, K., King, M. & Ashworth, M. (1994). Controlled evaluation of brief intervention by general practitioners to reduce chronic use of benzodiazepines. *British Journal of General Practice*, **44**, 408-12.

Basson, R. (2001). Female sexual response: the role of drugs in the management of sexual dysfunction. *American College of Obstetricians and Gynecologists*, **98**, 350-3.

Bastian, H., Glasziou, P. & Chalmers, I. (2010). Seventy-five trials and eleven systematic reviews a day: how will we ever keep up? *PLoS Medicine*, **7**, e1000326.

Bateman, A. & Fonagy, P. (1999). The effectiveness of partial hospitalization in the treatment of borderline personality disorder: a randomised controlled trial. *American Journal of Psychiatry*, **156**, 1563-9.

Bateman, A. & Fonagy, P. (2000) Effectiveness of psychotherapeutic treatment of personality disorder. *British Journal of Psychiatry*, **177**, 138-43.

Bateman, A. & Fonagy, P. (2009). Randomized controlled trial of outpatient mentalization-based treatment versus structured clinical management for borderline personality disorder. *American Journal of Psychiatry*, **166**, 1355-64.

Bauer, M. & Dopfmer, S. (1999). Lithium augmentation in treatment-resistant depression: meta-analysis of placebo-controlled studies. *Journal of Clinical Psychopharmacology*, **19**(5), 427-34.

Baumann, P., Nil, R. et al. (1996). A double-blind, placebo-controlled trial of citalopram with and without lithium in the treatment of therapy-resistant depressive patients: a clinical, pharmacokinetic, and pharmacogenetic investigation. *Journal of Clinical Psychopharmacology*, **16**(4), 307–14.

Baxter, L. R., Jr., Liston, E. H. & Schwartz, J. M. et al. (1986). Prolongation of the antidepressant response to partial sleep deprivation by lithium. *Psychiatry Research* **19**(1), 17–23.

Bayard, M., McIntyre, J., Hill, K. R. & Woodside, J., Jr. (2004). Alcohol withdrawal syndrome. *American Family Physician*, **69**, 1443–50.

Beauchemin, K. M. & Hays, P. (1997). Phototherapy is a useful adjunct in the treatment of depressed inpatients. *Acta Psychiatrica Scandinavica*, **95**(5), 424–7.

Beck, A. T. (2006). How an anomalous finding led to a new system of psychotherapy. *Nature Medicine*, **12**, 1139–41.

Beckwith, L. (1988). Intervention with disadvantaged parents of sick preterm infants. *Psychiatry*, **51**, 242–7.

Beidel, D. C., Turner, S. M. & Morris, T. L. (2000). Behavioural treatment of childhood social phobia. *Journal of Consulting Clinical Psychology*, **68**, 1072–80.

Bellack, A. & DiClemente, C. (1999). Treating substance abuse among patients with schizophrenia. *Psychiatric Services*, **50**, 75–80.

Bellack, A. S., Bennett, M. E., Gearon, J. S., Brown, C. H. & Yang, Y. (2006). A randomized clinical trial of a new behavioral treatment for drug abuse in people with severe and persistent mental illness. *Archives of General Psychiatry*, **63**, 426–32.

Benedetti, F., Barbini, B., Lucca, A., Campori, E., Colombo, C. & Smeraldi, E. (1997). Sleep deprivation hastens the antidepressant action of fluoxetine. *European Archives of Psychiatry and Clinical Neuroscience*, **247** (2), 100–3.

Benedetti, F., Colombo, C., Barbini, B., Campori, E. & Smeraldi, E. (1999). Ongoing lithium treatment prevents relapse after total sleep deprivation. *Journal of Clinical Psychopharmacology*, **19**(3), 240–5.

Benedetti, F., Colombo, C., Barbini, B., Campori, E. & Smeraldi, E. (2001). Morning sunlight reduces length of hospitalization in bipolar depression. *Journal of Affective Disorders*, **62**(3), 221–3.

Benoit, D. & Coolbear, J. (1998). Post-traumatic feeding disorders in infancy: behavioral predicting treatment outcome. *Infant Mental Health Journal*, **19**, 409–91.

Benson, H. & Klipper, M. Z. (2000). *The Relaxation Response*. New York: Harper Collins.

Berger, W., Mendlowicz, M. V., Marques-Portella, C. et al. (2009). Pharmacologic alternatives to antidepressants in post-traumatic stress disorder: a systematic review. *Progress in Neuropsychopharmacology & Biological Psychiatry*, **17**, 169–80.

Bergeron, R., Ravindran, A. V., Chaput, Y. et al. (2002). Sertraline and fluoxetine treatment of obsessive-compulsive disorder: results of a double-blind, 6-month treatment study. *Journal of Clinical Psychopharmacology*, **22** 148–54.

Bergh, C., Brodin, U., Lindberg, G. & Södersten, P. (2002). Randomized controlled trial of a treatment for anorexia and bulimia nervosa. *Proceedings of the National Academy of Sciences*, **99**(14), 9486-91.

Bernstein, G. A., Hektner, J. M., Borchardt, C. M. & McMillan, M. H. (2001). Treatment of school refusal: one-year follow-up. *Journal of Child and Adolescent Psychiatry*, **40**, 206-13.

Bernstein, I. C. (1964). Anorexia nervosa treated successfully with electroshock therapy and subsequently followed by pregnancy. *American Journal of Psychiatry*, **120**, 1021-5.

Beumont, P. J. V., Russell, J. D. & Touyz, S. (1993). Treatment of anorexia nervosa. *Lancet* **341**, 1635-40.

Beumont, P. J., Arthur, B., Russel, J. D. & Touyz, S. W. & Stephen, W. (1994). Excessive physical activity in dieting disorder patients: proposals for a supervised exercise program. *International Journal of Eating Disorders*, **20**(2), 211-13.

Beumont, P., Hay, P. & Beumont, D. (2004). Australian and New Zealand clinical practice guidelines for the treatment of anorexia nervosa. *Australia and New Zealand Journal of Psychiatry*, **38** (9), 659-70.

Bickman, L. (1996). A continuum of care: more is not always better. *American Psychologist*, **51**, 698-701.

Biederman, J. Newcorn, J. & Sprich, S. (1991). Comorbidity of attention deficit hyperactivity disorder with conduct, depressive, anxiety and other disorders. *American Journal of Psychiatry*, **148**, 564-77.

Bienvenu, O., Onyike, C. & Stein, M. et al. (2006). Agoraphobia in adults: incidence and longitudinal relationship with panic. *British Journal of Psychiatry*, **188**, 432-8.

Birks, J. & Flicker, L. (2003). Selegiline for Alzheimer's disease. *Cochrane Database of Systematic Reviews*, 1.

Birks, J., Grimley Evans, J. Iakovidou, V. & Tsolaki, M. (2000). Rivastigmine for Alzheimer's disease. *Cochrane Database of Systematic Reviews*, 4.

Birks, J., Grimley, E. V. & Van Dongen, M. (2002). *Ginkgo biloba* for cognitive impairment and dementia. *Cochrane Database of Systematic Reviews*, **4**, CD00312.

Birmaher, B., Brent, D. A. & Benson, R. S. (1998). Summary of the practice parameters for the assessment and treatment of children and adolescents with depressive disorders. *Journal of American Academy of Child and Adolescent Psychiatry*, **37**, 1234-8.

Birmaher, B., Brent, D. A., Kolko, D. et al. (2000). Clinical outcome after short-term psychotherapy for adolescents with major depressive disorder. *Archives of General Psychiatry*, **57**, 29-36.

Birmaher, B., Axelson, D. A., Monk, K. et al. (2003). Fluoxetine for treatment of childhood anxiety disorders. *Journal of the American Academy of Child and Adolescent Psychiatry*, **42**, 415-23.

Birmingham, C. L., Guitierrez, E., Jonat, L. & Beumont, P. (2004). Randomized controlled trial of warming in anorexia nervosa. *International Journal of Eating Disorders*, **35**(2), 234-8.

Bissada, H., Tasca, G. A., Barber, A. M. & Bradwin, J. (2008). Olanzapine in the treatment of low body weight and obsessive thinking in women with anorexia nervosa: a randomized, double-blind placebo-controlled trial. *American Journal of Psychiatry*, **165**, 1281–8.

Bisson, J. I., Tavakoly, B., Witteveen, A. B. et al. (2010). TENTS guidelines: development of post-disaster psychosocial care guidelines through a Delphi process. *British Journal of Psychiatry*, **196**, 69–74.

Black, B. & Uhde, T. W. (1994). Treatment of elective mutism with Fluoxetine: a double-blind placebo-controlled study. *Journal of the American Academy of Child and Adolescent Psychiatry*, **33**, 1000–6.

Black,. L. Cullen,. C, Dicken,. P. & Turnbull J. (1998). Anger control. *British Journal of Hospital Medicine*, **39**, 325–9.

Black, M. M., Dubowitz, H., Hutcheson, J., Berenson-Howard, J. & Starr, R. H. (1995). A randomized clinical trial of home intervention for children with failure to thrive. *Pediatrics*, **95**, 807–14.

Blagg, N. R. & Yule, W. (1984). The behavioural treatment of school refusal. *Behavioural Research Therapy*, **22**, 119–27.

Blanchard, R. (1993). Varieties of autogynephilia and their relationship to gender dysphoria. *Archives of Sexual Behavior*, **22**(3), 241–51.

Blanchard, R. & Steiner, B. W. (eds) (1990). *Clinical Management of Gender Identity Disorders in Children and Adults*. Washington DC: American Psychiatric Press.

Blanchard, R., Clemmensen, L. H. & Steiner, B. W. (1983). Gender reorientation and psychosocial adjustment in male-to-female transsexuals. *Archives of Sexual Behavior*, **12**(6), 503–9.

Blanchard, R., Steiner, B. W., Clemmensen, L. H. & Dickey, R. (1989). Prediction of regrets in postoperative transsexuals. *Canadian Journal of Psychiatry*, **34**, 43–5.

Blanco, C., Heimberg, R. G., Schneier, F. R. et al. (2010). A placebo-controlled trial of phenelzine, cognitive behavioral group therapy, and their combination for social anxiety disorder. *Archives of General Psychiatry*, **67**, 286–95.

Blanco, C., Schneier, F. R., Schmidt, A. et al. (2003). Pharmacological treatment of social anxiety disorder: a meta-analysis. *Depression and Anxiety*, **18**, 29–40.

Blondal, T., Franzon, M. & Westin, A. (1997). A double-blind randomized trial of nicotine nasal spray as an aid in smoking cessation. *European Respiratory Journal*, **10**, 1585–90.

Bloomquist, M. L. & Schnell, S. V. (2002). *Helping Children with Aggression and Conduct Problems*. New York: Guilford.

Blouin, A. G., Blouin, J. H. et al. (1996). Light therapy in bulimia nervosa: a double-blind, placebo-controlled study. *Psychiatry Research*, **60**(1), 1–9.

Blum, N., St. John, D., Stuart, S. et al. (2008). Systems Training for Emotional Predictability and Problem Solving (STEPPS) for outpatients with borderline personality disorder: a randomized controlled trial and 1-year follow-up. *American Journal of Psychiatry*, **165**, 468–478.

Blumenthal, J. A., Babyak, M. A., Moore, K. A. et al. (1999). Effects of exercise training on older patients with major depression. *Archives of Internal Medicine*, **159**(19), 2349–56.

Bodlund, O. & Kullgren, G. (1996). Transsexualism: general outcome and prognostic factors: a five-year follow-up study of nineteen transsexuals in the process of changing sex. *Archives of Sexual Behavior*, **25**, 303–16.

Bolliger, C. T., Zellweger, J. P., Danielsson, T. *et al.* (2000). Smoking reduction with oral nicotine inhalers: double blind, randomised clinical trial of efficacy and safety. *British Medical Journal*, **321**, 329–33.

Bondy, A. & Frost, L. (1996). Educational approaches in pre-school: behavior techniques in a public school setting. In: E. Schopler & G. B. Mesibov, eds. *Learning and Cognition in Autism, Current Issues in Autism*. New York: Plenum Press.

Bora, R., Leaning, S., Moores, A. & Roberts, G. (2010). Life coaching for mental health recovery: the emerging practice of recovery coaching. *Advances in Psychiatric Treatment*, **16**, 459–67.

Borduin, C. M., Mann, B. J., Cone, L. T. et al. (1995). Multisystemic treatment of serious juvenile offenders: long-term prevention of criminality and violence. *Journal of Consulting and Clinical Psychology*, **63**, 569–78.

Bornovalova, M. A. & Daughters, S. B. (2007). How does Dialectical Behavior Therapy facilitate treatment retention among individuals with comorbid borderline personality disorder and substance use disorders? *Clinical Psychology Review*, **27**, 923–43.

Bouza, C., Angeles, M., Munoz, A. & Amate, J. M. (2004). Efficacy and safety of naltrexone and acamprosate in the treatment of alcohol dependence: a systematic review. *Addiction*, **99**, 811–28.

Bowden-Jones, O., Iqbal, M. Z., Tyrer, P. et al. (2004). Prevalence of personality disorder in alcohol and drug services and associated co-morbidity. *Addiction*, **99**, 1306–14.

Bowen, S., Witkiewitz, K., Dillworth, T. M. et al. (2006). Mindfulness meditation and substance use in an incarcerated population. *Psychology of Addictive Behaviors*, **20**, 343–7.

Bower, P. & Gilbody, S. (2005). Stepped care in psychological therapies: access, effectiveness and efficiency. Narrative literature review. *British Journal of Psychiatry*, **186**, 11–7.

Bradwejn, J., Ahokas, A., Stein, D. J., Salinas, E., Emilien, G., Whitaker, T. (2005). Venlafaxine extended-release capsules in panic disorder: flexible-dose, double-blind, placebo-controlled study. *British Journal of Psychiatry*, **187**, 352–9.

Brady, K. T. & Sonne, S. C. (1999). The role of stress in alcohol use, alcoholism treatment, and relapse. *Alcohol Research & Health*, **23** (4), 263–71.

Brady, K., Pearlstein, T., Asnis, G. M. et al. (2000). Efficacy and safety of sertraline treatment of posttraumatic stress disorder: a randomized controlled trial. *Journal of the American Medical Association*, **283**, 1837–44.

Braun, D. L., Sunday, S. R., Fornari, V. M. & Halmi, K. A. (1999). Bright light therapy decreases winter binge frequency in women with bulimia nervosa: a double-blind, placebo-controlled study. *Comprehensive Psychiatry*, **40**(6), 442–8.

Breitbart, W., Marotta, R., Platt, M. et al., (1996). A double-blind trial of haloperidol, chlorpromazine and lorazepam in the treatment of delirium in hospitalized AIDS patients. *American Journal of Psychiatry*, **153**, 231–7.

Brent, D. A., Holder, D., Kolko, D. et al. (1997). A clinical psychotherapy trial for adolescent depression comparing cognitive, family, and supportive therapy. *Archives of General Psychiatry*, **54**, 877–85.

Brent, D. A., Kolko, D., Birmaher, B. *et al.* (1998). Predictors of treatment efficacy in a clinical trial of three psychosocial treatments for adolescent depression. *Journal of the American Academy of Child and Adolescent Psychiatry*, **37**, 906–14.

Brent, D., Emslie, G., Clark, G. et al. (2008). Switching to another SSRI or to venlafaxine with or without cognitive behavioral therapy for adolescents with SSRI-resistant depression: the TORDIA randomized controlled trial. *Journal of the American Medical Association*, **299**, 901–13.

Brestan, E. V. & Eyberg, S. M. (1998). Effective psychosocial treatments of conduct-disordered children and adolescents: 29 years, 82 studies, and 5272 kids. *Journal of Clinical Child Psychology*, **27**, 180–9.

Brewer, J. A., Sinha, R., Chen, J. A. et al. (2009). Mindfulness training and stress reactivity in substance abuse: results from a randomized, controlled stage I pilot study. *Substance Abuse*, **30**, 306–17.

Bridge, J., Iyenar, S., Salary, C. et al. (2007). Clinical response and risk for reported suicidal ideation and suicide attempts in pediatric antidepressant treatment: a meta-analysis of randomized controlled trials. *Journal of the American Medical Association*, **297**, 1583–96.

Britton, A. & Russell, R. (2004). Multidisciplinary team interventions for delirium in patients with chronic cognitive impairment. *Cochrane Database of Systematic Reviews*, **2**, CD000395.

Brodaty, H., Ames, D. & Snowdon, J. (2003). A randomized placebo-controlled trial of risperidone for the treatment of aggression, agitation, and psychosis of dementia. *Journal of Clinical Psychiatry*, **64**, 134–43.

Bronskill, S. E., Anderson, G. M., Sykora, K. et al. (2004). Neuroleptic drug therapy in older adults newly admitted to nursing homes: incidence, dose, and specialist contact. *Journal of the American Geriatric Society*, **52**, 749–55.

Browder, D. M., Bambara, L. M. & Belfiore, P. J. (1997). Using a person-centred approach in community-based institutions for adults with developmental disabilities. *Journal of Behavioral Education*, **7**, 519–28.

Brown, G. W., Birley, J. L. & Wing, J. (1972). Influence of family life on the course of schizophrenic disorders: a replication. *British Journal of Psychiatry*, **121**, 241–58.

Brown, S. & Yalom, I. D. (1977). Interactional group therapy with alcoholics. *Journal of Studies on Alcoholism*, **38**, 426–56.

Brownley, K. A., Berkman, N. D., Sedway, J. A., Lohr, K. N. & Bulik., C. M. (2007). Binge eating disorder treatment: a systematic review of randomized controlled trials. *International Journal of Eating Disorders*, **40**, 337–48.

Bruce, S. E., Vasile, R. G., Goisman, R. M. et al. (2003). Are benzodiazepines still the medication of choice for patients with panic disorder with or without agoraphobia? *American Journal of Psychiatry*, **160**(8), 1432–8.

Bryant, R. A., Mastrodomenico, J., Felmingham, K. L. et al. (2008). Treatment of acute stress disorder: a randomized controlled trial. *Archives of General Psychiatry*, **65**, 659–67.

Bryant-Waugh, R., Markham, L., Kreipe, R. E. & Walsh, B. T. (2010). Feeding and eating disorders in childhood. *The International Journal of Eating Disorders*, **43**(2), 98–111.

Brylewski, J. & Duggan, L. (2004). Antipsychotic medication for challenging behaviour in people with learning disability. *Cochrane Database of Systematic Reviews*, **3**, CD000377.

Budd, S. & Brown, W. (1974). Effect of reorientation technique on postcardiotomy delirium. *Nursing Research*, **23**, 341–8.

Budney, A. J. & Higgins, S. T. (1998). *A Community Reinforcement Plus Vouchers Approach: Treating Cocaine Addiction*. Rockville, MD: NIDA.

Budney, A. J. & Moore, B. A. (2002). Development and consequences of cannabis dependence. *Journal of Clinical Pharmacology*, **42**, 28S–33S.

Budney, A. J., Radonovich, K. J., Higgins, S. T. & Wong, C. J. (1998). Adults seeking treatment for marijuana dependence: a comparison to cocaine-dependent treatment seekers. *Experimental and Clinical Psychopharmacology*, **6**, 419–26.

Budney, A. J., Higgins, S. T., Radonovich, K. J. & Novy, P. L. (2000). Adding voucher-based incentives to coping skills and motivational enhancement improves outcomes during treatment for marijuana dependence. *Journal of Consulting and Clinical Psychology*, **68**, 1051–61.

Budney, A. J., Moore, B. A. & Vandrey, R. (2003). Health consequences of marijuana use. In: J. Brick, ed. *Medical Consequences of Drug Abuse*. London: Haworth Press, pp. 171–218.

Budney, A. J., Hughes, J. R., Moore, B. A. & Vandrey, R. (2004). Review of the validity and significance of cannabis withdrawal syndrome. *American Journal of Psychiatry*, **161**, 1967–77.

Budney, A. J., Moore, B. A., Rocha, H. & Higgins, S. T. (2006). Voucher-based incentives and behavior therapy for adult marijuana dependence. *Journal of Consulting and Clinical Psychology*, **74**, 307–16.

Budney, A. J., Vandrey, R. G., Hughes, J. R., Moore, B. A. & Bahrenburg, B. (2007). Oral delta-9-tetrahydrocannabinol suppresses withdrawal symptoms. *Drug and Alcohol Dependence*, **86**, 22–9.

Buitelaar, J. K., Van der Gaag, R. J., Cohen-Kettenis, P. & Melman, C. T. M. (2001). A randomized controlled trial of risperidone in the treatment of aggression in hospitalized adolescents with subaverage cognitive abilities. *Journal of Clinical Psychiatry*, **62**, 239–48.

Bullock, M. L., Kiresuk, T. J., Sherman, R. E. et al. (2002). A large randomized placebo controlled study of auricular acupuncture for alcohol dependence. *Journal of Substance Abuse Treatment*, **22**, 71–7.

Burke, B. L., Arkowitz, H. & Menchola, M. (2003) The efficacy of motivational interviewing: a meta-analysis of controlled clinical trials. *Journal of Consulting & Clinical Psychology*, **71**, 843–61.

Burns, B. J., Farmer, E. M. Z., Angold, A., Costello, E. J. & Behar, L. (1996). A randomized trial of case management for youths with serious emotional disturbance. *Journal of Clinical Child Psychology*, **25**, 476–86.

Busato, W. & Galindo, C. C. (2004). Topical anaesthetic use for treating premature ejaculation: a double-blind, randomized, placebo-controlled study. *BJU International*, **93**, 1018–21.

Butler, A. C., Chapman, J. E., Forman, E. M. & Beck, A. T. et al. (2006). The empirical status of cognitive-behavioral therapy: a review of meta-analyses. *Clinical Psychology Review*, **26**, 17–31.

Butler, G., Fennell, M., Robson, P. & Gelder, M. (1991). Comparison of behavior therapy and cognitive behavior therapy in the treatment of generalized anxiety disorder. *Journal of Consulting and Clinical Psychology*, **59**, 167–75.

Bxarone, P., Poewe, W., Albrecht, S. et al. (2010). Pramipexole for the treatment of depressive symptoms in patients with Parkinson's disease: a randomised, double-blind, placebo-controlled trial. *Lancet Neurology*, **9**, 573–80.

Byford, S., Barrett, B., Roberts, C. et al. (2007). Economic evaluation of a randomised controlled trial for anorexia nervosa in adolescents. *British Journal of Psychiatry*, **191**, 436–40.

Bystritsky, A., Ackerman, D. L., Rosen, R. M. et al. (2004). Augmentation of serotonin reuptake inhibitors in refractory obsessive-compulsive disorder using adjunctive olanzapine: a placebo-controlled trial. *Journal of Clinical Psychiatry*, **65**, 565–8.

Cachelin, F. M., Striegel-Moore, R. H., Elder, K. A., Pike, K. M., Wilfley, D. E. & Fairburn, C. G. (1999). Natural course of a community sample of women with binge eating disorder. *International Journal of Eating Disorders*, **25**, 45–54.

Caligiuri, M. R., Jeste, D. V. & Lacro, J. P. (2000). Antipsychotic-induced movement disorders in the elderly: epidemiology and treatment recommendations. *Drugs Aging*, **17**, 363–84.

Candy, J., Cawley, R. H., Balfour, F. H. G. et al. (1972). Feasibility study for a controlled trial of formal psychotherapy. *Psychological Medicine*, **2**, 345–8.

Carlbring, P., Nilsson-Ihrfelt, E., Waara, J. et al. (2005). Treatment of panic disorder: live therapy vs. self-help via the Internet. *Behavior Research Therapy*, **43** (10), 1321–33.

Carlson, C. L., Pelham, W. E., Milich, R. & Dixon, J. (1992). Single and combined effects of methylphenidate and behavior therapy on the classroom performance of children with attention-deficit hyperactivity disorder. *Journal of Abnormal Child Psychology*, **20**, 213–32.

Carlson, L. E., Speca, M., Patel, K. D. & Goodey, E. (2004). Mindfulness-based stress reduction in relation to quality of life, mood, symptoms of stress and levels of cortisol, dehydroepiandrosterone sulfate (DHEAS) and melatonin in breast and prostate cancer outpatients. *Psychoneuroendocrinology*, **29**, 448–74.

Carnwath, T. & Hardman, J. (1998). Randomised double-blind comparison of lofexidine and clonidine in the outpatient treatment of opiate withdrawal. *Drug and Alcohol Dependence*, **50**, 251–4.

Caro, J., Getsios, D., Migliaccio-Walle, K., Ishak, J., El-Hadi, W. & the AHEAD Study Group (2003). Rational choice of cholinesterase inhibitor for the treatment of Alzheimer's disease in Canada: a comparative economic analysis. *BioMed Central Geriatrics*, **3**(1), 6.

Carpenter, L. L., Yasmin, S. & Price, L. H. (2002). A double-blind, placebo-controlled study of antidepressant augmentation with mirtazapine. *Biological Psychiatry*, **51**, 183-8.

Carr, A. (2004). *The Easy Way to Stop Smoking*. New York: Sterling.

Carrey, N., Mendella, P., McMaster, F. et al. (2002). Developmental psychopharmacology. In: S. Kutcher, ed. *Practical Child and Adolescent Psychopharmacology*. Cambridge: Cambridge University Press.

Carroll, K. C. (2000). Science-based therapies for drug dependence. *The Economics of Neuroscience*, **2**, 41-7.

Carroll, K. M. (1997). Integrating psychotherapy and pharmacotherapy to improve drug abuse outcomes. *Journal of Addictive Behaviors*, **22**, 233-45.

Carroll, K. M. (1998). *A Cognitive-Behavioural Approach: Treating Cocaine Addiction*. Rockville, MD: National Institute on Drug Abuse.

Carroll, K. M., Ball, S. A., Nich, C. et al. (2001). Targeting behavioral therapies to enhance naltrexone treatment of opioid dependence: efficacy of contingency management and significant other involvement. *Archives of General Psychiatry*, **58**(8), 755-61.

Carroll, K. M., Rounsaville, B. & Keller, D. (1991). Relapse prevention strategies for the treatment of cocaine abuse. *American Journal of Drug and Alcohol Abuse*, **17**, 249-65.

Carroll, K. M., Nich, C., Ball, S. A., McCance, E. & Rounsaville, B. J. (1998). Treatment of cocaine and alcohol dependence with psychotherapy and disulfiram. *Addiction*, **93**, 713-27.

Carroll, K. M., Fenton, L. R., Ball, S. A. et al. (2004). Efficacy of disulfiram and cognitive behavior therapy in a cocaine-dependent outpatient: a randomised placebo-controlled trial. *Archives of General Psychiatry*, **61**, 264-72.

Carroll, K. M., Easton, C. J., Nich, C. et al. (2006). The use of contingency management and motivational/skills-building therapy to treat young adults with marijuana dependence. *Journal of Consulting & Clinical Psychology*, **74**, 955-66.

Carson, C. C., Rajfer, J., Eardley, I. et al. (2004). The efficacy and safety of Tadalafil: an update. *BJU International*, **93**, 1276-81.

Caruso, S., Agnello, C., Intelisano, G., Farina, M., Di Mari, L. & Cianci, A. (2004). Placebo-controlled study of the efficacy and safety of daily apomorphine SL intake in premenopausal women affected by hypoactive sexual desire disorder and sexual arousal disorder. *Urology*, 2004, **63**, 955-9.

Casacalenda, N. & Boulenger, J. P. (1998). Pharmacologic treatments effective in both generalized anxiety disorder and major depressive disorder: clinical and theoretical implications. *Canadian Journal of Psychiatry*, **43**, 722-30.

Casey, P. (2009). Adjustment disorder: epidemiology, diagnosis and treatment. *CNS Drugs*, **23**, 927-38.

Casey, P. R., Tyrer, P. & Platt, S. (1985). The relationship between social functioning and psychiatric symptomatology in primary care. *Social Psychiatry*, **20**, 5–9.

Casey, R. J. & Berman, J. S. (1985). The outcome of psychotherapy with children. *Psychological Bulletin*, **98**, 388–400.

Casey, S. D., Perrin, C. J., Lesser, A. D., Perrin, S. H., Casey, C. L. & Reed, G. K. (2009). Using descriptive assessment in the treatment of bite acceptance and food refusal. *Behavior Modification*, **33**(5), 537–58.

Chakos, M., Lieberman, J., Hoffman, E., Bradford, D. & Sheitman, B. (2001). Effectiveness of second-generation antipsychotics in patients with treatment-resistant schizophrenia: a review and meta-analysis of randomized trials. *American Journal of Psychiatry*, **158**, 518–26.

Chamberlain, P. & Reid, J. B. (1998) Comparison of two community alternatives to incarceration for chronic juvenile offenders. *Journal of Consulting and Clinical Psychology*, **66**, 624–33.

Chamberlain, P. & Rosicky, J. G. (1995). The effectiveness of family therapy in the treatment of adolescents with conduct disorders and delinquency. *Journal of Marital and Family Therapy*, **21**, 441–59.

Chamberlain, P. (1990). Comparative evaluation of specialized foster-care for seriously delinquent youths: a first step. *Community Alternatives: International Journal of Family Care*, **2**, 21–36.

Chamberlain, P. (2003). *Treating Chronic Juvenile Offenders: Advances Made Through the Oregon Multidimensional Treatment Foster Care Model.* Washington, DC: American Psychological Association.

Chan, A. W. (1985). Alcoholism and epilepsy. *Epilepsia*, **26**, 323–33.

Chanen, A. M., Jackson, H. J., McCutcheon, L. K. et al. (2008). Early intervention for adolescents with borderline personality disorder using cognitive analytic therapy: randomised controlled trial. *British Journal of Psychiatry*, **193**, 477–84.

Channon, S., de Silva, P., Hemsley, D. & Perkins, R. (1989). A controlled trial of cognitive-behavioural and behavioural treatment of anorexia nervosa. *Behaviour Research and Therapy*, **27**, 529–35.

Chanpattana, W., Chakrabhand, M. L., Sackeim, H. A. et al. (1999). Continuation ECT in treatment-resistant schizophrenia: a controlled study. *Journal of ECT*, **15**, 178–92.

Chatham, M. A. (1978). The effect of family involvement on patients' manifestations of postcardiotomy psychosis. *Heart & Lung*, **7**, 995–9.

Chatoor, I. (2002). Feeding disorders in infants and toddlers: diagnosis and treatment. *Child & Adolescent Psychiatric Clinics of North America*, **11**, 163–83.

Chatoor, I. (2003). Food refusal by infants and young children: diagnosis and treatment. *Child and Adolescent Psychiatry Clinics of North America*, **11**, 163–83.

Chavira, D. A. & Stein, M. B. (2002). Phenomenology of social phobia. In D. J. Stein & E. Hollander, eds. *The American Psychiatric Publishing Textbook of Anxiety Disorders*. Washington

DC: American Psychiatric Publishing, Inc., pp. 289–300.

Chesley, E. B. & Kreipe, R. E. (2003). Anorexia nervosa and the internet. *Eating Disorder Review*, July/August.

Chial, H. J., Camilleri, M., Williams, D. E., Litzinger, K. & Perrault, J. (2003). Rumination syndrome in children and adolescents: diagnosis, treatment, and prognosis. *Pediatrics*, **111**, 158–62.

Chick, J., Howlett, H., Morgan, M. Y. & Ritson, B. (2000). United Kingdom Multi-centre Acamprosate Study (UKMAS): a 6-month prospective study of acamprosate versus placebo in preventing relapse after withdrawal from alcohol. *Alcohol and Alcoholism*, **35**, 176–87.

Childress, A. R., Hole, A. V., Ehrman, R. N., Robbins, S. J., McLellan, A. T. & O'Brien, C. P. (1993). Cue reactivity and cue reactivity interventions in drug dependence. In: L. S. Onken, J. D. Blaine & J. J. Boren, eds. *Behavioural Treatments for Drug Abuse and Dependence*, pp. 73–95. Rockville, MD: National Institute on Drug Abuse.

Christie, D. (2007). Cognitive behavioural approaches. In: B. Lask & R. Bryant-Waugh, eds. *Anorexia Nervosa and Related Eating Disorders in Childhood and Adolescence*, 3rd edn. Hove, East Sussex: Psychology Press/Taylor and Francis Group, pp. 229–55.

Chung, M. Y., Min, K. H., Jun, Y. J. et al. (2004). Efficacy and tolerability of mirtazapine and sertraline in Korean veterans with posttraumatic stress disorder: a randomized open label trial. *Human Psychopharmacology*, **19**, 489–94.

Cicchetti, D., Toth, S. L. & Rogosch, F. A. (1999). The efficacy of toddler–parent psychotherapy to increase attachment security in off-spring of depressed mothers. *Attachment and Human Development*, **1**, 34–66.

Cicchetti, D., Rogosch, F. A. & Toth, S. L. (2006). Fostering secure attachment in infants in maltreating families through preventive interventions. *Development and Psychopathology*, **18**, 623–49.

Cipriani, A., Furukawa, T. A., Salanti, G. et al. (2009). Comparative efficacy and acceptability of 12 new-generation antidepressants: a multiple-treatments meta-analysis. *Lancet*, **373**, 746–58.

Clare, L., Woods, R. T., Moniz Cook, E. D., Orrell, M. & Spector, A. (2003). Cognitive rehabilitation and cognitive training for early-stage Alzheimer's disease and vascular dementia. *Cochrane Database of Systematic Reviews*, **4**, CD003260.

Clark, A. (2004). Incidences of new prescribing by British child and adolescent psychiatrists: a prospective study over 12 months. *Journal of Psychopharmacology*, **18**, 115–20.

Clark, D. M., Salkovskis, P. M., Hackmann, A., Wells, A., Ludgate, J. & Gelder, M. (1999). Brief cognitive therapy for panic disorder: a randomised controlled trial. *Journal of Consulting & Clinical Psychology*, **67**, 583–9.

Clark, D. M., Ehlers, A., McManus, F. et al. (2003). Cognitive therapy versus fluoxetine in generalized social phobia: a randomized placebo-controlled trial. *Journal of Consulting and Clinical Psychology*, **71**, 1058–67.

Clarke, G. N., Hawkins, W., Murphy, M. et al. (1995). Targeted prevention of unipolar depressive disorder in an at risk sample of high school adolescents: a randomized trial of a group cognitive interview. *Journal of the American Academy of Child and Adolescent Psychiatry*, **34**, 312–21.

Clarke, G. N., Rohde, P., Lewinsohn, P. M., Hops, H. & Seeley, J. R. (1999). Cognitive-behavioral treatment of adolescent depression: efficacy of acute group treatment and booster sessions. *Journal of American Academy of Child and Adolescent Psychiatry*, **38**, 272–9.

Clarkin, J. F., Levy, K. N., Lenzenweger, M. F. & Kernberg, O. F. (2007). Evaluating three treatments for borderline personality disorder: a multiwave study. *American Journal of Psychiatry*, **164**, 922–8.

Claudino, A. M., Hay, P., Lima, M. S., Bacaltchuk, J., Schmidt, U. & Treasure, J. (2006). Antidepressants for anorexia nervosa. *Cochrane Database of Systematic Reviews*, **1**, CD004365.

Clausen, J. M., Landsverk, J., Ganger, W., Chadwick, D. & Litrownik, A. (1998). Mental health problems of children in foster care. *Journal of Child & Family Studies*, **7**, 283–96.

Cloitre, M., Cohen, L. R., Koenen, K. C. & Han, H. (2002). Skills training in affective and interpersonal regulation followed by exposure: a phase-based treatment for PTSD related to childhood abuse. *Journal of Consult Clinical Psychology*, **70**, 1067–74.

Clomipramine Collaborative Study Group (1991). Clomipramine in the treatment of patients with obsessive-compulsive disorder. *Archives of General Psychiatry*, **48**, 754–6.

Coffey, C. E., Carlin, J. B., Degenhardt, L., Lynskey, M. T., Sanci, L. & Patton, G. C. (2002). Cannabis dependence in young adults: an Australian population study. *Addiction*, **97**, 187–94.

Cohen, J., Deblinger, E., Mannarino, A. P. & Steer, R. A. (2004). A multisite, randomised controlled trial for children with sexual abuse-related PTSD symptoms. *Journal of the American Academy of Child and Adolescent Psychiatry*, **43**, 393–402.

Cohen-Kettenis, P. T., Delemarre-van de Waal, H. A. & Gooren, L. J. (2008). The treatment of adolescent transsexuals: changing insights. *Journal of Sexual Medicine*, **5**, 1892–7.

Cole, M. G., Primeau, F. & McCusker, J. (1996). Effectiveness of interventions to prevent delirium in hospitalized patients: a systematic review. *Canadian Medical Association Journal*, **155**, 1263–8.

Colombo, C., Lucca, A., Benedetti, F., Barbini, B., Campori, E. & Smeraldi, E. (2000). Total sleep deprivation combined with lithium and light therapy in the treatment of bipolar depression: replication of main effects and interaction. *Psychiatry Research*, **95**(1), 43–53.

Compton, S. N., March, J. S., Brent, D., Albano, A. M., Weersing, V. R. & Curry, J. (2004). Cognitive-behavioral psychotherapy for anxiety and depressive disorders in children and adolescents: an evidence-based medicine review. *Journal of the American Academy of Child and Adolescent Psychiatry*, **48**, 930–59.

Connor, D. F. & Rubin, J. (2010). Guanfacine extended release in the treatment of attention deficit hyperactivity disorder in children and adolescents. *Drugs Today*, **46**, 299–314.

Conners, K., Casat, C. D. & Gualtieri, C. et al. (1996). Bupropion hydrochloride in attention deficit disorder with hyperactivity. *Journal of the American Academy of Child and Adolescent Psychiatry*, **35**, 1314.

Connor, D. F., Glatt, S. J., Lopez, I. D., Jackson, D. & Melloni, R. H. (2002). Psychopharmacology and aggression. I: A meta-analysis of stimulant effects on overt/covert aggression-related behaviors in ADHD. *Journal of the American Academy of Child & Adolescent Psychiatry*, **41**, 253–61.

Connors, G. J., Tonigan, J. S. & Miller, W. R. (2001). A longitudinal model of A.A. affiliation, participation, and outcome: retrospective study of the Project MATCH outpatient and aftercare samples. *Journal of Studies on Alcohol*, **62**, 817–25.

Cook, C. C. H., Hallwood, P. M. & Thomson, A. D. (1998). B-vitamin deficiency and neuro-psychiatric syndromes in alcohol misuse. *Alcohol & Alcoholism*, **33**, 317–36.

Cooke, R. A., Chambers, J. B, Singh, R. et al. (1994). QT interval in anorexia nervosa. *British Heart Journal*, **72**(1), 69–73.

Cooper, P. J., Coker, S. & Fleming, C. et al. (1996). An evaluation of the efficacy of supervised cognitive behavioral self-help bulimia nervosa. *Journal of Psychosomatic Research*, **40**, 281–7.

Cooper, P. J., Murray, L., Wilson, A. & Romaniuk, H. (2003). Controlled trial of the short- and long-term effect of psychological treatment of post-partum depression. 1. Impact on maternal mood. *British Journal of Psychiatry*, **182**, 412–19.

Copeland, J., Swift, W., Roffman, R. & Stephens, R. S. (2001). A randomized controlled trial of brief cognitive-behavioral interventions for cannabis use disorder. *Journal of Substance Abuse Treatment*, **21**, 55–64.

Cordioli, A., Heldt, E., Bochi, D. B. et al. (2003). Cognitive-behavioural group therapy in obsessive-compulsive disorder: a randomised clinical trial. *Psychotherapy and Psychosomatics*, **72**, 211.

Correll, C. (2008). Antipsychotic use in children and adolescents: minimizing adverse effects to maximize outcomes. *Journal of the American Academy of Child and Adolescent Psychiatry*, **47**, 9–20.

Correll, C., Manu, P., Olshansky, V., Napolitano, B., Kane, J. M. & Malhortra A. K. (2009). Cardiometabolic risk of second-generation antipsychotic medications during first-time use in children and adolescents. *Journal of the American Medical Association*, **302**, 1765–73.

Cosgrove, G. R. (2000). Surgery for psychiatric disorders. *CNS Spectrums*, **5**(10), 43–52.

Costello, E. & Angold, A. (1995). Epidemiology. In: J. March, ed. *Anxiety Disorders in Children and Adolescents*. New York: Guilford Press, pp. 109–24.

Cottraux, J., Mollard, E., Bouvard, M. et al. (1990). A controlled study of fluvoxamine and exposure in obsessive-compulsive disorder. *International Clinical Psychopharmacology*, **5**, 17–30.

Couturier, J. & Lock, J. (2007) A review of medication use for children and adolescents with eating disorders. *Journal of* the Canadian Academy of Child and Adolescent Psychiatry, **16**, 173–6.

Covey, L. S. & Glassman, A. H. (1991). A meta-analysis of double-blind placebo controlled trials of clonidine for smoking cessation. British Journal of Addiction, **86**, 991–8.

Craft, M., Ismail, I. A., Krisnamurti, D. et al. (1987). Lithium in the treatment of aggression in mentally handicapped patients: a double-blind trial. British Journal of Psychiatry, **150**, 685–9.

Craske, M. G. (1999). Anxiety Disorders: Psychological Approaches to Theory and Treatment. Boulder, CO: Westview Press.

Craske, M., DeCola, J., Sachs, A. & Pontillo, D. et al. (2003). Panic control treatment for agoraphobia. Journal of Anxiety Disorders, **17**, 321–33.

Crisp, A. H., Callender, J. S., Halek, C. & Hsu, L. K. G. (1992). Long-term mortality in anorexia nervosa: a 20-year follow-up of the St. George's and Aberdeen cohorts. British Journal of Psychiatry, **161**, 104–7.

Crisp, A. H. and Kalucy, R. S. (1973). The effect of leucotomy in intractable adolescent weight phobia (primary anorexia nervosa). Postgraduate Medical Journal, **49**, 883–93.

Crisp, A. H., Norton, K., Gowers, S. et al. (1991). A controlled study of the effect of therapies aimed at adolescent and family psychopathology in anorexia nervosa. British Journal of Psychiatry, **159**, 325–33.

Crits-Christoph, P., Siqueland, L., Blaine, J. et al. (1999). Psychosocial treatments for cocaine dependence: results of the National Institute on Drug Abuse Collaborative Cocaine Study. Archives of General Psychiatry, **56**, 495–502.

Crow, S. & Schmidt, U. (2008). Complex treatments for eating disorders. In: P. Tyrer & K. R. Silk, eds. Cambridge Textbook of Effective Treatments in Psychiatry. Cambridge: Cambridge University Press, pp. 647–55.

Crow, S. J., Mitchell, J. E., Roerig, J. D. & Steffen, K. (2009). What potential role is there for medication treatment in anorexia nervosa? International Journal of Eating Disorders, **42**, 1–8.

Crumrine, P. K., Feldman, H. M., Teodori, J., Handen, B. L. & Alvin, R. M. (1987). The use of methylphenidate in children with seizures and attention deficit disorder. Annals of Neurology, **B**, 441–2.

Curran, H. V., Collins, R., Fletcher, S., Kee, S. C., Woods, B. & Iliffe, S. (2003). Older adults and withdrawal from benzodiazepine hypnotics in general practice: effects on cognitive function, sleep, mood and quality of life. Psychological Medicine, **33**, 1223–37.

Curtis, N. M., Ronan, K. R. & Borduin, C. M. (2004). Multisystemic therapy: a meta-analysis of outcome studies. Journal of Family Psychology, **18**, 411–19.

D'Silva, K., Duggan, C. & Mccarthy, L. (2004). Does treatment really make psychopaths worse? A review of the evidence. Journal of Personality Disorders, **18**, 163–77.

Daiuto, A., Baucom, D., Epstein, N. & Dutton, S. (1998). The application of behavioral couples therapy to the assessment and treatment of agoraphobia: implications of empirical research. Clinical Psychology Review, **18**, 663–87.

Dam, M., Tonin, P., De Boni, A. et al. (1996). Effects of fluoxetine and maprotiline on functional recovery in post-stroke hemiplegic patients undergoing rehabilitation therapy. *Stroke*, **27**, 1211–14.

Dare, C., Eisler, I., Russell, G., Treasure, J. & Dodge, L. (2001). Psychological therapies for adults with anorexia nervosa: randomized controlled trial of out-patient treatments. *British Journal of Psychiatry*, **178**, 216–21.

Daubenmier, J.J. (2003). A comparison of Hatha yoga and aerobic exercise on women's body satisfaction. Dissertation Abstracts International: Section B: The Sciences & Engineering, 63(9-B).

Davenport, C. W. (1986). A follow-up study of 10 feminine boys. *Archives of Sexual Behavior*, **15**, 511–7.

Davidson, J., Kudler, H., Smith, R. et al. (1990). Treatment of posttraumatic stress disorder with amitriptyline and placebo. *Archives of General Psychiatry*, **47**, 259–66.

Davidson, J. R., Potts, N., Richichi, E. et al. (1993). Treatment of social phobia with clonazepam and placebo. *Journal of Clinical Psychopharmacology*, **13**, 423–8.

Davidson, J., Pearlstein, T., Londborg, P. et al. (2001). Efficacy of sertraline in preventing relapse of posttraumatic stress disorder: results of a 28-week double-blind, placebo-controlled study. *American Journal of Psychiatry*, **158**, 1974–81.

Davidson, J. R. T., Foa, E. B., Huppert, J. D. et al. (2004). Fluoxetine comprehensive cognitive behavioral therapy, and placebo in generalized social phobia. *Archives of General Psychiatry*, **61**, 1005–13.

Davidson, J., Rothbaum, B. O., Tucker, P., Asnis, G., Benattia, I. & Musgnung, J. J. et al. (2006a). Venlafaxine extended release in posttraumatic stress disorder: a sertraline- and placebo-controlled study. *Journal of Clinical Psychopharmacology*, **26**(3), 259–67.

Davidson, J., Baldwin, D., Stein, D. J. et al. (2006b). Treatment of posttraumatic stress disorder with venlafaxine extended release: a 6-month randomized controlled trial. *Archives of General Psychiatry*, **63**(10), 1158–65.

Davidson, K. & Tyrer, P. (1996). Cognitive therapy for antisocial and borderline personality disorders: single case study series. *British Journal of Clinical Psychology*, **35**, 413–29.

Davidson, K., Norrie, J., Tyrer, P. et al. (2006). The effectiveness of cognitive behavior therapy for borderline personality disorder: results from the borderline personality disorder study of cognitive therapy (BOSCOT) trial. *Journal of Personality Disorders*, **20**, 450–65.

Davis, J., Barter, J. & Kane, J. M. (1989). Antipsychotic drugs. In: H. I. Kaplan & B. J. Sadock, eds. *Comprehensive Textbook of Psychiatry V. Baltimore*, Williams and Wilkins, pp. 1591–626.

Davis, J. M., Wang, Z. & Janicak, P. G. et al. (1993). A quantitative analysis of clinical drug trials for the treatment of affective disorders. *Psychopharmacology Bulletin*, **29**, 175–81.

Davis, J. M., Chen, N. & Glick, I. D. (2003). A meta-analysis of the efficacy of second-generation antipsychotics.

Archives of General Psychiatry, **60**, 553–64.

Davis, R., Olmsted, M. P., Rockert, W. (1990). Brief group psychoeducation for bulimia nervosa: assessing the clinical significance of change. *Journal of Consulting and Clinical Psychology*, **58**(6), 882–5.

Davis, R., Olmsted, M., Rockert, W. Marques, T. & Dolhanty, J. (1997). Group psychoeducation for bulimia nervosa with and without additional psychotherapy process sessions. *International Journal of Eating Disorders*, **22** (1), 25–34.

Davis, W. T., Campbell, L., Tax, J. & Lieber, C. S. (2002). A trial of "standard" outpatient alcoholism treatment vs. a minimal treatment control. *Journal of Substance Abuse Treatment*, **23**, 9–19.

Dawson, G., Rogers, S., Munson, J. et al. (2010). Randomized, controlled trial of an intervention for toddlers with autism: the Early Start Denver model. *Pediatrics*, **125**, e7–e23.

de Beurs, E., Lange, A., van Dyck, R. & Koele, P. (1995). Respiratory training prior to exposure in vivo in the treatment of panic disorder with agoraphobia: efficacy and predictors of outcome. *Australian and NZ Journal of Psychiatry*, **29**(1), 104–13.

De Deyn, P. P, Rabheru, K., Rasmussen, A. et al. (1999). A randomized trial of risperidone, placebo, and haloperidol for behavioural symptoms of dementia. *Neurology*, **53**, 946–55.

De Deyn, P. P., Katz, I. R., Brodaty, H., Lyons, B., Greenspan, A. & Burns, A. et al. (2005). Management of agitation, aggression, and psychosis associated with dementia: a pooled analysis including three randomized, placebo-controlled double-blind trials in nursing home residents treated with risperidone. *Clinical Neurology and Neurosurgery*, **107**, 497–508.

de Lima, M. S., de Oliveira Soares, B. G., Reisser, A. A. & Farrell, M. (2002). Pharmacological treatment of cocaine dependence: a systematic review. *Addiction*, **97**, 931–49.

DeRubeis, R., Hollon, S. D., Amsterdam, J. D. et al. (2005). Cognitive therapy vs. medications in the treatment of moderate to severe depression. *Archives of General Psychiatry*, **62**(4), 409–16.

Deb, S., Lyons, I., Koutzoukis, C., Ali, I., & Mccarthy, G. et al. (1999). Rate of psychiatric illness one year after traumatic brain injury. *American Journal of Psychiatry*, **156**, 374–8.

Deblinger, E., Steer, R. & Lippmann, J. (1999). Two-year follow-up study of cognitive behavioural therapy for sexually abused children suffering post-traumatic stress symptoms. *Child Abuse and Neglect*, **23**, 1371–8.

Degun-Mather, M. (2003). Ego-state therapy in the treatment of a complex eating disorder. *Contemporary Hypnosis*, **20**, 165–73.

Delate, T., Gelenberg, A. J., Simmons, V. A. & Motheral, B. R. (2004). Trends in the use of antidepressants in a national sample of commercially insured pediatric patients, 1998 to 2002. *Psychiatric Services*, **55**, 387–91.

DelBello, M., Schwiers, M. L., Rosenberg, H. L. & Strakowski, S. M. (2002). A double-blind, randomized, placebo-controlled study of quetiapine a adjunctive treatment for adolescent mania. *Journal of the American Academy of Child and Adolescent Psychiatry*, **41**, 1216–23.

DelBello, M., Kowatch, R., Adler, C. *et al.* (2006). A double-blind randomized pilot study comparing quetiapine and divalproex for adolescent mania. *Journal of the American Academy of Child and Adolescent Psychiatry*, **45**, 305–13.

De Leon, G. (2004). Therapeutic communities. In: M. Galanter and H. D. Kleber, eds. *Textbook of Substance Abuse Treatment*, 3rd ed. Washington, D.C.: American Psychiatric Press, pp. 485–501.

Denis, C., Fatseas, M., Lavie, E. & Auriacombe, M. (2006a). Pharmacological interventions for benzodiazepine mono-dependence management in out patient settings. *Cochrane Database of Systematic Reviews*, **3**, CD005194.

Denis, C., Lavie, E., Fatseas, M. & Auriacombe, M. (2006b). Psychotherapeutic interventions for cannabis abuse and/or dependence in outpatient settings. *Cochrane Database of Systematic Reviews*, **3**, CD005336. doi: 10.1002/14651858.CD005336.

Department of Health (2002). *Mental Health Policy Implementation Guide: Dual Diagnosis Good Practice Guide*. London: Department of Health.

Department of Health (2003a). Prescription costs analysis (PCA 2003 online). http://www.publications.doh.gov.uk/stats/pca2003.pdf

Department of Health (2003b). Selective serotonin reuptake inhibitors – use in children and adolescents with major depressive disorder. http://www.dhsspsni.gov.uk/hssmd49-03.pdf

Diamond-Raab, L. & Orrell-Valente, J. K. (2002). Art therapy, psychodrama, and verbal therapy. An integrative model of group therapy in the treatment of adolescents with anorexia nervosa and bulimia nervosa. *Child and Adolescent Psychiatry Clinics of North America*, **11**, 343–64.

Dibble, L. & Tandon, R. (1992). Post-ECT myoclonic jerks in a depressed patient with bulimia. *Convulsive Therapy*, **8**(4), 285–9.

Dickerson Mayes, S., Calhoun, S. L., Krecko, V. F., Vesell, H. P. & Hu, J. (2001). Outcome following child psychiatric hospitalization. *Journal of Behavioral Health Services & Research*, **28**, 96–103.

DiMascio, A., Weissman, M. M., Prusoff, B. A., Neu, C., Zwilling, M. & Klerman, G. L. (1979). Differential symptom reduction by drugs and psychotherapy in acute depression. *Archives of General Psychiatry*, **36**, 1450–6.

Dimidjian, S., Hollon, S. D., Dobson, K. S. et al. (2006). Randomized trial of behavioral activation, cognitive therapy, and antidepressant medication in the acute treatment of adults with major depression. *Journal of Consulting and Clinical Psychology*, **74**, 658–70.

Dingemans, A. E., Bruna, M. J. & van Furth E. F. (2002). Binge eating disorder: a review. *International Journal of Obesity*, **26**, 299–307.

Dodge, E., Hodes, M., Eisler, I. & Dare, C. (1995). Family therapy for bulimia nervosa in adolescents: an exploratory study. *Journal of Family Therapy*, **17**, 59–77.

Doering, S., Horz, S., Rentrop, M. et al. (2010). Transference-focused psychotherapy v. treatment by community psychotherapists for borderline personality disorder: randomised controlled trial. *British Journal of Psychiatry*, **196**, 389–95.

Dolan, L. J., Kellam, S. G., Brown C. H. *et al.* (1993). The short-term impact of two classroom-based preventive interventions on aggressive and shy behaviors and poor achievement. *Journal of Applied Developmental Psychology*, **14**, 317–45.

Doody, R. S., Geldmacher, D. S., Gordon, B., Perdomo, C. A., Pratt, R. D. & the Donepezil Study Group (2001). Open-label, multicenter, phase 3 extension study of the safety and efficacy of donepezil in patients with Alzheimer disease. *Archives of Neurology*, **58**, 427–33.

Dorey, G., Speakman, M., Feneley, R., Swinkels, A., Dunn, C. & Ewings, P. (2004). Randomised controlled trial of pelvic floor muscle exercises and manometric biofeedback for erectile dysfunction. *British Journal of General Practice*, **54**, 819–25.

Dozier, M., Stovall, K. C., Albus, K. & Bates, B. (2001). Attachment for infants in foster care: the role of caregiver state of mind. *Child Development*, **72**, 1467–77.

Dozier, M., Peloso, E., Lindhiem, O. et al. (2006). Developing evidence-based interventions for foster children: an example of a randomized clinical trial with infants and toddlers. *Journal of Social Issues*, **62**, 767–85.

Dubicka, B., Hadley, S. & Roberts, C. (2006). Suicidal behaviour in youths with depression treated with new-generation antidepressants: meta-analysis. *British Journal of Psychiatry*, **189**, 393–8.

Dudley, W. H. & Williams, J. G. (1972). Electroconvulsive therapy in delirium tremens. *Comprehensive Psychiatry*, **13**, 357–60.

Dula, E. S., Bukofzer, R., Perdok, R. J. & George, M. (2001). Apomorphine Study Group: double-blind, cross-over comparison of 3 mg apomorphine SL with placebo and with 4 mg apomorphine SL in male erectile dysfunction. *European Urology*, **39**, 558–64.

Durlak, J. A., Fuhrman, T. & Lampman, C. (1991). Effectiveness of cognitive behaviour therapy for maladaptive children: a meta-analysis. *Psychological Bulletin*, **110**, 204–14.

Dush, D. M., Hirt, M. L. & Schroeder, H. E. (1989). Self-statement modification in the treatment of child behavior disorders: a meta-analysis. *Psychological Bulletin*, **106**, 97–106.

Eaden, J., Abrams, K., Shears, J. & Mayberry, J. (2006). Randomized controlled trial comparing the efficacy of a video and information leaflet versus information leaflet alone on patient knowledge about surveillance and cancer risk in ulcerative colitis. *Inflammatory Bowel Diseases*, **8**, 407–12.

Ebmeier, K. P., Donaghey, C. & Steele, J. D. (2006). Recent developments and current controversies in depression. *Lancet*, **367**, 153–67.

Eckerberg, B. (2002). Treatment of sleep problems in families with young children: effects of treatment on family well-being. *Acta Paediatrica*, **93**, 126–34.

Eddy, J. M., Reid, J. B., Stoolmiller, M. & Fetrow, R. A. (2003). Outcomes during middle school for an elementary school-based preventive intervention for conduct problems: follow-up results from a randomized trial. *Behavior Therapy*, **34**, 535–52.

Eisler, I. (2005). The empirical and theoretical base of family therapy and multiple family day therapy for adolescent anorexia nervosa. *Journal of Family Therapy*, **27**, 104–31.

Eisler, I., Dare, C., Hodes, M., Russell, G. F. M., Dodge, E. & Le Grange, D. (2000). Family therapy for adolescent anorexia nervosa: the results of a controlled comparison of two family interventions. *Journal of Child Psychology and Psychiatry*, **41**, 727–36.

Eisler, L., Simic, M., Russell, G. & Dare, C. (2007). A randomized controlled treatment trial of two forms of family therapy in adolescent anorexia nervosa: a five-year follow-up. *Journal of Child Psychology Psychiatry*, **48**, 552–60.

Elkin, I., Shea, M. T., Watkins, J. T. et al. (1989). National Institute of Mental Health treatment of depression collaborative research program: general effectiveness of treatments. *Archives of General Psychiatry*, **46**, 971–82.

Elsenga, S. & van den Hoofdakker, R. H. (1982). Clinical effects of sleep deprivation and clomipramine in endogenous depression. *Journal of Psychiatric Research*, **17**(4), 361–74.

Emerson, E., Mason, H., Swarbrick, R., Mason, L. & Hatton, C. (2001) The prevalence of challenging behaviors: a total population study. *Research in Developmental Disabilities*, **22**, 77–93.

Emmelkamp, P. M., Benner, A., Kuipers, A., Feiertag, G. A., Koster, H. C. & van

Apeldoorn, F. J. (2006). Comparison of brief dynamic and cognitive-behavioural therapies in avoidant personality disorder. *British Journal of Psychiatry*, **189**, 60–4.

Emrick, C. D. & Tonigan, J. S. (2004). Alcoholics Anonymous and other 12-Step groups. In: M. Galanter & H. D. Kleber, eds. *The American Psychiatric Publishing Textbook of Substance Abuse Treatment*, 3rd edn. Washington, D.C.: American Psychiatric Press, pp. 485–501.

Emslie, G. J., Heiligenstein, J. H., Wagner, K. D. et al. (2002). Fluoxetine for acute treatment of depression in children and adolescents: a placebo-controlled, randomized clinical trial. *Journal of the American Academy of Child and Adolescent Psychiatry*, **41**, 1205–15.

Eranti, S., Mogg, A., Pluck, G., Landau, S. et al. (2007). A randomized controlled trial with 6-month follow up of repetitive transcranial magnetic stimulation and electroconvulsive therapy for severe depression. *American Journal of Psychiatry*, **164**, 73–81.

Erkinjuntti, T., Kurz, A., Gauthier, S., Bullock, R., Lilienfeld, S. & Damaraju C. V. (2002). Efficacy of galantamine in probable vascular dementia and Alzheimer's disease combined with cerebrovascular disease: a randomized trial. *The Lancet*, **359**, 1283–90.

Ernst, E. & Pittler, M. H. (1998). Yohimbine for erectile dysfunction: a systematic review and meta-analysis of randomized clinical trials. *Journal of Urology*, **159**(2), 433–6.

Erzegovesi, S., Guglielmo, E., Siliprandi, F. & Bellodi, L. (2005). Low-dose in obsessive-compulsive risperidone augmentation of fluvoxamine treatment disorder: a double-blind, placebo-controlled study. *European Neuropsychopharmacology*, **15**, 69–74.

European Monitoring Center for Drugs and Drug Addiction (2003). *Annual Report 2003: The State of the Drugs Problem in the Acceding and Candidate Countries to the European Union.* Luxembourg: Office of the Official Publications of the European Communities.

Evans, M. E., Armstrong, M. I., Kuppinger, A. D., Huz, S. & McNulty, T. L. (1998). Preliminary outcomes of an experimental study comparing treatment foster care and family-centered intensive case management. In: M. H. Epstein, K. Kutash & A. Duchnowski, eds. *Outcomes for Children and Youth with Emotional and Behavioral Disorders and their Families: Programs and Evaluation Best Practices.* Austin, TX: PRO-ED, pp. 543–80.

Evans, M. D., Hollon, S. D., DeRubeis, R. J. et al. (1992). Differential relapse following cognitive therapy and pharmacotherapy for depression. *Archives of General Psychiatry*, **49**, 802–8.

Eyberg, S. M. (1988). Parent–Child Interaction Therapy: Integration of traditional and behavioral concerns. *Child and Family Behavior Therapy*, **10**, 33–48.

Faggiano, F., Vigna-Taglianti, F., Versino, E. & Lemma, P. (2003). Methadone maintenance at different dosages for opioid dependence. In: *Cochrane Database Systematic Review*, **3**, CD002208. Oxford: Update Software Ltd.

Fahlen, T., Nilsson, H. L., Borg, K., Humble, M. & Pauli, U. et al. (1995).

Social phobia: the clinical efficacy and tolerability of the monoamine-oxidase-A and serotonin uptake inhibitor brofaromine: a double-blind placebo-controlled study. *Acta Psychiatrica Scandinavica*, **92**, 351–8.

Fairburn, C. G. (1981). A cognitive behavioral approach to the treatment of bulimia. *Psychological Medicine*, **11**, 707–11.

Fairburn, C. (1997). Interpersonal psychotherapy for bulimia nervosa. In: D. M. Garner & P. E. Garfinkel, eds. *The Handbook of Treatment for Eating Disorders*, 2nd edn. New York: Guilford Press, pp. 278–94.

Fairburn, C. G. & Bohn, K. (2005). Eating Disorder Not Otherwise Specified (EDNOS): an example of the troublesome 'Not Otherwise Specified (NOS)' category in DSM-IV. *Behaviour Research and Therapy*, **43**, 691–701.

Fairburn, C. & Cooper, Z. (2011). Eating disorders, DSM-5 and clinical reality. *British Journal of Psychiatry*, **198**, 8–10.

Fairburn, C. G., Cooper, Z., Doll, H. A. et al. (2000). The natural course of bulimia nervosa and binge eating disorder in young women. *Archives of General Psychiatry*, **57**, 659–65.

Fairburn, C. G., Cooper, Z. & Shafran, R. et al. (2003). Cognitive behaviour therapy for eating disorders: a "transdiagnostic" theory and treatment. *Behaviour Research and Therapy*, **41**, 509–28.

Fairburn, C. G., Cooper, Z., Doll, H. A. et al. (2009). Transdiagnostic cognitive behavioral therapy for patients with eating disorders: a two-site trial with 60-week follow-up. *American Journal of Psychiatry*, **166**, 311–9.

Fallon, B. A., Petkova, E., Skritskaya, N. et al. (2008). A double-masked, placebo-controlled study of fluoxetine for hypochondriasis. *Journal of Clinical Psychopharmacology*, **28**, 638–45.

Farre, M., Mas, A., Torrens, M., Moreno, V. & Cami, J. (2002). Retention rate and illicit opioid use during methadone maintenance intervention: a meta-analysis. *Drug and Alcohol Dependence*, **65**, 283–90.

Farrell, J. M., Shaw, I. A. & Webber, M. A. (2009). A schema-focused approach to group psychotherapy for outpatients with borderline personality disorder. *Journal of Behavior Therapy & Experimental Psychology*, **40**, 317–28.

Fava, M., Alpert, J. et al. (2002). Double-blind study of high-dose fluoxetine versus lithium or desipramine augmentation of fluoxetine in partial responders and nonresponders to fluoxetine. *Journal of Clinical Psychopharmacology*, **22**(4), 379–87.

Fedoroff, I. C. & Taylor, S. (2001). Psychological and pharmacological treatments of social phobia: a meta-analysis. *Journal of Clinical Psychopharmacology*, **21**, 311–24.

Ferber, R. & Kryger, M. (1995). *Principles and Practice of Sleep Medicine in the Child*. Philadelphia: W. B. Saunders Company, pp. 79–89 & 99–106.

Ferreri, M., Lavergne, F., Berlin, I., Payan, C. & Puech, A. J. (2001). Benefits from mianserin augmentation of fluoxetine in patients with major depression non-responders to fluoxetine alone. *Acta Psychiatrica Scandinavica*, **103**, 66–72.

Field, T. (2002). Massage therapy. *Medical Clinics of North America*, **86**(1), 163–171.

Field, T., Schanberg, S., Kuhn, C., Fierro, K., Henteleff, T., Mueller, C., Yando, R. & Burman, I. (1998). Bulimic adolescents benefit from massage therapy. *Adolescence*, **33**, 554–63.

Fineberg, N. A. & Galem, T. M. (2005). Evidence-based pharmacotherapy of obsessive-compulsive disorder. *International Journal of Neuropsychopharmacology*, **8**, 107–29.

Fink, H. A., MacDonald, R., Rutks-Indulis, R., Nelson, D. B. & Wilt, T. J. (2002). Sildenafil for male erectile dysfunction: a systematic review and meta-analysis. *Archives of Internal Medicine*, **162**, 1349–60.

Fiore, M. C., Smith, S. S., Jorenby, D. E. & Baker, T. B. (1994). The effectiveness of the nicotine patch for smoking cessation: a meta-analysis. *Journal of the American Medical Association*, **271**, 1940–7.

Fiore, M. C., Bailey, W. C., Cohen, S. J. *et al.* (2000). *Clinical Practice Guideline: Treating Tobacco Use and Dependence*. US Department of Health and Human Services. Rockville, MD: US Public Health Service.

Fisher, W. W., Adelinis, J. D., Volkert, V. M., Keeney, K. M., Neidert, P. L. & Hovanetz, A. (2005). Assessing preferences for positive and negative reinforcement during treatment of destructive behavior with functional communication training. *Research in Developmental Disabilities*, **26**, 153–68.

Fleming, M. F., Mundt, M. P., French, M. F. *et al.* (2002). Brief physician advice for problem drinkers: long-term efficacy and benefit-cost analysis. *Alcoholism, Clinical and Experimental Research*, **26**, 36–43.

Foa, E. B., Kozak, M. J., Steketee, G. S. & McCarthy, P. R. (1992). Treatment of depressive and obsessive-compulsive symptoms in OCD by imipramine and behaviour therapy. *British Journal of Clinical Psychology*, **31** (Pt 3), 279–92.

Foa, E. B., Dancu, C. V., Hembree, E. A. et al. (1999). A comparison of exposure therapy, stress inoculation training, and their combination for reducing post-traumatic stress disorder in female assault victims. *Journal of Consulting and Clinical Psychology*, **67**, 194–200.

Foa, E. B., Liebowitz, M. R., Kozak, M. J. et al. (2005). Randomized placebo-controlled trial of exposure and ritual prevention, clomipramine, and their combination in the treatment of obsessive–compulsive disorder. *American Journal of Psychiatry*, **162**, 151–61.

Folkerts, H. W., Michael, N., Tolle, R. et al. (1997). Electroconvulsive therapy vs. paroxetine in treatment-resistant depression: a randomized study. *Acta Psychiatrica Scandinavica*, **96**, 334–42.

Fontaine, C. S., Hynan, L. S., Koch, K., Martin-Cook, K., Svetlik, D. & Weiner, M. F. (2003). A double-blind comparison of olanzapine versus risperidone in the acute treatment of dementia-related behavioral disturbances in extended care facilities. *Journal of Clinical Psychiatry*, **64**, 726–30.

Forbes, D., Creamer, M., Bisson, J. I. et al. (2010). A guide to guidelines for the treatment of PTSD and related conditions. *Journal of Traumatic Stress*, **23**, 537–52.

Foxcroft, D. R., Ireland, D., Lister-Sharp, D. J., Lowe, G. & Breen, R. (2003). Longer-term primary prevention for alcohol misuse in young people: a systematic review. *Addiction*, **98**, 397–411.

Frangou, S., Lewis, M. & McCrone, P. (2006). Efficacy of ethyl-eicosapentaenoic acid in bipolar depression: randomised, double-blind, placebo-controlled study. *British Journal of Psychiatry* **188**, 46–50.

Frank, E., Kupfer, D. J., Perel, T. M. et al. (1990). Three-year outcomes for maintenance therapies in recurrent depression. *Archives of General Psychiatry*, **47**, 1093–9.

Frankel, F., Cantwell, D. P. & Myatt, R. (1996). Helping ostracized children: social skills training and parent support for socially rejected children. In: E. D. Hibbs & P. S. Jensen, eds. *Psychosocial Treatments for Child and Adolescent Disorders: Empirically Based Strategies for Clinical Practice*. Washington, DC: American Psychological Association, pp. 595–617.

Franzen, U., Backmund, H. & Gerlinghoff, M. (2004). Day treatment group programme for eating disorders: reasons for drop-out. *European Eating Disorders Review*, **12**, 153–8.

Freestone, M. H., Ladouceur, R., Gagnon, F. et al. (1997). Cognitive-behavioral treatment of obsessive thoughts: a controlled study. *Journal of Consulting and Clinical Psychology*, **65**, 405–13.

Fridell, M. (2003). Psychosocial treatment for drug dependence. In: M. Berglund, S. Thelander & E. Jonsson, eds. *Treating Alcohol and Drug Abuse: An Evidence Based Review*. Berlin: Wiley-VCH GmbH & Co.

Friedman, J. H. (2010). Parkinson's disease psychosis 2010: a review article *Parkinsonism and Related Disorders* **16**, 553–60.

Fruehwald, S., Gatterbauer, E., Rhak, P. & Baumhackl, U. (2003). Early fluoxetine treatment of post-stroke depression: a 3-month double-blind, placebo-controlled study with an open-label long-term follow up. *Journal of Neurology*, **250**, 347–51.

Furukawa, T. A., Watanabe, N. & Churchill, R. (2007). Combined psycho-therapy plus antidepressants for panic disorder with or without agoraphobia. *Cochrane Database of Systematic Reviews*, **1**, CD004364.

Gagiano, C., Read, S., Thorpe, L. et al. (2005). Short- and long-term efficacy and safety of risperidone in adults with disruptive behavior disorders. *Psychopharmacology (Berlin)*, **179**, 629–36.

Galanter, M., Dermatis, H., Glickman, L. et al. (2004). Network therapy: decreased secondary opioid use during buprenorphine maintenance. *Journal of Substance Abuse Treatment*, **26**, 313–18.

Gallagher-Heather, M., Rabbin, B. A. & McCloskey, M. S. (2004). A brief group cognitive-behavioural intervention for social phobia in childhood. *Journal of Anxiety Disorders*, **18**, 459–79.

Gamberini, M., Bolliger, D., Lurati Buse, G. A. et al. (2009). Rivastigmine for the prevention of postoperative delirium in elderly patients undergoing elective cardiac surgery: a randomized controlled trial. *Critical Care Medicine*, **37**, 762–8.

Garbutt, J. C., West, S. L., Carey, T. S., Lohr, K. N. & Crews, F. T. (1999). Pharmacological treatment of alcohol dependence: a review of the evidence. *Journal of the American Medical Association*, **281**, 1318–25.

Garbutt, J. C., Kranzler, H. R., O'Malley, S. S. et al. (2005). Efficacy and tolerability of long-acting injectable naltrexone for alcohol dependence: a randomized controlled trial. *Journal of the American Medical Association*, **293**, 1617–25.

Garcia-Palacios, A., Hoffman, H., Carlin, A., Furness, T. A., III & Botella, C. (2002). Virtual reality in the treatment of spider phobia: a controlled study. *Behaviour Research and Therapy*, **40**(9), 983–93.

Gareri, P., Cotroneo, A., Lacava, R. et al. (2004). Comparison of the efficacy of new and conventional antipsychotic drugs in the treatment of behavioral and psychological symptoms of dementia (BPSD). *Archives of Gerontology Geriatric Supplement*, **9**, 207–15.

Garety, P. A., Fowler, D.G., Freeman, D., Bebbinton, P., Dunn, G. & Kuipers, E. (2008). Cognitive-behavioural therapy and family intervention for relapse Prevention and symptom reduction in psychosis: randomised controlled trial. *British journal of psychiatry*, **192**, 412–23.

Garner, D. M. & Needleman, L. D. (1997). Sequencing and integration of treatments. In: D. M. Garner & P. E. Garfinkel, eds. *Handbook of Treatment for Eating Disorders*. New York: Guilford Press, pp. 50–66.

Garner, D. M. & Vitousek, P. K. M. (1997). Cognitive-behavioral therapy for anorexia nervosa. In: D. M. Garner & P. E. Garfinkel, eds. *The Handbook of Treatment for Eating Disorders*, 2nd edn. New York: Guilford Press, pp. 94–144.

Garnok-Jones, K. P. & Keating, G. M. (2010). Spotlight on atomoxetine in attention deficit hyperactivity disorder in children and adolescents. *CNS Drugs*, **24**, 85–8.

Garrett, C. J. (1997). Recovery from anorexia nervosa: a sociological perspective. *International Journal of Eating Disorders*, **21**, 261–72.

Garssen, B., de Ruiter, C. & Van Dyck, R. (1992). Breathing retraining: a rational placebo? *Clinical Psychology Review*, **12** (2), 141–53.

Geddes, J., Freemantle, N., Harrison, P. & Bebbington, P. (2000). Atypical antispychotics in the treatment of schizophrenia: systematic overview and meta-regression analysis. *British Medical Journal*, **321**, 1371–6.

Geddes, J. R., Rendell, J. M. & Goodwin, G. M. et al. (2003). BALANCE: a large simple trial of maintenance treatment for bipolar disorder. *World Psychiatry*, **1**, 48–51.

Geddes, J. R., Goodwin, G. M., Huffman, R., Paska, W., Evoniuk, G. & Leadbetter, R. (2009). Additional clinical trail data and a retrospective pooled analysis of response rates across all randomized trials conducted by GSK. *Bipolar Disorders*, **8** (Suppl. 1), 32.

Geddes, J. R., Goodwin, G. M., Rendell, J. et al. (2010). Lithium plus valproate combination therapy versus monotherapy for relapse prevention in bipolar I disorder (BALANCE): a randomised open-label trial. *Lancet*, **375**, 385–95.

Geist, R., Heinmaa, M., Stephens, D., Davis, R. & Katzman, D. K. (2000). Comparison of family therapy and family group psychoeducation in adolescents with anorexia nervosa. *Canadian Journal of Psychiatry*, **45**, 173–8.

Gelernter, C. S., Uhde, T. W., Cimbolic, P. et al. (1991). Cognitive-behavioral and pharmacological treatments of social phobia: a controlled study. *Archives of General Psychiatry*, **48**, 938–45.

Geller, D., Biederman, J., Stewart, E. et al. (2003). Which SSRI? A meta-analysis of pharmacotherapy trials in paediatric obsessive compulsive disorder. *American Journal of Psychiatry*, **160**, 1919–28.

George, M. S., Lisanby, S. H. & Sackeim, H. A. et al. (1999). Transcranial Magnetic Stimulation: applications in neuropsychiatry. *Archives of General Psychiatry*, **56**, 300–11.

George, M. S., Nahas, Z., Kozel, F. A. et al. (2003). Mechanisms and the current state of transcranial magnetic stimulation. *CNS Spectrums*, **8**(7), 496–514.

George, M. S., Rush, A. J., Marangell, L. B. et al. (2005). A one year comparison of vagus nerve stimulation with treatment as usual for treatment-resistant depression. *Biological Psychiatry*, **58**(5), 364–73.

George, T. P., Verrico, C. D. & Roth, R. H. (1998). Effects of repeated nicotine pretreatment on mesoprefontal dopaminergic and behavioral responses to acute footshock stress. *Brain Research*, **801**, 36–49.

George, T. P., Chawarski, M. C., Pakes, J., Carroll, K. M., Kosten, T. R. & Schottenfeld, R. S. (2000). Disulfiram versus placebo for cocaine dependence in buprenorphine-maintained subjects: a preliminary trial. *Biological Psychiatry*, **47**, 1080–6.

Gevensleben, H., Holl, B., Albrecht, B. et al (2010). Neurofeedback training in children with ADHD: 6-month follow-up o a randomised controlled trial. *European Child & Adolescent Psychiatry*, **19**, 715–24.

Ghazi-Noori, S., Chung, T. H., Deane, K. H. O. et al. (2003). Therapies for depression in Parkinson's disease. *Cochrane Database of Systematic Reviews*, 3, CD003465. Oxford: Update Software Ltd.

Ghaziuddin, N., Kutcher, S. P., Knapp, P. & American Academy of Child and Adolescent Psychiatry Work Group on Quality Issues (2004). Summary of the practice parameter for the use of electroconvulsive therapy with adolescents. *Journal of American Academy of Child Adolescent Psychiatry*, **43**, 119–22.

Gibbons, M. B., Crits-Christoph, P., Levinson, J. et al. (2002). Therapist interventions in the interpersonal and cognitive therapy sessions of the Treatment of Depression Collaborative Research Program. *American Journal of Psychotherapy*, **56**, 3–26.

Gibbons, R. D., Brown, C. H., Hur, K. et al. (2007). Early evidence on the effects of regulators' suicidality warnings on SSRI prescriptions and suicide in children and adolescents. *American Journal of Psychiatry*, **164**, 1356–63.

Giesen-Bloo, J., van Dyck, R., Spinhoven, P. et al. (2006). Outpatient psychotherapy for borderline personality disorder: randomized trial of schema-focused therapy vs. transference-focused psychotherapy. *Archives of General Psychiatry*, **63**, 649–58.

Gijsman, H. J., Geddes, J. R., Rendell, J. M., Nolen, W. A. & Goodwin, G. M. (2004). Antidepressants for bipolar depression: a systematic review of randomized controlled trials. *American Journal of Psychiatry*, **161**, 1537–47.

Giovino, G. A. (2002). Epidemiology of tobacco use in the United States. *Oncogene*, **21**, 7326–40.

Gleeson, J., Cotton, S., Alvarez-Jimenez, M. et al. (2009.) A randomized controlled trial of relapse prevention therapy for first-episode psychosis patients. *Journal of Clinical Psychiatry*, **70**, 477–86.

Gogtay, N. & Rapoport, J. (2008). Clozapine use in children and adolescents. *Expert Opinion in Pharmacotherapy*, **9**, 459–65.

Goldberg, S. C., Halmi, K. A., Eckert, E. D., Casper, R. C. & Davis, J. M. (1979). Cyproheptadine in anorexia nervosa. *British Journal of Psychiatry*, **134**, 67–70.

Goldner, E. M., Birmingham, C. L. & Smye, V. (1997). Addressing treatment refusal in anorexia nervosa: clinical, ethical and legal considerations. In: D. M. Garner & P. E. Garfinkel, eds. *Handbook of Treatment for Eating Disorders*, 2nd edn. New York: Guilford Press.

Goldstein, I., Lue, T. F., Padma-Nathan, H., Rosen, R. C., Steers, W. D., Wicker, P. A., for the Sildenafil Study Group (1998). Oral sildenafil in the treatment of erectile dysfunction. *New England Journal of Medicine*, **338**, 1397–404.

Goldstein, M., Peters, L., Baillie, A., McVeigh, P., Minshall, G. & Fitzjames, D. (2010). The effectiveness of a day program for the treatment of adolescent anorexia nervosa. *International Journal of Eating Disorders*. doi: 10.1002/eat.20789.

Gonzalez, G., Sevarino, K., Sofuoglu, M. et al. (2003). Tiagabine increases cocaine-free urines in cocaine-dependent methadone-treated patients: results of a randomized pilot study. *Addiction*, **98**, 1625–32.

Goodwin, F. K., Murphy, D. L., Bunney Jr., W. E. et al. (1969). Lithium-carbonate treatment in depression and mania: a longitudinal double-blind study. *Archives of General Psychiatry*, **21**(4), 486–96.

Goodyer, I. M., Herbert, J. & Tamplin, A. (2003). Psychoendocrine antecedents of persistent first-episode major depression in adolescents: a community-based longitudinal enquiry. *Psychological Medicine*, **33**, 601–10.

Gordon, C. T., State, R. C., Nelson, J. E., Hamburger, S. D. & Rapoport, J. L. (1993). A double-blind comparison of clomipramine, desipramine, and placebo in the treatment of autistic disorder. *Archives of General Psychiatry*, **50**, 441–7.

Gossop, M., Marsden, J., Stewart, D. & Kidd, T. (2003). The National Treatment Outcome Research Study (NTORS): 4–5 year follow-up results. *Addiction*, **98**, 291–303.

Gould, R. A., Otto, M. W., Pollack, M. H. & Yap, L. (1997a). Cognitive behavioural and pharmacological treatment of generalised anxiety disorder: a preliminary meta-analysis. *Behavior Therapy*, **28**, 285–305.

Gould, R. A., Buckminster, S., Pollack, M. H., Otto, M. & Yap, L. (1997b). Cognitive-behavioral and pharmacological treatment for social phobia: a meta-analysis. *Clinical Psychology: Science and Practice*, **4**, 291–306.

Gowers, S. & Bryant-Waugh, R. (2004). Management of child and adolescent eating disorders: the current evidence base and future directions. *Journal of Child Psychology and Psychiatry*, **45**, 63–83.

Gowers, S., Norton, K., Halek, C., & Crisp, A. H. (1994). Outcome of outpatient psychotherapy in a random allocation treatment study of anorexia nervosa. *International Journal of Eating Disorders*, **15**, 65–77.

Gowers, S. G., Clark, A., Roberts, C. et al. (2007). Clinical effectiveness of treatments for anorexia nervosa in adolescents: randomised controlled trial. *British Journal of Psychiatry*, **191**, 427–35.

Gowers, S., Claxton, M., Rowlands, L. et al. (2010). Drug prescribing in child and adolescent eating disorder services. *Child and Adolescent Mental Health*, **15**, 18–22.

Graham, A. W. & Fleming, M. S. (1998). Brief interventions. In: A. W. Graham, T. K. Schultz & B. B. Wilford, eds. *Principles of Addiction Medicine*, 2nd edn. Chevy Chase, MD: American Society of Addiction Medicine, Inc, pp. 615–30.

Graham, P. (1998). *Cognitive-Behaviour Therapy for Children and Adolescents.* Cambridge: Cambridge University Press.

Grandison, M. K. & Boudinot, F. D. (2000). Age related changes in protein binding of drugs: implications for therapy. *Clinical Pharmacokinetics*, **38**, 271–90.

Grandmaison, E. & Simard, M. (2003). Critical review of memory stimulation programs in Alzheimer's disease. *The Journal of Neuropsychiatry and Clinical Neurosciences*, **15**, 130–44.

Grant, B. F., Stinson, F. S., Dawson, D. A. et al. (2004). Prevalence and co-occurrence of substance use disorders and independent mood and anxiety disorders: results from the National Epidemiologic Survey on Alcohol and Related Conditions. *Archives of General Psychiatry*, **61**, 807-16.

Gray, C. A. (1995). Teaching children with autism to 'read' social situations. In: A. Quill, ed. *Teaching Children with Autism: Strategies to Enhance Communication and Socialization*. New York: Delmar, pp. 219-42.

Gray, R., Leese, M., Bindman, J. et al. (2006). Adherence therapy for people with schizophrenia: European multicentre randomized controlled trial. *British Journal of Psychiatry*, **189**, 508-14.

Greater London Alcohol and Drug Alliance (2004). *An evidence base for the London crack cocaine strategy: a consultation document prepared for the Greater London Alcohol and Drug Alliance*. London: Greater London Authority.

Green, J. M. (2003). Are attachment disorders best seen as social impairment syndromes? *Attachment and Human Development*, **5**, 259-64.

Green, J. M. & Goldwyn, R. (2002). Annotation: Attachment disorganisation and psychopathology: new findings in attachment research and their potential implications for developmental psychopathology in childhood. *Journal of Child Psychology and Psychiatry*, **43**, 835-46.

Green, J., Jacobs, B., Beecham, J. et al. (2007). Inpatient treatment in child and adolescent psychiatry: a prospective study of health gain and costs. *Journal of Child Psychology and Psychiatry*, **48**, 1259-67.

Green, J., Charman, T., McConachie, H. et al. and the PACT Consortium (2010). Parent-mediated communication-focused treatment for preschool children with autism (MRC Pact); a randomised controlled trial. *The Lancet*, **375**(9732), 2152-60.

Green, R. (1978). Sexual identity of 37 children raised by homosexual or transsexual parents. *American Journal of Psychiatry*, **135**, 692-7.

Green, R. (1998). Sexual functioning in post-operative transsexuals: male-to-female and female-to-male. *International Journal of Impotence Research*, **10** (Suppl 1), S22-4.

Greenberg, B. D., George, M. S., Martin, J. D. et al (1997). Effect of prefrontal repetitive transcranial magnetic stimulation in obsessive-compulsive disorder: a preliminary study. *American Journal of Psychiatry*, **154**, 867-9.

Greenberg, P. E., Sisitsky, T., Kessler, R. C. et al. (1999). The economic burden of anxiety disorders in the 1990s. *Journal of Clinical Psychiatry*, **60**(7), 427-35.

Greenblatt, M., Grosser, G. H., Wechsler, H. et al. (1964). Differential response of hospitalized depressed patients to somatic therapy. *American Journal of Psychology*, **120**, 935-43.

Gregory, S., Shawcross, C. R. & Gill, D. et al. (1985). The Nottingham ECT Study: a double-blind comparison of bilateral, unilateral and stimulated ECT in depressive illness. *British Journal of Psychiatry*, **146**, 520-4.

Greist, J. H., Jefferson, J. W., Kobak, K. A. et al. (1995). A 1 year double-blind placebo-controlled fixed dose study of sertraline in the treatment of obsessive-compulsive disorder. *International Clinical Psychopharmacology*, **10**, 57-65.

Greist, J. H., Marks, I. M., Baer, L. et al. (2002) Behavior therapy for obsessive-compulsive disorder guided by a computer or by a clinician compared with relaxation as a control. *Journal of Clinical Psychiatry*, **63**, 138-45.

Grella, C. E., Anglin, M. D. & Wugalter, S. E. (1997). Patterns and predictors of cocaine and crack use by clients in standard and enhanced methadone maintenance treatment. *American Journal of Drug and Alcohol Abuse*, **23**, 15-42.

Gresham, F. M. & Nagle, R. J. (1980). Social skills training with children: Responsiveness to modelling and coaching as a function of peer orientation. *Journal of Consulting and Clinical Psychology*, **48**, 718-29.

Griffiths, R. A., Hadzi-Pavlovic, D. & Channon-Little, L. (1996). The short-term follow-up effects of hypnobehavioural and cognitive behavioural treatment for bulimia nervosa. *European Eating Disorder Review*, **4**(1), 12-31.

Grigoriadis, D., Kennedy, S. H. et al. (2003). A comparison of anti-depressant response in younger and older women. *Journal of Clinical Psychopharmacology*, **23**(4), 405-7.

Gros, D. F. & Antony, M. M. (2006). The assessment and treatment of specific phobias: a review. *Current Psychiatry Reports*, **8**(4), 298-303.

Grossman, P., Niemann, L., Schmidt, S. & Walach, H. (2004). Mindfulness-based stress reduction and health benefits: a meta-analysis. *Journal of Psychosomatic Research*, **57**, 35-43.

Guastella, A. J., Dadds, M. R., Lovibond, P. F., Mitchell, P. & Richardson, R. (2007). A randomized controlled trial of the effect of D-cycloserine on exposure therapy for spider fear. *Journal of Psychiatric Research*, **41**, 466-71.

Gurney, V. W. & Halmi, K. A. (2001). An eating disorder curriculum for primary care providers. *International Journal of Eating Disorder*, **30**, 209-12.

Haessler, F., Glaser, T. & Beneke, L. J. et al. (2007). Zuclopenthixol in aggressive challenging behaviour in learning disability: discontinuation study. *British Journal of Psychiatry*, **190**, 447-8.

Haigh, R. & Treasure, J. L. (2003). Investigating the Needs of Carers in the Area of Eating Disorders: Development of the Carers' Needs Assessment Measure (CaNAM). *European Eating Disorder Review*, **11**, 125-41.

Hajak, G., Muller, W. E., Wittchen, H. U., Pittrow, D. & Kirch, W. (2003). Abuse and dependence potential for the non-benzodiazepine hypnotics zolpidem and zopiclone: a review of case reports and epidemiological data. *Addiction*, **98**, 1371-8.

Hall, A. & Crisp, A. H. (1987). Brief psychotherapy in the treatment of anorexia nervosa: outcome at one year. *British Journal of Psychiatry*, **151**, 185-91.

Hallstrom, C., Treasaden, I., Edwards, J. G. & Lader, M. (1981). Diazepam, propranolol and their combination in the management of chronic anxiety. *British Journal of Psychiatry*, **139**, 417-21.

Halmi, K. A., Eckert, E., LaDu, T. J. & Cohen, J. (1986). Anorexia nervosa: treatment efficacy of cyproheptadine and amitriptyline. *Archives of General Psychiatry*, **43**(2), 177-81.

Hampson, R. B. & Beavers, R. W. (1996). Family therapy and outcome: relationships between therapist and family styles. *Contemporary Family Therapy*, **18**, 345-70.

Han, C. & Kim, Y. (2004). A double-blind trial of risperidone and haloperidol for the treatment of delirium. *Psychosomatics*, **45**, 297–301.

Han, J. S., Trachtenberg, A. I. & Lowinson, J. H. (2004). Acupuncture. In: J. H. Lowinson, P. Ruiz, R. B. Millman & J. G. Langrod, eds. *Substance Abuse: A Comprehensive Textbook*, 4th edn. Philadelphia, PA: Lippincott Williams & Wilkins.

Handen, B. L., Sahl, R. & Hardan, A. Y. (2008). Guanfacine in children with autism and/or intellectual disabilities. *Journal of Developmental and Behavioral Pediatrics*, **29**, 303–8.

Haney, M., Ward, A. S., Comer, S. D., Foltin, R. W. & Fischman, M. W. (1999). Abstinence symptoms following smoked marijuana in humans. *Psychopharmacology*, **14**, 395–404.

Haney, M., Hart, C. L., Vosburg, S. K., Nasser, J., Bennett, A., Zubaran, C. & Foltin, R. W. (2004). Marijuana withdrawal in humans: effects of oral THC or Divalproex. *Neuropsychopharmacology*, **29**, 158–70.

Hansen, V., Lund, E. & Smith-Sivertsen, T. (1998). Self-reported mental distress under the shifting daylight in the high north. *Psychological Medicine*, **28**, 447–52.

Harmon, R. J. & Riggs, P. D. (1996). Clonidine for posttraumatic stress disorder in preschool children. *Journal of the American Academy of Child and Adolescent Psychiatry*, **35**, 1247–9.

Hart, S., Field, T., Hernandez-Reif, M. & Nearing, G. (2001). Anorexia nervosa symptoms are reduced by massage therapy. *Eating Disorders*, **9**, 289–99.

Hawley, C. J., Tattersall, M., Dellaportas, C. & Hallstrom, C. (1994). Comparison of long-term benzodiazepine users in three settings. *British Journal of Psychiatry*, **165**, 792–6.

Haug, T. T., Blomhoff, S., Hellstrøm, K., et al. (2003). Exposure therapy and sertraline in social phobia: 1-year follow-up of a randomised controlled trial. *British Journal of Psychiatry*, **182**, 312–18.

Hay, P. J. & Bacaltchuk, J. (2008). Bulimia nervosa. *Clinical Evidence* (Online) June 12, pii: 1009.

Hay, P. P., Bacaltchuk, J., Stefano, S. & Kashyap, P. (2009). Psychological treatments for bulimia nervosa and binging. *Cochrane Database of Systematic Reviews*, **7**(4), CD000562.

Hazell, P. (2006). Drug therapy for attention-deficit/hyperactivity disorder-like symptoms in autistic disorder. *Journal of Paediatrics and Child Health*, **43**, 19–24.

Hazell, P. L. & Stuart, J. E. (2003). A randomized controlled trial of clonidine added to psychostimulant medication for hyperactive and aggressive children. *Journal of the American Academy of Child & Adolescent Psychiatry*, **42**, 886–94.

Hazell, P., O'Connell, D., Heathcote, D. & Henry, D. A. (2009). Tricyclic drugs for depression in children and adolescents. *Cochrane Depression, Anxiety and Neurosis Group Cochrane Database of Systematic Reviews*, **1**, 2009.

Health Technology Board for Scotland (2002). Health Technology Assessment Advice 3: Prevention of Relapse in Alcohol Dependence. HTBS.

Heather, N., Bowie, A., Ashton, H. et al. (2004). Randomized controlled trial of two brief interventions against long-term benzodiazepine use: outcome of intervention. *Addiction Research Theory*, **12**, 141-54.

Hedges, D.W., Reimherr, F.W., Hoopes, S.P. et al. (2003). Treatment of bulimia nervosa with topiramate in a randomized, double-blind, placebo-controlled trial, part 2: improvement in psychiatric measures. *Journal of Clinical Psychiatry*, **64**(12), 1449-54.

Heim, C., Newport, D.J., Bonsall, R., Miller, A.H. & Nemeroff, C.B. (2001). Altered pituitary-adrenal axis responses to provocative challenge tests in adult survivors of childhood abuse. *American Journal of Psychiatry*, **158**, 575-81.

Heimberg, R.G. (2002). Cognitive-behavioral therapy for social anxiety disorder: current status and future directions. *Biological Psychiatry*, **51**, 101-8.

Heimberg, R.G., Liebowitz, M.R., Hope, D.A. et al. (1998). Cognitive behavioral group therapy vs. phenelzine for social phobia. *Archives of General Psychiatry*, **55**, 1133-41.

Heldt, E.M., Gisele, G., Kipper, L., Blaya, C., Isolan, L. & Otto, M.W. (2006). One-year follow-up of pharmacotherapy-resistant patients with panic disorder treated with cognitive-behavior therapy: outcome and predictors of remission. *Behaviour Research and Therapy*, **44**(5), 657-65.

Hellstrom, K., Fellenius, J. & Ost, L.G. (1996). One versus five sessions of applied tension in the treatment of blood phobia. *Behaviour Research and Therapy*, **34**(2), 101-12.

Henggeler, S.W., Melton, G.B. & Smith, L.A. (1992). Family preservation using multisystemic therapy: an effective alternative to incarcerating serious juvenile offenders. *Journal of Consulting and Clinical Psychology*, **60**, 953-61.

Henggeler, S.W., Schoenwald, S.K., Borduin, C.M., Rowland, M.D. & Cunningham, P.B. (1998). *Multisystemic Treatment of Antisocial Behavior in Children and Adolescents*. New York: Guilford.

Herbert, J.D., Gaudiano, B.A., Rheingold, A.A. et al. (2009). Cognitive behavior therapy for generalized social anxiety disorder in adolescents: a randomized controlled trial. *Journal of Anxiety Disorders*, **23**, 167-77.

Herpertz, S.C., Zanarini, M., Schulz, C.S. et al. (2007). World Federation of Societies of Biological Psychiatry (WFSBP) Guidelines for Biological Treatment of Personality Disorders. *The World Journal of Biological Psychiatry*, **8**, 212-44.

Herpetz-Dahlmann, B. & Remschmidt, H. (1993). Depression and psychosocial adjustment in adolescent anorexia nervosa: a controlled 3-year follow-up study. *European Child and Adolescent Psychiatry*, **2**, 146-54.

Herrmann, N. & Lanctôt, K. (2006). Atypical antipsychotics for neuropsychiatric symptoms of dementia: malignant or maligned? *Drug Safety*, **29**, 833-43.

Herrmann, N. & Lanctôt, K.L. (2007). Pharmacologic management of neuropsychiatric symptoms of Alzheimer disease. *Canadian Journal of Psychiatry*, **52**, 630-46.

Herrmann, N., Lanctot, K.L., Eryavec, G. & Khan, L.R. (2004a). Noradrenergic activity is associated with response to pindolol in aggressive Alzheimer's disease patients. *Journal of Psychopharmacology*, **18**, 215-20.

Herrmann, N., Mamdani, M. & Lanctôt, K. L. et al. (2004b). Atypical antipsychotics and risk of cerebrovascular accidents. *American Journal of Psychiatry*, **161**, 1113-15.

Herzog, T., Hartmann, A. & Falk, C. (1996). Total symptom-oriented and psychodynamic concept in inpatient treatment of anorexia nervosa: a quasi-experimental comparative study of 40 admission episodes. *Psychotherapie Psychosomatische Medizin und Psychologie*, **46**, 11-22.

Hesse, M. (2009). Integrated psychological treatment for substance use and co-morbid anxiety or depression vs. treatment for substance use alone: a systematic review of the published literature. *BMC Psychiatry*, **9**, 6.

Hetrick, S. E., Purcell, R., Garner, B. & Parslow, R. (2010). Combined pharmacotherapy and psychological therapies for post traumatic stress disorder (PTSD). *Cochrane Database of Systematic Reviews*, **7**, CD007316.

Higgins, S. T., Wong, C. J., Badger, G. J., Haug-Ogden, D. E. & Dantona, R. L. (2000). Contingent reinforcement increases cocaine abstinence during outpatient treatment and one year follow-up. *Journal of Consulting and Clinical Psychology*, **68**, 64-72.

Hill, K. P. & Sofuoglu, M. (2007). Biological treatments for amfetamine dependence: recent progress. *CNS Drugs*, **21**, 851-69.

Hirsch, S. & Leff, J. (1971). Parental abnormalities of verbal communication in the transmission of schizophrenia. *Psychological Medicine*, **1**(2), 118-27.

Hoffman, K. T., Marvin, R. S., Cooper, G. & Powell, B. (2006). Changing toddlers' and preschoolers' attachment classifications: The Circle of Security intervention. *Journal of Consulting and Clinical Psychology*, **74**, 1017-26.

Hofmann, S. G. (2004). Cognitive mediation of treatment change in social phobia. *Journal of Consulting and Clinical Psychology*, **72**, 393-9.

Hofmann, S. G., Meuret, A. E., Smits, J. A. et al. (2006). Augmentation of exposure therapy with D-cycloserine for social anxiety disorder. *Archives of General Psychiatry*, **63**, 298-304.

Hogarty, G. E., Ulrich, R. F., Mussare, F. & Aristigueta, N. (1976). Drug discontinuation among long term, successfully maintained schizophrenic outpatients. *Diseases of the Nervous System*, **37**, 494-500.

Hogervorst, E., Williams, J., Budge, M., Riedel, W. & Jolles, J. (2000). The nature of the effect of female gonadal hormone replacement therapy on cognitive function in post-menopausal women: a meta-analysis. *Neuroscience*, **101**, 485-512.

Hohagen, F., Winkelmann, G., Rasche-Ruchle, H. et al. (1998). Combination of behaviour therapy with fluvoxamine in comparison with behaviour therapy and placebo: results of a multicentre study. *British Journal of Psychiatry*, Suppl **35**, 71-8.

Hohman, C., Hamon, R., Batshaw, M. L. et al. (1988). Transient postnatal elevation of serotonin levels in mouse neocortex. *Brain Research*, **47**, 163-6.

Holder, H., Longabaugh, R., Miller, W. R. & Rubonis, A. V. (1991) The cost-effectiveness of treatment for alcoholism: a first approximation. *Journal of Studies on Alcohol*, **52**, 517–40.

Holder, H. D., Cisler, R. A., Longabaugh, R., Stout, R. L., Treno, A. J. & Zweben, A. (2000). Alcoholism treatment and medical care costs from Project MATCH. *Addiction*, **95**, 999–1013.

Hollander, E., Baldini Rossi, N., Sood, E. & Pallanti, S. (2003). Risperidone augmentation in treatment-resistant obsessive-compulsive disorder: a double-blind, placebo-controlled study. *International Journal of Neuropsychopharmacology*, **6**, 397–401.

Hollander, E., Phillips, A., Chaplin, W. et al. (2005). A placebo controlled crossover trial of liquid fluoxetine on repetitive behaviors in childhood and adolescent autism. *Neuropsychopharmacology*, **30**, 582–9.

Hollon, S. D., DeRubeis, R., Shelton, C. et al. (2005). Prevention of relapse following cognitive therapy vs. medications in moderate to severe depression. *Archives of General Psychiatry*, **62**(4), 417–22.

Honer, W. G., Thornton, A. E., Chen, E. Y. et al. (2006). Clozapine alone versus clozapine and risperid one with refractory schizophrenia. *New England Journal of Medicine*, **354**, 472–82.

Hoopes, S. P., Reimherr, F. W., Hedges, D. W. et al. (2003). Treatment of bulimia nervosa with topiramate in a randomized, double-blind, placebo-controlled trial, part 1: improvement in binge and purge measures. *Journal of Clinical Psychiatry*, **64**(11), 1335–41.

Hope, D. A., Heimberg, R. G. & Bruch, M. A. (1995). Dismantling

cognitive-behavioral group therapy for social phobia. *Behaviour Research and Therapy*, **33**, 637–50.

Horikawa, N., Yamazaki, T., Miyamoto, K. et al. (2003). Treatment for delirium with risperidone: results of a prospective open trial with 10 patients. *General Hospital Psychiatry*, **25**, 289–92.

Horowitz, J., Wolitzky, K. & Powers, M. (2005). *Psychosocial Treatments for Specific Phobias: A Meta-analysis*. Washington, DC.

Howard, R. J., Juszczak, Ballard, C. G., et al. (2007). Donezepil for the treatment of agitation in Alzheimer's disease. *New England Journal of Medicine*, **357**, 1382–92.

Howard, R. J., Juszczak, E., Ballard, C. G. et al. (2008). Donepezil for the treatment of agitation in Alzheimer's disease. *New England Journal of Medicine*, **357**, 1382–92.

Howlin, P. & Rutter, M. (1987). *Treatment of Autistic Children*. Chichester: Wiley.

Howlin, P. (2010). Evaluating psychological treatments for children with autism-spectrum disorders. *Advances in Psychiatric Treatment*, **16**, 133–40.

Howlin, P., Gordon, K., Pasco, G. & Charman, T. (2007). A group randomised, controlled trial of the Picture Exchange Communication System for children with autism. *Journal of Child Psychology and Psychiatry*, **48**, 473–8.

Howlin, P., Magiati, I. & Charman, T (2009). Systematic review of early intensive behavioural interventions for children with autism. *American Journal of Mental Retardation*, **114**, 23–41.

Hughes, J. R. (1991). Long-term use o nicotine-replacement therapy. In

S. M. Henningfield, ed. *New Developments in Nicotine-Delivery Systems.* New York: Carlton, pp. 64–71.

Hughes, J. R. (1994). An algorithm for smoking cessation. *Archives of Family Medicine,* **3**, 280–5.

Humphreys, K. (2003). Alcoholics Anonymous and 12-Step alcoholism treatment programs. In: M. Galanter, ed. *Recent Developments in Alcoholism, Vol 16: Research on Alcoholism Treatment.* New York: Kluwer Academic/Plenum, pp. 149–64.

Humphreys, K. & Moos, R. H. (2001). Can encouraging substance abuse patients to participate in self-help groups reduce demand for health care? A quasi-experimental study. *Alcoholism: Clinical and Experimental Research,* **25**, 711–16.

Humphreys, K., Mankowski, E. S., Moos, R. H. & Finney, J. W. (1999). Do enhanced friendship networks and active coping mediate the effect of self-help groups on substance abuse? *Annals of Behavioral Medicine,* **21**, 54–60.

Humphreys, K., Wing, S., McCarty, D. et al. (2004). Self-help organizations for alcohol and drug problems: toward evidence-based practice and policy. *Journal of Substance Abuse Treatment,* **26**, 151–8.

Huppert, J. D. & Franklin, M. E. (2006). Cognitive behavioral therapy for obsessive-compulsive disorder: an update. *Current Psychiatry Reports,* **7**, 268–73.

Hurt, R. D., Sachs, D. P. L., Glover, E. D. et al. (1997). A comparison of sustained-release bupropion and placebo for smoking cessation. *New England Journal of Medicine,* **337**, 1195–202.

Hymel, S., Wagner, E. & Butler, L. J. (1990). Reputational bias: view from the peer group. In: S. R. Asher & J. D. Coie, eds. *Peer Rejection in Childhood.* Cambridge: Cambridge University Press, pp. 156–88.

Illich, I. (1975). *Medical Nemesis. The Expropriation of Health.* London: Marion Boyars.

Ingenhoven, T., Lafay, P., Rinne, T., Passchier, J. & Duivenvoorden, H. (2010). Effectiveness of pharmacotherapy for severe personality disorders: meta-analyses of randomized controlled trials. *Journal of Clinical Psychiatry,* **71**, 14–25.

Insel, T. (1995). The development of brain and behavior. In: F. Bloom & D. Kupfer, eds. *Psychopharmacology: The Fourth Generation of Progress.* New York: Raven Press.

Institute of Medicine (1990). *Broadening the Base of Treatment for Alcohol Problems.* Washington, D.C.: National Academy Press (retrieved from http://www.nap.edu).

International Psychogeriatric Association (1998). *Behavioural and Psychological Symptoms of Dementia.* Chicago: International Psychogeriatric Association.

International Psychogeriatric Association (2002). Behavioural and Psychological Symptoms of Dementia (pp. 1–20). http://www.ipa-online.org/ipaonlinev3/ipaprograms/bpsdarchives/bpsdrev/6BPSDfinal.pdf: International Psychogeriatric Association.

Ipser, J. C., Kariuki, C. M. & Stein, D. J. (2008). Pharmacotherapy for social anxiety disorder: a systematic review. *Expert Reviews in Neurotherapeutics,* **8**, 235–57.

Irvin, J. E., Bowers, C. A., Dunn, M. E. & Wang, M. C. (1999). Efficacy of relapse prevention: a meta-analytic review. *Journal of Consulting and Clinical Psychology*, **67**, 563–70.

Izzo, A. A. (2004). Drug interactions with St. John's Wort (*Hypericum perforatum*): a review of the clinical evidence. *International Journal of Clinical Pharmacology Therapy*, **42**, 139–48.

Jackson, H. J., McGorry, P. D., Killackey, E. et al. (2008). Acute-phase and 1-year follow-up results of a randomized controlled trial of CBT versus befriending for first-episode psychosis: the ACE project. *Psychological Medicine*, **38**, 725–35.

Jacobi, C., Hayward, C., DeZwann, M., Karemer, H. C. & Agras, W. S. (2004). Coming to terms with risk factors for eating disorders: application of risk terminology and suggestions for a general taxonomy. *Psychological Bulletin*, **130** (1), 19–65.

Jacobs, B., Green, J., Kroll, L., Tobias, C., Dunn, G. & Briskman, J. (2009). The effect of inpatient care on measured Health Needs in children and adolescents. *Journal of Child Psychology and Psychiatry*, **50**, 1273–81.

Jacobson, N. D., Dobson, K. S., Truax, P. A. et al. (1996). A component analysis of cognitive-behavioral treatment for depression. *Journal of Consulting and Clinical Psychology*, **64**, 295–304.

Jacobson, N. S., Martell, C. R. & Dimidjian, S. et al. (2001). Behavioral activation treatment for depression: returning to contextual roots. *Clinical Psychology: Science and Practice*, **8**(3), 255–68.

Jacobson, S. W. & Frye, K. F. (1991). Effects of maternal social support on attachment: experimental evidence. *Child Development*, **62**, 572–82.

Jäger, B., Liedke, R., Künsebeck, H.-W., Lempa, W., Kersting, A. & Seide, L. (1996). Psychotherapy and bulimia nervosa: evaluation and long-term follow-up of two conflict-orientated treatment conditions. *Acta Psychiatrica Scandinavica*, **93**, 268–78.

Janowsky, D. S., Kraus, J. E., Barnhill, L. J. et al. (2003). Effects of topiramate on aggressive, self-injurious, and disruptive/destructive behaviors in the intellectually disabled: an open-label retrospective study. *Journal of Clinical Psychopharmacology*, **23**, 500–4.

Janowsky, D. S., Shetty, M., Barnhill, L. J. et al. (2005). Serotonergic antidepressant effects on aggressive, self-injurious and destructive/disruptive behaviours in intellectually disabled adults: a retrospective, open-label, naturalistic trial. *International Journal of Neuropsychopharmacology*, **8**, 37–48.

Jarrett, R. B., Schaffer, M., McIntire, D. et al. (1999). Treatment of atypical depression with cognitive therapy or phemelzein: a double-blind placebo-controlled trial. *Archives of General Psychiatry*, **56**, 431–7.

Jenike, M. A. (1998). Neurosurgical treatment of obsessive-compulsive disorder *British Journal of Psychiatry,* **35** (Suppl) 79–90.

Jeste, D. V., Caligiuri, M. P., Paulsen, J. S et al. (1995). Risk of tardive dyskinesia in older patients: a prospective longitudinal study of 266 outpatients. *Archive of General Psychiatry*, **52**, 756–65.

John, U., Veltrup, C., Driessen, M., Wetterling, T. & Dilling, H. (2003). Motivational intervention: an individual counselling vs. a group treatment approach for alcohol-dependent inpatients. *Alcohol & Alcoholism*, **38**, 263–9.

Johnson, R. E., Eissenberg, T., Stitzer, M. L., Strain, E. C., Liebson, I. A. & Bigelow, G. E. (1995). A placebo controlled clinical trial of buprenorphine as a treatment for opioid dependence. *Drug and Alcohol Dependence*, **40**, 17–25.

Johnson, R. E., Chutuape, M. A., Strain, E. C., Walsh, S. L., Stitzer, M. L. & Bigelow, G. E. (2000). A comparison of levomethadyl acetate, buprenorphine, and methadone for opioid dependence. *New England Journal of Medicine*, **343**, 1290–7.

Johnson, R. E., Strain, E. C. & Amass, L. (2003). Buprenorphine: how to use it right. *Drug and Alcohol Dependence*, **70** (2 Suppl), S59–77.

Johnston, L. D., O'Malley, P. M. & Bachman, J. G. (2002). *Monitoring the Future National Survey Results on Adolescent Drug Use: Overview of Key Findings* (NIH Publication No. 03-5374). Bethesda, MD: National Institute on Drug Abuse. 56.

Jones, C., Cormac, I., Silveira da Mota Neto, J. I. & Campbell, C. (2004). Cognitive behaviour therapy for schizophrenia. *The Cochrane Database of Systematic Reviews*, **4**, CD000524. pub2. doi: 10.1002/14651858.CD000524.pub2. Oxford: Update Software Ltd.

Jones, P. B., Barnes, T. R., Davies, L. et al. (2006). Randomized controlled trial of the effect on Quality of Life of second- vs. first-generation antipsychotic drugs in schizophrenia: Cost Utility of the Latest Antipsychotic Drugs in Schizophrenia Study (CUtLASS 1). *Archives of General Psychiatry*, **63**, 1079–87.

Jorenby, D. E., Leischow, S. J., Nides, M. A. et al. (1999). A controlled trial of sustained-release bupropion, a nicotine patch, or both for smoking cessation. *New England Journal of Medicine*, **340**, 685–91.

Jorenby, D. E., Hays, J. T., Rigotti, N. A. et al. (2006). Efficacy of varenicline, an α4β2 nicotinic acetylcholine receptor partial agonist, vs. placebo or sustained-release bupropion for smoking cessation: a randomized controlled trial. *Journal of the American Medical Association*, **296**, 56–63.

Josiassen, R. C., Joseph, A., Kohegyi, E. et al. (2005). Clozapine augmented with risperidone in the treatment of schizophrenia: a randomized, double-blind, placebo-controlled trial. *American Journal of Psychiatry*, **162**, 130–6.

Joyce, P. R., Mulder, R. T. et al. (2003). A differential response to nortriptyline and fluoxetine and melancholic depression: the importance of age and gender. *Acta Psychiatrica Scandinavica*, **108**, 20–3.

Joyce, P. R., McKenzie, J. M., Carter, J. D. et al. (2007). Temperament, character and personality disorders as predictors of response to interpersonal psychotherapy and cognitive behaviour therapy for depression. *British Journal of Psychiatry*, **190**, 503–8.

Juffer, F., Hoksbergen, A. C., Riksen-Walraven, J. M. & Kohnstamm, G. A. (1997). Early intervention in adoptive families: supporting maternal sensitive responsiveness, infant–mother attachment, and infant competence. *Journal of Child Psychology and Psychiatry*, **38**, 1039–50.

Juffer, F., Bakermans-Kranenburg, M. J. & van Ijzendoorn, M. H. (2005). The importance of parenting in the development of disorganized attachment: evidence from a preventative intervention study in adoptive families. *Journal of Child Psychology and Psychiatry*, **46**, 263–74.

Jureidini, J. N., Doecke, C. J., Mansfield, P. R. et al. (2004). Efficacy and safety of antidepressants for children and adolescents. *British Medical Journal*, **328**, 879–83.

Kabat-Zinn, J. (1990). *Full Catastrophe Living: Using the Wisdom of Your Body and Mind to Face Stress, Pain, and Illness*. New York: Delacorte.

Kächele, H., Kordy, H., Richard, M. & Research Group TR-EAT (2001). Therapy amount and outcome of inpatient psychodynamic treatment of eating disorders in Germany: Data from a multicenter study. *Psychotherapy Research*, **11**, 239–57.

Kadden, R. M. & Conney, N. L. (2005). Treating alcohol problems. In: G. A. Marlatt & D. M. Donovan, eds. *Relapse Prevention: Maintenance Strategies in the Treatment of Addictive Behaviors*. New York: Guilford Press, pp. 65–91.

Kadden, R., Carroll, K., Donovan, D. *et al.* (1994). *Cognitive-Behavioral Coping Skills Therapy Manual: A Clinical Research Guide for Therapists Treating Individuals with Alcohol Abuse and Dependence* (Project Match Monograph Series Vol. 3; NIH Publication No. 94-3724). Rockville, MD: National Institute on Alcohol and Alcoholism.

Kadden, R. M., Litt, M. D., Kabela-Cormier, E. & Petry, N. M. (2007). Abstinence rates following behavioral treatments for marijuana dependence. *Addictive Behaviors*, **32**, 1220–36.

Kafantaris, V., Coletti, D., Dicker, R., Padula, G. & Kane, J. M. (2003). Lithium treatment of acute mania in adolescents: a large open trial. *Journal of the American Academy of Child and Adolescent Psychiatry*, **42**, 1038–45.

Kafantaris, V., Coletti, D., Dicker, R. et al. (2004). Lithium treatment of acute mania in adolescents: a placebo-controlled discontinuation study. *Journal of the American Academy of Child and Adolescent Psychiatry*, **43**, 984–93.

Kahn, C. & Pike, K. (2001). In search of predictors of dropout from inpatient treatment for anorexia nervosa. *International Journal of Eating Disorders*, **30**, 237–44.

Kahn, R. J., McNair, D. M., Lipman, R. S. et al. (1986). Imipramine and chordiazepoxide in depressive and anxiety disorders: II. Efficacy in anxious outpatients. *Archives of General Psychiatry*, **43**, 79–85.

Kakko, J., Svanborg, K. D., Kreek, M. J. & Heilig, M. (2003). 1-year retention and social function after buprenorphine-assisted relapse prevention treatment for heroin dependence in Sweden: a randomised, placebo-controlled trial. *Lancet*, **361**, 662–8.

Kaminer, Y., Burleson, J. A. & Goldberger, R. (2002). Cognitive-behavioral coping skills and psychoeducation therapies for adolescent substance abuse. *Journal of Nervous & Mental Disease*, **190**, 737–45.

Kampman, K. M., Alterman, A. I. & Volpicelli, J. R. (2001a). Cocaine withdrawal symptoms and initial urine toxicology results predict treatment attrition in outpatient cocaine dependence treatment. *Psychology of Addictive Behavior*, **15**, 52–9.

Kampman, K. M., Volpicelli, J. R. & Mulvaney, F. (2001b). Effectiveness of propranolol for cocaine dependence treatment may depend on cocaine withdrawal symptom severity. *Drug and Alcohol Dependence*, **63**, 69–78.

Kampman, M., Keijsers, G. P. J., Hoogduin, C. A. L. & Hendriks, G.-J. (2002). A randomized, double-blind, placebo-controlled study of the effects of adjunctive paroxetine in panic disorder patients unsuccessfully treated with cognitive-behavioral therapy alone. *Journal of Clinical Psychiatry*, **63**(9), 772–7.

Kane, J. M., Honigfeld, G., Singer, J., Meltzer, H. & Group tCCS (1988). Clozapine for the treatment-resistant schizophrenic: a double-blind comparison versus chlorpromazine/benztropine. *Archives of General Psychiatry*, **45**, 789–96.

Kaplan, H. S. (1974). *The New Sex Therapy: Active Treatment of Sexual Dysfunctions*. New York: Brunner Mazel.

Kasari, C., Freeman, S. & Paparella, T. (2006). Joint attention and symbolic play in young children with autism: a randomized controlled intervention study. *Journal of Child Psychology and Psychiatry*, **47**, 611–20.

Kasari, C., Paparella, T., Freeman, S. & Jahromi, L. B. (2008). Language outcome and autism: randomized comparison of joint attention and play interventions. *Journal of Consulting and Clinical Psychology*, **76**, 125–37.

Kasper, S., Gastpar, M., Müller, W. E. et al. (2008). Efficacy of St. John's wort extract WS 5570 in acute treatment of mild depression: a reanalysis of data from controlled clinical trials. *European Archives of Psychiatry and Clinical Neuroscience*, **258**, 59–63.

Katon, W. J., Roy-Byrne, P., Russo J. & Cowley, D. (2002). Cost-effectiveness and cost offset of a collaborative care intervention for primary care patients with panic disorder. *Archives of General Psychiatry*, **95**, 1098–104.

Katona, C. L., Abou-Saleh, M. T. et al. (1995). Placebo-controlled trial of lithium augmentation of fluoxetine and lofepramine. *British Journal of Psychiatry*, **166**(1), 80–6.

Katz, R. J., De Veaugh-Geiss, J. & Landau, P. (1990). Clomipramine in obsessive-compulsive disorder. *Biological Psychiatry*, **28**, 401–14.

Katz, R. J., Lott, M. H., Arbus, P. et al. (1995). Pharmacotherapy of post-traumatic stress disorder with a novel psychotropic. *Anxiety*, **1**, 169–74.

Kaye, W. H., Nagata, T., Weltzin, T. E. et al. (2001). Double-blind placebo-controlled administration of fluoxetine in restricting- and restricting-purging-type anorexia nervosa. *Biological Psychiatry*, **49**(7), 644–52.

Kazanjian, A. & Rothon, D. A. (2002). *Acupuncture in the Management of Alcohol and Drug Dependence*. Vancouver, BC: British Columbia Office of Health Technology Assessment, University of British Columbia.

Kazdin, A. E. (1996). Dropping out of child therapy: issues for research and implications for practice. *Clinical Child Psychology and Psychiatry*, **1**, 133–56.

Kazdin, A. E. (2000). *Psychotherapy for Children and Adolescents: Directions for Research and Practice*. Oxford: Oxford University Press.

Kazdin, A. E. & Wassel, G. (1999). Barriers to treatment participation and therapeutic change among children referred for conduct disorder. *Journal of Clinical Child Psychology*, **28**, 160–72.

Kazdin, A. E., Bass, D., Ayers, W. A. & Rodgers, A. (1990). Empirical and clinical focus of child and adolescent psychotherapy research. *Journal of Consulting and Clinical Psychology*, **58**, 729–40.

Kearns, G. L. & Reed, M. D. (1989). Clinical pharmacokinetics in infants and children: a reappraisal. *Clinical Pharmacokinetics*, **17**, 29–67.

Keel, P. K., Fichter, M., Quadflieg, N. et al. (2004). Application of a latent class analysis to empirically define eating disorder phenotypes. *Archives of General Psychiatry*, **61**, 192–200.

Keller, M. B., McCullough, J. P., Klein, D. N. et al. (2000). A comparison of nefazodone, the cognitive behavioral-analysis system of psychotherapy, and their combination for the treatment of chronic depression. *New England Journal of Medicine*, **342**, 1462–70.

Kellner, C. H., Knapp, R., Husain, M. M et al. (2010). Bifrontal, bitemporal and right unilateral electrode placement in ECT: randomized trial. *British Journal of Psychiatry*, **196**, 226–34.

Kelly, D. & Mitchell-Heggs, N. (1973). Stereotactic limbic leucotomy: a follow-up study of thirty patients. *Postgraduate Medical Journal*, **49**, 852–65.

Kenardy, J. A., Dow, M. G., Johnston, D. W., Newman, M. G., Thomson, A. & Taylor, C. B. (2003). A comparison of delivery methods of cognitive-behavioral therapy for panic disorder: an international multicenter trial. *Journal of Consulting and Clinical Psychology*, **71**(6), 1068–75.

Kenardy, J. R. S. & Dob, R. (2005). Cognitive behaviour therapy for panic disorder: long-term follow-up. *Cognitive Behaviour Therapy*, 2003, **34**(2), 75–8.

Kendall, P. C. (ed.) (2000). *Child & Adolescent Therapy: Cognitive-Behavioral Procedures*. New York: Guilford Press.

Kendall, P. C., Flannery-Schroeder, E., Panichelli-Mindel, S. M. et al. (1997). Therapy for youths with anxiety disorders: a second randomised clinical trial. *Journal of Consulting and Clinical Psychology*, **65**, 366–80.

Kennedy, E. (2004). *Child and Adolescent Psychotherapy: A Systematic Review of Psychoanalytic Approaches*. London: North Central London Strategic Health Authority.

Kennedy, E., Kumar, A. & Datta, S. S. (2007). Antipsychotic medication for childhood-onset schizophrenia. *Cochrane Database of Systematic Reviews*, **3**, CD004027. doi: 10.1002/14651858.CD004027.pub2.

Kenwright, M. & Marks, I. (2004) Computer-aided self-help for phobia/panic: feasibility study. *British Journal of Psychiatry*, **179**, 456–9.

Kerwin, M. E. (1999). Empirically supported treatments in pediatric psychology: severe feeding problems. *Journal of Pediatric Psychology*, **24**, 193–214.

Keso, L. & Salaspuro, M. (1990). Inpatient treatment of employed alcoholics: a randomized clinical trial of Hazelden-type and traditional treatment. *Alcoholism: Clinical and Experimental Research*, **14**, 584–9.

Kessler, R. C., Stang, P., Wittchen, H. U., Stein, M. & Walters, E. E. (1999). Lifetime co-morbidities between social phobia and mood disorders in the US National Comorbidity Survey. *Psychological Medicine*, **29**, 555–67.

Kessler, R. C., Berglund, P., Demler O. (2005a). Lifetime prevalence and age-of-onset distributions of DSM-IV disorders in the National Comorbidity Survey Replication. *Archives of General Psychiatry*, **62**, 593–602.

Kessler, R. C., Chiu, W. T., Demler, O., Merikangas, K. R. & Walters, E. E. (2005b). Prevalence, severity, and comorbidity of 12-month DSM-IV disorders in the National Comorbidity Survey Replication. *Archives of General Psychiatry*, **62**, 617–27.

Kessler, R. C., Chiu, W. T., Jin, R., Ruscio, A. M., Shear, K. & Walters, E. E. (2006). The epidemiology of panic attacks, panic disorder, and agoraphobia in the National Comorbidity Survey Replication. *Archives of General Psychiatry*, **63**, 415–24.

Kho, K. H., Vreeswijk, M. F., Simpson, S. & Zwinderman, A. H. (2003). A meta-analysis of electroconvulsive therapy efficacy in depression. *Journal of ECT*, **19**(3), 139–47.

Kiefer, F., Jahn, H., Tarnaske, T. et al. (2003). Comparing and combining naltrexone and acamprosate in relapse prevention of alcoholism: a double-blind, placebo-controlled study. *Archives of General Psychiatry*, **60**, 92–99.

Kim, K. Y., Bader, G. M., Kotlyar, V. et al. (2003). Treatment of delirium in older adults with quetiapine. *Journal of Geriatric Psychiatry and Neurology*, **16**, 29–31.

King, B. H., Hollander, E., Sikich, L. et al. (2009). Lack of efficacy of citalopram in children with autism spectrum disorders and high levels of repetitive behavior: citalopram ineffective in children with autism. *Archives of General Psychiatry*, **66**, 583–90.

King, M., Holt, V. & Nazareth, I. (2007). Women's views of their sexual difficulties: agreement and disagreement with clinical diagnoses. *Archives of Sexual Behavior*, **36**, 281–8.

King, N., Tonge, B., Heyne, D. et al. (1998). Cognitive behavioural treatment of school-refusing children: a controlled evaluation. *Journal of the American Academy of Child and Adolescent Psychiatry*, **37**, 395–403.

King, V. L., Stoller, K. B., Hayes, M. et al. (2002). A multicenter randomized evaluation of methadone medical maintenance. *Drug and Alcohol Dependence*, **65**, 137–48.

Kingdon, D. G. & Turkington, D. (1995). *Cognitive Behavioral Therapy of Schizophrenia*. Psychology Press.

Kingdon, D., Tyrer, P., Seivewright, N., Ferguson, B. & Murphy, S. (1996). The Nottingham Study of Neurotic Disorder: influence of cognitive therapists on outcome. *British Journal of Psychiatry*, **169**, 93–97.

Kinsey, A. C., Pomeroy, W. B. & Martin, C. E. (1948). *Sexual Behaviour in the Human Male*. Philadelphia: Saunders.

Kirchmayer, U., Davoli, M., Verster, A. D., Amato, L., Ferri, M. & Perucci, C. A. (2002). A systematic review on the efficacy of naltrexone maintenance treatment in opioid dependence. *Addiction*, **97**, 1241–9.

Klein Velderman, M., Bakermans-Krenenburg, M. J., Juffer, F. & van Ijzendoorn, M. H. (2006). Effects of attachment-based interventions on maternal sensitivity and infant attachment: differential susceptibility of highly reactive infants. *Journal of Family Psychology*, **20**, 266–74.

Klein, R. G., Abikoff, H., Klass, E., Ganeles, D., Seese, L. M. & Pollack, S. (1997). Clinical efficacy of methylphenidate in conduct disorder with and without attention deficit hyperactivity disorder. *Archives of General Psychiatry*, **54**, 1073–9.

Klerman, G. L., Weissman, M. M., Rousaville, B. J. & Chevron, E. S. (1984). *Interpersonal Psychotherapy of Depression*. New York: Basic Books.

Klink van der J. J., Blonk, R. W., Schene, A. H. & van Dijk, F. J. (2003). Reducing long term sickness absence by an activating intervention in adjustment disorders: a cluster randomised controlled design. *Occupational & Environmental Medicine*, **60**, 429–37.

Kobak, K. A., Greist, J. H., Jefferson, J. W., Katzelnick, D. J. & Henk, H. J. (1998). Behavioral versus pharmacological treatments of obsessive compulsive disorder: a meta-analysis. *Psychopharmacology (Berlin)*, **136**, 205–16.

Kockott, G. & Fahrner, E. M. (1987). Transsexuals who have not undergone surgery: a follow-up study. *Archives of Sexual Behavior*, **16**, 511–22.

Kocsis, J. H., Gelenberg, A. J., Rothbaum, B. O. et al. (2009). Cognitive Behavioral Analysis System of Psychotherapy and brief supportive psychotherapy for augmentation of antidepressant nonresponse in chronic depression. *Archives of General Psychiatry*, **66**, 1178–88.

Kodak, T. & Piazza, C. C. (2008). Assessment and behavioral treatment of feeding and sleeping disorders in children with autism spectrum disorders. *Child and Adolescent Psychiatric Clinics of North America*, **17** (4), 887–905.

Koenigsberg, H. W., Reynolds, D. & Goodman, L. (2003). Risperidone in the treatment of schizotypal personality disorder. *Journal of Clinical Psychiatry*, **64**, 628–34.

Kolb, L. C., Burris, B. C. & Griffiths, S. (1984). Propranolol and clonidine in the treatment of the chronic post-traumatic stress disorders of war. In: B. A. Van der Kolk, ed. *Post-traumatic Stress Disorder. Psychological and Biological Sequelae*. Washington, DC: American Psychiatric Press, pp. 98–105.

Kolevzon, A., Mathewson, K. A. & Hollander, E. (2006). Selective serotonin reuptake inhibitors in autism: a review of efficacy and tolerability. *Journal of Clinical Psychiatry*, **67**, 407–14.

Kollins, S. H. (2008). A qualitative review of issues arising in the use of psycho stimulant medications in patients with ADHD and comorbid substance use disorders. *Current Medical Research and Opinion*, **24**, 1345–57.

Koran, L. M., Hanna, G. L., Hollander, E., Nestadt, G., Simpson, H. B., on behalf of the American Psychiatric Association (2007). Practice guideline for the treatment of patients with obsessive-compulsive disorder. *American Journal of Psychiatry*, **164** (7 Suppl), 5–53.

Kornstein, S. G., Schatzberg, A. F. et al. (2000). Gender differences in treatment response to sertraline versus imipramine in chronic depression. *American Journal of Psychiatry*, **157**(9), 1445–52.

Kosten, T. R. & O'Connor, P. G. (2003). Management of drug and alcohol withdrawal. *New England Journal of Medicine*, **348**, 1786–95.

Kosten, T. R. (2002). Pathophysiology and treatment of cocaine dependence. In C. Nemeroff, ed. *Neuropsychopharmacology: The Fifth Generation of Progress*. Baltimore, MD: Lippincott Williams & Wilkins, pp. 1461–73.

Kosten, T. R. (2003). Buprenorphine for opioid detoxification: a brief review. *Addictive Disorders and Their Treatment*, **2**, 107–12.

Kosten, T. R., Frank, J. B., Dan, E., McDougle, C. J. & Giller, E. L. (1991). Pharmacotherapy for posttraumatic stress disorder using phenelzine or imipramine. *Journal of Nervous and Mental Disease*, **179**, 366–70.

Kosten, T., Oliveto, A., Feingold, A. et al. (2003). Desipramine and contingency management for cocaine and opiate dependence in buprenorphine maintained patients. *Drug & Alcohol Dependence*, **70**, 315–25.

Kotler, L. A., Cohen, P., Davies, M., Pine, D. S. & Walsh, B. T. (2001). Longitudinal relationships between childhood, adolescent, and adult eating disorders. *Journal of the American Academy of Child & Adolescent Psychiatry*, **40**, 1434–40.

Kotler, L. A., Devlin, M. J., Davies, M. & Walsh, B. T. (2003). An open trial of fluoxetine for adolescents with bulimia nervosa. *Journal of Child and Adolescent Psychopharmacology*, **13**, 329–35.

Kovacs, M., Rush, A. J., Beck, A. T. & Hollon, S. T. (1981). Depressed outpatients treated with cognitive therapy or pharmacotherapy. *Archives of General Psychiatry*, **38**, 33–9.

Kowatch, R. A., Fristad, M., Birmaher, B. et al. and the Child Psychiatric Workgroup on Bipolar Disorder (2005). Treatment guidelines for children and adolescents with bipolar disorder. *Journal of the American Academy of Child and Adolescent Psychiatry*, **44**, 213–35.

Kranzler, H. R. & Van Kirk, J. (2001). Efficacy of naltrexone and acamprosate for alcoholism treatment: a meta-analysis. *Alcoholism: Clinical and Experimental Research*, **25**, 1335–41.

Kranzler, H. R., Armeli, S., Tennen, H. et al. (2003). Targeted naltrexone for early problem drinkers. *Journal of Clinical Psychopharmacology*, **23**, 294–304.

Krauth, C. (2002). How high are the costs of eating disorders – anorexia nervosa and bulimia nervosa – for German Society? *European Journal of Health Economics*, **3**, 244–50.

Krijn, M., Emmelkamp, P. M., Biemond, R., de Wilde, L. C., Schuemie, M. J. & van der Mast, C. A. (2004). Treatment of acrophobia in virtual reality: the role of immersion and presence. *Behaviour Research and Therapy*, **42**(2), 229–39.

Kripke, D. F., Mullaney, D. J., Klauber, M. R., Risch, S. C. & Gillin, J. C. (1992). Controlled trial of bright light for nonseasonal major depressive disorders. *Biological Psychiatry* **31**(2), 119–34.

Kristeller, J. L. & Hallett, C. B. (1999). An exploratory study of a meditation-based intervention for binge eating disorder. *Journal of Health Psychology* **4**(3), 357–63.

Kroenke, K. & Swindle, J. (2000). Cognitive-behavioral therapy for somatization and symptom syndromes: a critical review of controlled clinical trials. *Psychotherapy and Psychosomatics*, **69**, 205–15.

Kuiper, B. & Cohen-Kettenis, P. (1988). Sex reassignment surgery: a study of 141 Dutch transsexuals. *Archives of Sexual Behavior*, **17**, 439–57.

Kumar, V., Anand, R., Messina, J., Hartman, R. & Veach, J. (2000). An efficacy and safety analysis of Exelon in Alzheimer's disease patients with concurrent vascular risk factors. *European Journal of Neurology*, **7**, 159–69.

Kumra, S., Frazier, J. A., Jacobsen, L. K. et al. (1996). Childhood-onset schizophrenia: a double-blind clozapine-haloperidol comparison. *Archives of General Psychiatry*, **53**, 1090–7.

Kumra, S., Kranzler, H., Gerbino-Rosen, G. et al. (2007). Clozapine and "high-dose" olanzapine in refractory early-onset schizophrenia: a 12-week randomized and double-blind comparison. *Biological Psychiatry*, **63**, 524–9.

Kurlan, R., Cummings, J., Raman, R. & Thal, L. (2007). Quetiapine for agitation or psychosis in patients with dementia and parkinsonism: Alzheimer's Disease Cooperative Study Group. *Neurology*, **68**, 1356–63.

Kusel, A. B. (1999). Primary prevention of eating disorders through media literacy training of girls. *Dissertation Abstracts International B: The Sciences & Engineering*, **60**(4-B), 1859.

Kypri, K., Langley, J. D., Saunders, J. B., Cashell-Smith, M. L. & Herbison, P. (2008). Randomized controlled trial of web-based alcohol screening and brief intervention in primary care. *Archives of Internal Medicine*, **168**, 530–6.

Kypri, K., Sitharthan, T., Cunningham, J. A., Kavanagh, D. J. & Dean, J. I. (2005). Innovative approaches to intervention for problem drinking. *Current Opinion in Psychiatry*, **18**, 229–34.

Lacroix, I., Berrebi, A., Chaumerliac, C., Lapeyre-Mestre, M., Montastruc, J. L. & Damase-Michel, C. (2004). Buprenorphine in pregnant opioid-dependent women: first results of a prospective study. *Addiction*, **99**, 209–14.

Laederach-Hofmann, K., Graf, C., Horber, F et al. (1999). Imipramine and diet counseling with psychological support in the treatment of obese binge eaters: a randomized, placebo-controlled double-blind study. *International Journal of Eating Disorders*, **26**(3), 231–44.

Lam, R. W., Goldner, E. M. & Grewal, A. K (1996). Seasonality of symptoms in anorexia and bulimia nervosa. *International Journal of Eating Disorders*, **19**, 35–44.

Lam, R. W., Lee, S. K., Tam, E. M., Grewal, A. & Yatham, L. N. (2001). An open trial of light therapy for women with seasonal affective disorder and comorbid bulimia nervosa. *Journal of Clinical Psychiatry*, **62**(3), 164–8.

Lambourn, J. & Gill, D. (1978). A controlled comparison of simulated and real ECT. *British Journal of Psychiatry*, **133**, 514–19.

Lancaster, T. & Stead, L. F. (1999). Self help interventions for smoking cessation. *Cochrane Database Systematic Review*. Oxford: Update Software Ltd.

Lanctôt, K. L., Best, T. S., Mittmann, N. et al. (1998). Efficacy and safety of neuroleptics in behavioural disorders associated with dementia. *Journal of Clinical Psychiatry*, **59**, 550–61; quiz 562–3.

Landen, M., Walinder, J. & Lundstrom, B. (1996). Prevalence, incidence and sex ratio of transsexualism. *Acta Psychiatrica Scandinavica*, **93**, 221–3.

Landen, M., Walinder, J., Hambert, G. & Lundstrom, B. (1998). Factors predictive of regret in sex reassignment. *Acta Psychiatrica Scandinavica*, **97**, 284–9.

Larimer, M. E. & Cronce, J. M. (2002). Identification, prevention and treatment: a review of individual-focused strategies to reduce problematic alcohol consumption by college students. *Journal of Studies on Alcohol*, **Suppl. 14**, 148–63.

Lask, B. & Bryant-Waugh, R. (2007). *Anorexia Nervosa and Related Eating Disorders in Childhood and Adolescence*, 3nd edn. Hove, East Sussex: Psychology Press, Taylor and Francis Group.

Lasser, K., Boyd, J. W., Woolhandler, S. et al. (2000). Smoking and mental illness: a population-based prevalence study. *Journal of the American Medical Association*, **284**, 2606–10.

Laumann, E. O., Paik, A. & Rosen, R. C. (1999). Sexual dysfunction in the United States: prevalence and predictors. *Journal of the American Medical Association*, **281**, 537–44.

Laundreville, P., Bordes, M., Dicaire L. & Verrault, R. (1998). Behavioral approaches for reducing agitation in residents of long-term-care facilities: critical review and suggestions for future research. *International Psychogeriatrics*, **10**, 397–419.

Law, M. & Tang, J. L. (1995). An analysis of the effectiveness of interventions intended to help people stop smoking. *Archives of Internal Medicine*, **155**, 1933–41.

Le Grange, D., Crosby, R., Rathouz, P. & Leventhal, B. (2007). A randomized controlled comparison of family-based treatment and supportive psychotherapy for adolescent bulimia nervosa. *Archives of General Psychiatry*, **64**, 1049–56.

LeBlanc, L. A., Piazza, C. C. & Krug, M. A. (1997). Comparing methods for maintaining the safety of a child with pica. *Research in Developmental Disabilities*, **18**, 215–20.

Leggio, L., Kenna, G. A. & Swift, R. M. (2008). New developments for the pharmacological treatment of alcohol withdrawal syndrome: a focus on non-benzodiazepine GABAergic medications. *Progress in Neuropsychopharmacology and Biological Psychiatry*, **32**, 1106–17.

Lehman, A. F., Lieberman, J. A. & Dixon, L. B. (2004). Practice guideline for the treatment of patients with schizophrenia, second edition. *American Journal of Psychiatry*, **161** (Suppl. 2), 1–56.

Leichsenring, F. & Leibing, E. (2003). The effectiveness of psychodynamic therapy and cognitive behavior therapy in the treatment of personality disorders: a meta-analysis. *American Journal of Psychiatry*, **160**, 1223–32.

Lejoyeux, M., Solomon, J. & Ades, J. (1998). Benzodiazepine treatment for alcohol-dependent patients. *Alcohol and Alcoholism*, **33**, 563–75.

Letemendia, J. F., Delva, N. J., Rodenberg, M. et al. (1993). Therapeutic advantage of bifrontal electrode placement in ECT. *Psychological Medicine*, **23**, 349–60.

Leucht, S., Pitschel-Walz, G., Abraham, D. & Kissling, W. (1999). Efficacy and extrapyramidal side-effects of the new antipsychotics olanzapine, quetiapine, risperidone, and sertindole compared to conventional antipsychotics and placebo: a meta-analysis of randomized controlled trials. *Schizophrenia Research*, **35**, 51–68.

Leucht, S., Barnes, T. R., Kissling, W., Engel, R. R., Correll, C. & Kane, J. M. (2003). Relapse prevention in schizophrenia with new-generation antipsychotics: a systematic review and exploratory meta-analysis of randomized, controlled trials. *American Journal of Psychiatry*, **160**, 1209–22.

Leucht, S., Corves, C., Arbter, D., Engel, R. R., Li, C. & Davis, J. M. (2009). Second-generation versus first-generation antipsychotic drugs for schizophrenia: a meta-analysis. *Lancet*, **373**, 31–41.

Levine, M. D., Marcus, M. D. & Moulton, P. (1996). Exercise in the treatment of binge-eating disorder. *International Journal of Eating Disorders*, **19**, 171–7.

Levine, S. B. & Shumaker, R. E. (1983). Increasingly Ruth: toward understanding sex reassignment. *Archives of Sexual Behavior*, **12**, 247–61.

Lewinsohn, P. M. & Clarke, G. N. (1999). Psychosocial treatments for adolescent depression. *Clinical Psychology Review*, **19**, 329–42.

Lewinsohn, P. M., Hops, H., Roberts, R. E., Seeley, J. R. & Andrew, J. A. (1993). Adolescent psychopathology, I: prevalence and incidence of depression and other DSM-III-R disorders in high school students. *Journal of Abnormal Psychology*, **103**, 133–44.

Lewis, S. W., Barnes, T. R., Davies, L. et al. (2006). Randomized controlled trial of effect of prescription of clozapine versus other second-generation antipsychotic drugs in resistant schizophrenia. *Schizophrenia Bulletin*, **32**, 715–23.

Licht, R. W & Quitzau, S. (2002). Treatment strategies in patients with major depression not responding to first-line sertraline treatment. *Psychopharmacology*, **161**, 143–51.

Liddle, H. A. (2004). Family-based therapies for adolescent alcohol and drug use: research contributions and future research needs. *Addiction*, **99** (Suppl. 2), 76–92.

Lidz, T., Flack, S. & Cornelison, A. (1965) *Schizophrenia and the Family*. New York: International Press.

Lieberman, A., Weston, D. & Pawl, J. (1991). Preventive intervention and outcome with anxiously attached dyads. *Child Development*, **62**, 199–209.

Lieberman, J.A., Stroup, T.S. & McEvoy, J.P. (2005). Effectiveness of antipsychotic drugs in patients with chronic schizophrenia. *New England Journal of Medicine*, **353**, 1209–23.

Liebowitz, M.R., Heimberg, R.G., Schneier, F.R. et al. (1999). Cognitive-behavioral group therapy versus phenelzine in social phobia: long-term outcome. *Depression and Anxiety*, **10**, 89–98.

Liebowitz, M.R., Schneier, F., Campeas, R. et al. (1992). Phenelzine vs. atenolol in social phobia: a placebo-controlled comparison. *Archives of General Psychiatry*, **49**, 290–300.

Liebowitz, M.R., Gelenberg, A.J. & Munjack, D. (2005). Venlafaxine extended release vs. placebo and paroxetine in social anxiety disorder. *Archives of General Psychiatry*, **62**, 190–8.

Liebrenz, M., Boesch, L., Stohler, R. et al. (2010). Benzodiazepine dependence: when abstinence is not an option. *Addiction*, **105**, 1877–8.

Lief, H.I. & Hubschman, L. (1993). Orgasm in the postoperative transsexual. *Archives of Sexual Behavior*, **22**, 145–55.

Linde, K., Ramirez, G., Mulrow, C.D., Pauls, A., Weidenhammer, W. & Melchart, D. (1996). St John's wort for depression: an overview and meta-analysis of randomised clinical trials. *British Medical Journal*, **313**(7052), 253–8.

Linde, K., Berner, M., Egger, M. & Mulrow, C. (2005). St John's wort for depression: meta-analysis of randomised controlled trials. *British Journal of Psychiatry*, **186**, 99–107.

Lindemalm, G., Korlin, D. & Uddenberg, N. (1986). Long-term follow-up of "sex change" in 13 male-to-female transsexuals. *Archives of Sexual Behavior*, **15**, 187–210.

Lindemalm, G., Korlin, D. & Uddenberg, N. (1987). Prognostic factors vs. outcome in male-to-female transsexualism: a follow-up study of 13 cases. *Acta Psychiatrica Scandinavica*, **75**, 268–74.

Linehan, M.M., Armstrong, H., Suarez, A, Allmon, D. & Heard, H.L. (1991). Cognitive-behavioural treatment of chronically parasuicidal borderline patients. *Archives of General Psychiatry*, **48**, 1060–64.

Linehan, M.M., Schmidt, H. 3rd., Dimeff, L.A., Craft, J.C., Kanter, J. & Comtois, K.A. (1999). Dialectical behavior therapy for patients with borderline personality disorder and drug-dependence. *American Journal on Addictions*, **8**, 279–92.

Linehan, M.M., Comtois, K.A., Murray, A.M. et al. (2006). Two-year randomized controlled trial and follow-up of dialectical behavior therapy vs. therapy by experts for suicidal behaviors and borderline personality disorder. *Archives of General Psychiatry*, **63**, 757–66.

Ling, W., Wesson, D.R., Charuvastra, C. & Klett, C.J. (1996). A controlled trial comparing buprenorphine and methadone maintenance in opioid dependence. *Archives of General Psychiatry*, **53**, 401–7.

Lingford-Hughes, A.R., Welch, S. & Nutt, D.J. (2004). Evidence-based guidelines for the pharmacological management of substance misuse, addiction and comorbidity: recommendations from the British Association for

Psychopharmacology. *Journal of Psychopharmacology*, **18**, 293–335.

Linscheid, T. R. & Murphy, L. B. (1999). Feeding disorders of infancy and early childhood. In: S. D. Nether, ed. *Child and Adolescent Psychological Disorders: A Comprehensive Textbook*. New York: Oxford University Press, pp. 139–55.

Lochman, J. E. & Wells, K. C. (1996). A social-cognitive intervention with aggressive children: prevention effects and contextual implementation issues. In: R. Peters & R. J. Mcmahon, eds. *Prevention and Early Intervention: Childhood Disorders, Substance Use and Delinquency*. Thousand Oaks, CA: Sage, pp. 111–43.

Lock, J. & Fitzpatrick, K. K. (2009). Advances in psychotherapy for children and adolescents with eating disorders. *American Journal of Psychotherapy*, **63**, 287–303.

Lock, J., Le Grange, D., Agras, W. S. & Dare, C. (2001). *Treatment Manual for Anorexia Nervosa: A Family-Based Approach*. New York: Guilford Publications, Inc.

Loeb, K. L., Walsh, B. T., Lock, J. et al. (2007). Open trial of family-based treatment for full and partial anorexia nervosa in adolescence: evidence of successful dissemination. *Journal of the American Academy of Child and Adolescent Psychiatry*, **46**, 792–800.

Lonergan, E. T., Cameron, M. & Luxenberg, J. et al. (2004). Valproic acid for agitation in dementia. *Cochrane Database of Systematic Reviews*, CD003945. Oxford: Update Software Ltd.

Lonergan, E., Luxenberg, J., Areosa Sastre, A. (2009). Benzodiazepines for delirium. *Cochrane Database of Systematic Reviews*, Oct **7**(4), CD006379.

Lorig, K. R. & Holman, H. (2003). Self-management education: history, definition, outcomes, and mechanisms. *Annals of Behavior Medicine*, **26**, 1–7.

Lovaas, O. I. (2002). *Teaching Individuals with Developmental Delays: Basic Intervention Techniques*. Austin, Texas: Pro-Ed.

Loy, C. & Schneider, L. (2006). Galantamine for Alzheimer's disease and mild cognitive impairment. *Cochrane Database of Systematic Reviews*, 1.

Luty, S. E., Carter, J. D., McKenzie, J. M. et al. (2007). Christchurch Psychotherapy of Depression Study: a randomised controlled trial of interpersonal psychotherapy and cognitive behaviour therapy. *British Journal of Psychiatry*, **190**, 496–502.

Lyketsos, C. G., DelCampo, L., Steinberg, M. et al. (2003). Treating depression in Alzheimer's disease: efficacy and safety of sertraline therapy, and the benefits of depression reduction: the DIADS. *Archives of General Psychiatry*, **60**, 737–46.

Lyons-Ruth, K., Connell, D. B., Grunebaum, H. U. & Botein, S. (1990). Infants at social risk: maternal depression and family support services. *Child Development*, **61**, 85–98.

Ma, H. & Teasdale, J. D. (2004). Mindfulness-based cognitive therapy for depression: replication and exploration of differential relapse prevention effects. *Journal of Consulting and Clinical Psychology*, **72**(1), 31–40.

Macey, M. L., Thompson, M., Santosh, P. J & Wong, I. C. K. (2005). Effects of the committee on safety of medicines advice on antidepressant prescribing to children and adolescents in the UK. *Drug Safety*, **28**, 1151-7.

Mackenzie, A., Funderburk, F. R. & Allen, R. P. (1999). Sleep, anxiety, and depression in abstinent and drinking alcoholics. *Substance Use and Misuse*, **34**, 347-61.

Mackin, P., Bishop, D., Watkinson, H., Gallagher, P. & Ferrier, I. N. (2007). Metabolic disease and cardiovascular risk in people treated with antipsychotics in the community. *British Journal of Psychiatry*, **191**, 23-9.

Maggioni, A. & Lifschitz, F. (1995). Nutritional management of failure to thrive. *Pediatric Clinics of North America*, **42**, 791-810.

Mains, J. A. & Scogin, F. R. (2003). The effectiveness of self-administered treatments: a practice-friendly review of the research. *Journal of Clinical Psychology*, **59**, 237-46.

Malouf, R. & Birks, J. (2004). Donepezil for vascular cognitive impairment. *Cochrane Database of Systematic Reviews*, 1, CD004395.

Manassis, K., Mendlowitz, S. L., Scapillato, D. et al. (2002). Group and individual cognitive-behavioural therapy for childhood anxiety disorders: a randomised trial. *Journal of the American Academy of Child and Adolescent Psychiatry*, **41**, 1423-30.

Mancini, C., Van-Ameringen, M., Oakman, R. & Farvolden, P. (1999). Serotonergic agents in the treatment of social phobia in children and adolescents: a case series. *Depression and Anxiety*, **10**(1), 33-9.

Mann, K., Lehert, P. & Morgan, M. Y. (2004). The efficacy of acamprosate in the maintenance of abstinence in alcohol-depending individuals: results of a meta-analysis. *Alcoholism: Clinical Experimental Research*, **28**, 51-63.

Mantovani, A., Stanford, A. D., Bulow, P. & Lisanby, S. H. (2008). Focal brain stimulation approaches to psychiatric treatment. In: P. Tyrer & K. R. Silk, eds. *Cambridge Textbook of Effective Treatments in Psychiatry*. Cambridge: Cambridge University Press, pp. 83-97.

Marcaurelle, R., Belanger, C. & Marchand, A. (2003). Marital relationship and the treatment of panic disorder with agoraphobia: a critical review. *Clinical Psychology Review*, **23**, 247-76.

March, J. S., Amaya-Jackson, L., Murray, M. D., Cathryn, M. & Schulte, A. (1998). Cognitive behavioural psychotherapy for children and adolescents with post-traumatic stress disorder after a single incident stressor. *Journal of the American Academy of Child & Adolescent Psychiatry*, **37**, 585-93.

Marcus, R. N., Owen, R., Kamen, L. et al. (2009). A placebo-controlled, fixed-dose study of aripiprazole in children and adolescents with irritability associated with autistic disorder. *Journal of the American Academy of Child and Adolescent Psychiatry*, **48**, 1110-19.

Marder, S. R., Essock, S. M., Miller, A. L. et al. (2002). The Mount Sinai conference on the pharmacology of schizophrenia. *Schizophrenia Bulletin*, **28**, 5-16.

Marder, S. R., Essock, S. M., Miller, A. L. et al. (2004). Physical health monitoring of patients with schizophrenia.

American Journal of Psychiatry, **161**, 1334–49.

Margolese, H. C. (2000). The male menopause and mood: testosterone decline and depression in the aging male: is there a link? *Journal of Geriatric Psychiatry and Neurology*, **13** (2), 93–101.

Mariani, J. & Levin, F. (2007). Treatment strategies for co-occurring ADHD and substance use disorders. *American Journal on Addictions*, **16**, 45–56.

Marks, I. M., Swinson, R. P. & Basoglu, M. et al. (1993). Alprazolam and exposure alone and combined in panic disorder with agoraphobia: a controlled study in London and Toronto. *British Journal of Psychiatry*, **162**, 776–87.

Marks, I. M., Kenwright, M., McDonough, M., Whittaker, M. & Mataix-Cols, D. (2004). Saving clinicians' time by delegating routine aspects of therapy to a computer: a randomized controlled trial in phobia/panic disorder. *Psychological Medicine*, **34**(1), 9–17.

Marks, L. S. (2003). Editorial comment 1. *Urology*, **62**, 125–6.

Marlatt, G. A. (2002). Buddhist philosophy and the treatment of addictive behavior. *Cognitive & Behavioral Practice*, **9**(1), 44–50.

Marlatt, G. A. & Gordon, J. R. (1985). *Relapse Prevention: Maintenance Strategies in the Treatment of Addictive Behaviors*. New York: Guilford.

Marlatt, G. A. & Witkiewitz, K. (2002). Harm reduction approaches to alcohol use: health promotion, prevention, and treatment. *Addictive Behaviors*, **27**, 867–86.

Marlatt, G. A., Pagano, R., Rose, D. & Marques, J. (1984). Effect of meditation and relaxation training upon alcohol use in male social drinkers. In: D. Shapiro & R. Walsh, eds. *Meditation: Classic and Contemporary Perspectives*. New York: Aldine, pp. 105–120.

Marrazzi, M. A., Bacon, J. P., Kinzie, J. & Luby, E. D. (1995). Naltrexone use in the treatment of anorexia nervosa and bulimia nervosa. *International Clinical Psychopharmacology*, **10**, 163–72.

Marshall, R. D., Beebe, K. L., Oldham, M. & Zaninelli, R. (2001). Efficacy and safety of paroxetine treatment for chronic PTSD: a fixed-dose, placebo-controlled study. *American Journal of Psychiatry*, **158**(12), 1982–8.

Martell, C. R., Dimidjian, S., Mulick, P. S., Roberts, L. J. & Wagner, A. (2003). Clinical applications of behavioral discussion. Panel Discussion, 37th Annual Convention, Association for Advancement of Behavior Therapy, Reno, Nevada.

Martin, J. L. R., Barbanoj, M. J., Schlaepfer, T. E. et al. (2003). Repetitive transcranial magnetic stimulation for the treatment of depression: systematic review and meta-analysis. *British Journal of Psychiatry*, **182**, 480–91.

Martin, J. L. R., Barbanoj, M. J., Schlaepfer, T. E. et al. (2004). Transcranial magnetic stimulation for treating depression [Review]. *The Cochrane Database of Systematic Reviews*, 1. Oxford: Update Softward Ltd.

Martins, J. G. (2009). EPA but not DHA appears to be responsible for the efficacy of omega-3 long chain polyunsaturated fatty acid supplementation in depression: evidence from a meta analysis of randomized controlled trials

Journal of the American College of Nutrition, **28**, 525–42.

Marziali, E. & Monroe-Blum, H. (1995). An interpersonal approach to group psychotherapy with borderline personality disorder. *Journal of Personality Disorders*, **9**, 179–89.

Mason, B. J., Goodman, A. M., Chabac, S. & Lehert, P. (2006). Effect of oral acamprosate on abstinence in patients with alcohol dependence in a double-blind, placebo-controlled trial: the role of patient motivation. *Journal of Psychiatric Research*, **40**, 383–93.

Masters, W. H. & Johnson, V. E. (1970). *Human Sexual Inadequacy*. Boston: Little Brown.

Mataix-Cols, D. & Marks, I. M. (2006). Self-help with minimal therapist contact for obsessive-compulsive disorder: a review. *European Psychiatry*, **21**, 75–80.

Mate-Kole, C., Freschi, M. & Robin, A. (1988). Aspects of psychiatric symptoms at different stages in the treatment of transsexualism. *British Journal of Psychiatry*, **152**, 550–3.

Mate-Kole, C., Freschi, M. & Robin, A. (1990). A controlled study of psychological and social change after surgical gender reassignment in selected male transsexuals. *British Journal of Psychiatry*, **157**, 261–4.

Mather, A. S., Rodriguez, C., Guthrie, M. F., McHarg, A. M., Reid, I. C. & McMurdo, M. E. (2002). Effects of exercise on depressive symptoms in older adults with poorly responsive depressive disorder: randomised controlled trial. *British Journal of Psychiatry*, **180**, 411–5.

Mattick, R. P., Breen, C., Kimber, J. & Dovoli, M. (2002a). Methadone maintenance therapy versus no opioid replacement therapy for opioid dependence. *Cochrane Database Systematic Reviews*, **4**, CD002209. Oxford: Update Software Ltd.

Mattick, R. P., Kimber, J., Breen, C. & Davoli, M. (2002b). Buprenorphine maintenance versus placebo or methadone maintenance for opioid dependence. *Cochrane Database of Systematic Reviews*, **4**. Oxford: Update Software Ltd.

Mayberg, H. S., Lozano, A. M., Voon, V. et al. (2005). Deep brain stimulation for treatment-resistant depression. *Neuron*, **45**, 651–60.

Mayo-Smith, M. F. (1997). Pharmacological management of alcohol withdrawal: a meta-analysis and evidence-based practice guideline. American Society of Addiction Medicine Working Group on Pharmacological Management of Alcohol Withdrawal. *Journal of the American Medical Association*, **278**, 144–51.

Mayou, R., Kirmayer, L. J., Simon, G., Kroenke, K. & Sharpe, M. (2005). Somatoform disorders: time for a new approach in DSM-V. *American Journal of Psychiatry*, **162**, 847–55.

McBride, N., Farringdon, F., Midford, R., Meuleners, L. & Phillips, M. (2004). Harm minimization in school drug education: final results of the School Health and Alcohol Harm Reduction Project (SHAHRP). *Addiction*, **99**, 278–91.

McCambridge, J. & Strang, J. (2004). The efficacy of single-session motivational interviewing in reducing drug consumption and perceptions of drug-related risk and harm among young people: results from a multi-site cluster randomized trial. *Addiction*, **99**, 39–52.

McCann, J., Stein, A., Fairburn, C. G. & Dunger, D. B. (1994). Eating habits and attitudes of mothers of children with non-organic failure to thrive. *British Medical Journal*, **70**, 234–6.

McCann, U. D. & Agras, W. S. (1990). Successful treatment of non-purging bulimia nervosa with desipramine: a double-blind placebo-controlled study [see comments]. *American Journal of Psychiatry*, **147**(11), 1509–13.

McCarney, R., Fisher, P., Iliffe, S. et al. (2008). *Ginkgo biloba* for mild to moderate dementia in a community setting: a pragmatic, randomised, parallel-group, double-blind, placebo-controlled trial. *International Journal of Geriatric Psychiatry*, **23**, 1222–30.

McCarthy, O. & Carr, A. (2002). Prevention of bullying. In: A. Carr, ed. *Prevention: What Works with Children and Adolescents? A Critical Review of Psychological Prevention Programmes for Children, Adolescents and their Families*. Hove, East Sussex: Brunner-Routledge, pp. 205–21.

McCracken, J. T., McGough, J., Shah, B. et al. and Research Units on Pediatric Psychopharmacology Autism Network. (2002). Risperidone in children with autism and serious behavioral problems. *New England Journal of Medicine*, **347**, 314–21.

McCrady, B. S., Epstein, E. E. & Hirsch, L. S. (1999). Maintaining change after conjoint behavioral alcohol treatment for men: outcomes at 6 months. *Addiction*, **94**, 1381–96.

McCullough, J. P. (2000). *Treatment of Chronic Depression: Cognitive Behavioral Analysis System of Psychotherapy*. New York: Guilford Press.

McDougle, C. J., Naylor, S. T., Cohen, D. J., Volkmar, F. R., Heninger, G. R. & Price, L. H. (1996). A double-blind, placebo-controlled study of fluvoxamine in adults with autistic disorder. *Archives of General Psychiatry*, **53**, 1001–8.

McElroy, S. L., Casuto, L. S., Nelson, E. B. et al. (2000). Placebo-controlled trial of sertraline in the treatment of binge eating disorder. *American Journal of Psychiatry*, **157**(6), 1004–6.

McElroy, S. L., Hudson, J. I., Capece, J. A. et al. (2007). Topiramate for the treatment of binge eating disorder associated with obesity: a placebo-controlled study. *Biological Psychiatry*, **61**, 1039–48.

McEvoy, J. P., Lieberman, J. A., Stroup, T. S. et al. (2006). Effectiveness of clozapine versus olanzapine, quetiapine, and risperidone in patients with chronic schizophrenia who did not respond to prior atypical antipsychotic treatment. *American Journal of Psychiatry*, **163**, 600–10.

McGuire, H. & Hawton, K. (2003). Interventions for vaginismus. *Cochrane Database of Systematic Reviews*, **1**, P:CD001760.

McGurk, S. R., Twamley, E. W., Sitzer, D. I et al. (2007). A meta-analysis of cognitive remediation in schizophrenia. *American Journal of Psychiatry*, **164**, 1791–802.

McIver, S., McGartland, M. & O'Halloran P. (2009). 'Overeating is not about the food': women describe their experience of a yoga treatment for binge eating. *Qualitative Health Research*, **19**, 1234–45.

McKay, J. R., Alterman, A. I., Cacciola, J. S., O'Brien, C. P., Koppenhave, J. M. & Shepard, D. S. (1999). Continuing care for cocaine dependence: comprehensive 2-year outcomes. *Journal of Consulting and Clinical Psychology*, **67**, 420–7.

McKeehan, M. B. & Martin, D. (2002). Assessment and treatment of anxiety disorders and co-morbid alcohol/other drug dependency. *Alcoholism Treatment Quarterly*, **20**, 45–59.

McKeith, I. G. (2006). Consensus guidelines for the clinical and pathologic diagnosis of dementia with Lewy bodies (DLB): report of the Consortium on DLB International Workshop. *Journal of Alzheimer's Disease*, **9** (3 Suppl), 417–23.

McKeith, I. G., Galasko, D., Kosaka, K. et al. (1996). Consensus guidelines for the clinical and pathological diagnosis of dementia with Lewy bodies (DLB): report of the Consortium on DLB International Workshop. *Neurology*, **47**, 1113–24.

McKeith, I., Del Ser, T., Spano, P. et al. (2000). Efficacy of rivastigmine in dementia with Lewy bodies: a randomised, double-blind, placebo-controlled international study. *Lancet*, **356**, 2031–6.

McKellar, J., Stewart, E. & Humphreys, K. (2003). Alcoholics Anonymous involvement and positive alcohol-related outcomes: cause, consequence, or just a correlate? A prospective 2-year study of 2,319 alcohol-dependent men. *Journal of Consulting and Clinical Psychology*, **71**, 302–8.

McLellan, A. T., Arndt, I. O., Metzger, D. S., Woody, G. E. & O'Brien, C. P. (1993). The effects of psychosocial services in substance abuse treatment. *Journal of the American Medical Association*, **269**, 1953–9.

McMain, S. F., Links, P. S., Gnam, W. H. et al. (2009). A randomized trial of dialectical behavior therapy versus general psychiatric management for borderline personality disorder. *American Journal of Psychiatry*, **166**, 1365–74.

McShane, R., Areosa Sastre, A. & Minakaran, N. (2006). Memantine for dementia. *Cochrane Database of Systematic Reviews*, 2.

Medical Research Council (1985). Clinical trial of the treatment of depressive illness. *British Medical Journal*, **5439**, 881–6.

Meehan, K. M., Wang, H., David, S. R. et al. (2002). Comparison of rapidly acting intramuscular olanzapine, lorazepam, and placebo: a double-blind, randomized study in acutely agitated patients with dementia. *Neuropsychopharmacology*, **26**, 494–504.

Mehler, P. S. & Weiner, K. L. (1993). Anorexia nervosa and total parenteral nutrition. *International Journal of Eating Disorders*, **14**, 297–304.

Meltzer, H., Gatward, R., Goodman, R. & Ford, T. (2003). Mental health of children and adolescents in Great Britain. *International Review of Psychiatry*, **15**, 185–7.

Melvin, G. A., Tonge, B. J., King, N. J., Heyne, D., Gordon, M. S. & Klimkeit, E. D. (2006). A comparison of cognitive-behavioural therapy, sertraline, and their combination for adolescent depression. *Journal of the American Academy of Child and Adolescent Psychiatry*, **45**, 1151–61.

Menza, M. A., Murray, G. B., Holmes, V. F. et al. (1998). Controlled study of extra-pyramidal reactions in the management of delirious, medically ill patients: intra-venous haloperidol versus intravenous haloperidol plus benzodia-zepines. *Heart and Lung*, **17**, 238–41.

Menza, M. A., Murray, G. B., Holmes, V. F. & Rafuls, W. A. (1988). Controlled study of extrapyramidal reactions in the management of delirious, medically ill patients: intravenous haloperidol versus intravenous haloperidol plus ben-zodiazepines. *Heart Lung*, **17**, 238–41.

Meuleman, E. J. H. (2003). Investigations in erectile dysfunction. *Current Opinions in Urology*, **13**, 411–16.

Meythaler, J. M., Bruner, R. C., Johnson, A. & Thomas, A. (2002). Amantadine to improve neurorecovery in traumatic brain injury-associated diffuse axonal injury: a pilot double-blind randomized trial. *Journal of Head Trauma Rehabilitation*, **17**, 300–13.

MHRA (2003). http://www.mhra.gov.uk/news/2003.htm#ssri, Vol. 2004: Medicines and Healthcare products Regulatory Agency.

Michelson, D., Allen, A. J., Busner, J. et al. (2002). Once-daily atomoxetine treat-ment for children and adolescents with attention deficit hyperactivity disorder: a randomized, placebo-controlled study. *American Journal of Psychiatry*, **159**, 1896–901.

Miklowitz, D. J. (2008). Adjunctive psycho-therapy for bipolar disorder: state of the evidence. *American Journal of Psychiatry*, **165**, 1408–19.

Miklowitz, D. J., Axelson, D. A., Birmaher, B. et al. (2008). Family-focused treatment for adolescents with bipolar disorder: results of a 2-year randomized trial. *Archives of General Psychiatry*, **65**, 1053–61.

Milano, W., Siano, C., Putrella, C. & Capasso, A. (2005). Treatment of buli-mia nervosa with fluvoxamine: a randomized controlled trial. *Advances in Therapeutics*, **22**, 278–83.

Milisen, K., Foreman, M. D., Abraham, I. L. et al. (2001). A nurse-led interdisciplinary intervention program for delirium in eld-erly hip-fracture patients. *Journal of the American Geriatrics Society*, **49**, 523–32.

Miller, W. R., Zweben, A., DiClemente, C. C. & Rychtarik, R. G. (1992). *Motivational Enhancement Therapy Manual: A Clinical Research Guide for Therapists Treating Individuals with Alcohol Abuse and Dependence* (NIAA Project Match Monograph Series Vol. 2). Rockville, MD: National Institute on Alcohol and Alcoholism.

Miller, D. D., Caroff, S. N., Davis, S. M. et.al. (2008) Extrapyramidal side-effects of antipsychotics in a randomised trial. *British Journal of Psychiatry*, **198**, 279–88.

Miller, A. L., Hall, C. S., Buchanan, R. W. et al. (2004). The Texas Medication Algorithm Project antipsychotic algo-rithm for schizophrenia: 2003 update *Journal of Clinical Psychiatry*, **65**, 500–8

Miller, W. R. & Rollnick, S. (1991) *Motivational Interviewing: Preparing People to Change Addictive Behavior* New York: Guilford Press.

Miller, W. R. & Sanchez, V. C. (1993) Motivating young adults for treatmen and life-style change. In: G. Howard ed. *Issues in Alcohol Use and Misuse by Young Adults*. South Bend, IN University of Notre Dame Press.

Miller, W. R. & Wilbourne, P. L. (2002). Mesa Grande: a methodological analysis of clinical trials of treatments for alcohol use disorders. *Addiction*, **97**, 265–77.

Milsap, R. L. & Szefler, S. J. (1986). Special pharmacokinetic considerations in children. In: W. E. Evans, J. J. Schentag & W. J. Jusko, eds. *Applied Pharmacokinetic Principles of Therapeutic Drug Monitoring*. Spokane, WA: Applied Therapeutics Inc., pp. 294–330.

Mindell, J. A. & Owens, J. A. (2010). *A Clinical Guide to Pediatric Sleep: Diagnosis and Management of Sleep Problems*, 2nd edn. Philadelphia: Wolters Kluwer/Lippincott Williams and Wilkins.

Mindell, J. A., Kuhn, B., Lewin, D. S., Meltzer, L. J. & Sadeh, A. (2006). Behavioral treatment of bedtime problems and night waking in infants and young children. *Journal of Sleep and Sleep Disorders Research*, **29**(10), 1263–76.

Minnis, H., Green, J., O'Connor, T. & Liew, A. (2009). Reactive Attachment Disorder and Attachment Patterns: evidence for the overlap. *Journal of Child Psychology & Psychiatry*, **50**(8), 931–42.

Minuchin, S., Rosman, B. I. & Baker, T. (1978). *Psychosomatic Families: Anorexia Nervosa in Context*. Cambridge, MA: Harvard University Press.

Mitchell, J. E., Fletcher, L., Hanson, K. et al. (2001). The relative efficacy of fluoxetine and manual-based self-help in the treatment of outpatients with bulimia nervosa. *Journal of Clinical Psychopharmacology*, **21**(3), 298–304.

Mitte, K., Noack, P., Steil, R. & Hautzinger, M. (2005). A meta-analytic review of the efficacy of drug treatment in generalized anxiety disorder. *Journal of Clinical Psychopharmacology*, **25**, 141–50.

Montague, D. K., Jarow, J., Broderick, G. A. et al. (2004). AUA guideline on the pharmacologic management of premature ejaculation. *Journal of Urology*, **172**, 290–4.

Monteiro, W. O., Noshirvani, H. F., Marks, I. M. & Lelliott, P. T. (1987). Anorgasmia from clomipramine in obsessive-compulsive disorder: a controlled trial. *British Journal of Psychiatry*, **151**, 107–12.

Montgomery, S. A., McIntyre, A., Osterheider, M. et al. (1993). A double-blind, placebo-controlled study of fluoxetine in patients with DSM-III-R obsessive-compulsive disorder: The Lilly European OCD Study Group. *European Neuropsychopharmacology*, **3**, 143–52.

Montgomery, S. A., Kasper, S., Stein, D. J., Bang Hedegaard, K. & Lemming, O. M. (2001). Citalopram 20 mg, 40 mg and 60 mg are all effective and well tolerated compared with placebo in obsessive-compulsive disorder. *International Clinical Psychopharmacology*, **16**, 75–86.

Montgomery, S. A., Nil, R., Durr-Pal, N., Loft, H. & Boulenger, J. P. (2005). A 24-week randomized, double-blind, placebo-controlled study of escitalopram for the prevention of generalized social anxiety disorder. *Journal of Clinical Psychiatry*, **66**, 1270–8.

Montgomery, S. A., Chatamra, K., Pauer, L., Whalen, E. & Baldinetti, F. (2008). Efficacy and safety of pregabalin in elderly people with generalised anxiety disorder. *British Journal of Psychiatry*, **193**, 389–94.

Monti, P.M., Abrams, D.B., Kadden, R.M. & Cooney, N.L. (1989). *Treating Alcohol Dependence: A Coping Skills Training Guide*. New York: Guilford Press.

Moore, B.A. & Budney, A.J. (2001). Tobacco smoking in marijuana dependent outpatients. *Journal of Substance Abuse*, **13**, 585–98.

Moore, B.A. & Budney, A.J. (2003). Relapse in outpatient treatment for marijuana dependence. *Journal of Substance Abuse Treatment*, **25**, 85–9.

Moos, R.H. & Moos, B.S. (2004). Long-term influence of duration and frequency of participation in Alcoholics Anonymous on individuals with alcohol use disorders. *Journal of Consulting and Clinical Psychology*, **72**, 81–90.

Moretti, R., Torre, P., Antonello, R.M., Cazzato, G. & Bava, A. (2003). Gabapentin for the treatment of behavioural alterations in dementia: preliminary 15-month investigation. *Drugs and Aging*, **20**, 1035–40.

Morgan, H.G., Purgold, J. & Welbourne, J. (1983). Management and outcome in anorexia nervosa: a standardized prognostic study. *British Journal of Psychiatry*, **143**, 282–7.

Morgan, J.F. & Crisp, A.H. (2002). Use of leucotomy for intractable anorexia nervosa: a long-term follow-up study. *International Journal of Eating Disorders*, **27**(3), 249–58.

Morgenstern, J. & Longabaugh, R. (2000). Cognitive behavioral treatment for alcohol dependence: a review of evidence for its hypothesized mechanisms of action. *Addiction*, **95**, 1475–90.

Morgenstern, J., Labouvie, E., McCrady, B.S., Kahler, C.W. & Frey, R.M. (1997). Affiliation with Alcoholics Anonymous after treatment: a study of its therapeutic effects and mechanism of action. *Journal of Consulting and Clinical Psychology*, **65**, 768–77.

Morgentaler, A. (1999). Male impotence. *Lancet*, **354**, 1713–18.

Morgenthaler, T.I., Owens, J., Alessi, C., Boehlecke, B., Brown, T.M. et al. (2006). Practice parameters for behavioral treatment of bedtime problems and night waking in infants and young children. *Sleep*, **29**(10), 1277–81.

Morishita, S. (2000). Treatment of anorexia nervosa with Naikan therapy. *International Medical Journal*, **7**(2), 151.

Morriss, R., Dowrick, C., Salmon, P. et al. (2007). Cluster randomised controlled trial of training practices in reattribution for medically unexplained symptoms. *British Journal of Psychiatry*, **191**, 536–42.

Morselli, P.L., Franco-Morselli, R., Bossi, L. et al. (1980). Clinical pharmacokinetics in newborn and infants: age related differences and therapeutic implications *Clinical Pharmacokinetics*, **5**, 485–527.

Morton, I. & Bleathman, C. (1991). The effectiveness of validation therapy in dementia: a pilot study. *International Journal of Geriatric Psychiatry*, **6** 327–30.

Moyer, A., Finney, J.W., Swearingen, C.E. & Vergun, P. (2002). Brief interventions for alcohol problems: a meta-analytic review of controlled investigations in treatment-seeking and non-treatment-seeking populations. *Addiction*, **97** 279–92.

Moynihan, R. & Mintzes, B. (2010). *Sex, Lies, and Pharmaceuticals: How Drug Companies Plan to Profit from Female Sexual Dysfunction*. Greystone Books.

MTA Cooperative Group (1999). A 14-month randomized clinical trial of treatment strategies for attention deficit hyperactivity disorder. *Archives of General Psychiatry*, **56**, 1073–85.

Muehlbacher, M., Nickel, M. K. & Nickel, C. (2005). Mirtazapine treatment of social phobia in women: a randomized, double-blind, placebo-controlled study. *Journal of Clinical Psychopharmacology*, **25**, 580–3.

Mueller, M. M., Piazza, C. C., Moore, J. W. & Kelley, M. E. (2003). Training parents to implement pediatric feeding protocols. *Journal of Applied Behavior Analysis*, **36**, 545–62.

Mufson, L. & Fairbanks, J. (1996). Interpersonal psychotherapy for depressed adolescents: a one year naturalistic follow-up study. *Journal of the American Academy of Child and Adolescent Psychiatry*, **35**, 1145–55.

Mufson, L., Moreau, M., Weissman, M. M. & Garfinkel, R. (1999). Efficacy of interpersonal psychotherapy for depressed adolescents. *Archives of General Psychiatry*, **56**, 573–9.

Mufson, L., Dorta, K. P., Wickramarante, P., Nomura, Y., Olfson, M. & Weissman, M. (2004). A randomized effectiveness trial of interpersonal psychotherapy for depressed adolescents. *Archives of General Psychiatry*, **61**, 577–84.

Mukaddes, N. M., Kaynak, F. N., Kinali, G., Besikci, H. & Issever, H. (2004). Psychoeducational treatment of children with autism and reactive attachment disorder. *Autism*, **8**, 101–9.

Mukherjee, S., Sackeim, H. A. & Schnur, D. B. (1994). Electroconvulsive therapy of acute manic episodes: a review of 50 years' experience. *American Journal of Psychiatry*, **151**, 169–76.

Mullen, P. D., Simons-Morton, D. G., Ramirez, G., Frankowski, R. F., Green, L. W. & Mains, D. A. (1997). A meta-analysis of trials evaluating patient education and counselling for three groups of preventive health behaviors. *Patient Educational Counseling*, **32**, 157–73.

Mundo, E., Bareggi, S. R., Pirola, R., Bellodi, L. & Smeraldi, E. (1997). Long-term pharmacotherapy of obsessive-compulsive disorder: a double-blind controlled study. *Journal of Clinical Psychopharmacology*, **17**, 4–10.

Murphy, S. & Tyrer, P. (1991). A double-blind comparison of the effects of gradual withdrawal of lorazepam, diazepam and bromazepam in benzodiazepine dependence. *British Journal of Psychiatry*, **158**, 511–16.

Murphy, T. J., Pagano, R. R. & Marlatt, G. A. (1986). Life-style modification with heavy alcohol drinkers: effects of aerobic exercise and meditation. *Addictive Behaviors*, **11**, 175–86.

Murphy, S. M., Owen, R. & Tyrer, P. (1989). Comparative assessment of efficacy and withdrawal symptoms after 6 and 12 weeks' treatment with diazepam or buspirone. *British Journal of Psychiatry*, **154**, 529–34.

Murray, L., Cooper, P. J., Wilson, A. & Romaniuk, H. (2003). Controlled trial of the short- and long-term effect of psychological treatment of post-partum depression. 2. Impact on the mother-child relationship and child outcome. *British Journal of Psychiatry*, **182**, 420–27.

Nakamura, J., Uchimura, N., Yamada, S. et al. (1997). Mianserin suppositories in the treatment of post-operative delirium. *Human Psychopharmacology*, **12**, 595–9.

National Clinical Guideline Centre for Acute and Chronic Conditions (2010). *Delirium: Diagnosis, Prevention and Management*. London: Royal College of Physicians.

National Collaborating Centre for Mental Health (2004). *Eating Disorders: Core Interventions in the Treatment and Management of Anorexia Nervosa, bulimia Nervosa and Related Eating Disorders*. London: British Psychological Society and Royal College of Psychiatrists.

National Collaborating Centre for Mental Health (2005a). *Depression in Children and Young People: Identification and Management in Primary, Community and Secondary care*. London: British Psychological Society and Royal College of Psychiatrists.

National Collaborating Centre for Mental Health (2005b). *Bipolar Disorder: The Management of Bipolar Disorder in Adults, Children and Adolescents*. London: British Psychological Society and Royal College of Psychiatrists.

National Collaborating Centre for Mental Health (2006a). *Obsessive Compulsive Disorder: Core Interventions in the Treatment of Obsessive Compulsive Disorder and Body Dysmorphic Disorder*. London: British Psychological Society and Royal College of Psychiatrists.

National Collaborating Centre for Mental Health (2006b). *Post-traumatic Stress Disorder (PTSD): The Management of PTSD in Adults and Children in Primary and Secondary Care*. London: British Psychological Society and Royal College of Psychiatrists.

National Collaborating Centre for Mental Health (2007). *Dementia: The NICE-SCIE Guideline on Supporting People with Dementia and their Carers in Health and Social Care*. London: British Psychological Society and Royal College of Psychiatrists.

National Collaborating Centre for Mental Health (2009a). *Depression: The Treatment and Management of Depression in Adults (Update)*. London: British Psychological Society and Royal College of Psychiatrists.

National Collaborating Centre for Mental Health (2009a). *Borderline Personality Disorder: The NICE Guideline on Treatment and Management*. London: British Psychological Society and Royal College of Psychiatrists.

National Collaborating Centre for Mental Health (2009b). *Antisocial Personality Disorder: Treatment, Management and Prevention*. London: British Psychological Society and Royal College of Psychiatrists.

National Collaborating Centre for Mental Health (2010). *Schizophrenia: Core Interventions in the Treatment and Management of Schizophrenia in Adult in Primary and Secondary Care (updated edition)*. London: British

Psychological Society and Royal College of Psychiatrists.

National Institute for Clinical Excellence (2000). Guidance on the use of methylphenidate for ADHD. http//www.nice.org.uk/pdf/Methylph-guidance13.pdf

National Institute for Clinical Excellence (2004). *Guideline on the use of zaleplon, zolpidem and zopiclone for the short term management of insomnia. Technology appraisal 77*. London: NICE.

National Institute for Health and Clinical Excellence (2007). *Management of anxiety (panic disorder with or without agoraphobia, and generalised anxiety disorder) in adults in primary, secondary and community care*. 2004 (amended 2007). London: NICE.

National Institute on Alcohol Abuse and Alcoholism (2000a). *Tenth Special Report to the U.S. Congress on Alcohol and Health, 2000*. Washington, DC: US Department of Health and Human Services.

National Institute on Alcohol Abuse and Alcoholism (2000b). *Alcohol Alert No. 49: New Advances in Alcoholism Treatment*. Rockville, MD: Author.

National Institute on Drug Abuse (2004). Scientifically based approaches to drug addiction treatment. In: *Principle of Drug Addiction Treatment: A Research Based Guide*. Rockville, MD: National Institute on Drug Abuse, pp. 1-7.

National Research Council (2001). *Educating Children with Autism. Committee on Educational Interventions for Children with Autism. Division of Behavioral and Social Sciences and Education*. National Research Council. Washington, DC: National Academy Press.

National Treatment Agency for Substance Misuse (2002). *Models of care for treatment of adult drug misusers: framework for developing local systems of effective drug misuse treatment in England*. London: National Treatment Agency for Substance Misuse.

Nazareth, I., Boynton, P. & King, M. (2003). Problems with sexual function in people attending London general practitioners: a cross sectional study. *British Medical Journal*, **327**, 423-6.

Nchito, M., Geissler, P. W., Mubila, L., Friis H. & Olsen, A. (2004). Effects of iron and multimicronutrient supplementation on geophagy: a two-by-two factorial study among Zambian schoolchildren in Lusaka. *Transactions of the Royal Society of Tropical Medicine and Hygiene*, **98**, 218-27.

Neal, L. A., Shapland, W. & Fox, C. et al. (1997). An open trial of moclobemide in the treatment of post-traumatic stress disorder. *International Clinical Psychopharmacology*, **12**, 231-7.

Neiderman, M., Zarody, M., Tattersall, M. & Lask, B. (2000). Enteric feeding in severe adolescent anorexia nervosa: a report of four cases. *International Journal of Eating Disorders*, **28**, 470-5.

Neiderman, M., Zarody, M., Tattersall, M. & Lask, B. (2000). Enteric feeding in severe adolescent anorexia nervosa: A report of four cases. *International Journal of Eating Disorders*, **28**, 470-475.

Nelson III, W. M. & Finch, A. J. (2000). Managing anger in youth: a cognitive-behavioral intervention approach. In: P. C. Kendall, ed. *Child & Adolescent*

Therapy: Cognitive-Behavioral Proce-dures, 2nd edn. New York: Guilford Press, pp. 129–170.

Neumark-Sztainer, D., Sherwood, N., Coller, T. & Hannan, P. (2000). Primary prevention of disordered eating among preadolescent girls: Feasibility and short-term effect of a community-based intervention. *Journal of the American Dietetic Association*, **100** (12), 1466–73.

Newton-Howes, G., Weaver, T. & Tyrer, P. (2008). Attitudes of staff towards patients with personality disorder in community health teams. *Australian and New Zealand Journal of Psychiatry*, **42**, 572–7.

Nierenberg, A. A., McLean, N. E. et al. (1995). Early non-response to fluoxetine as a predictor of poor eight-week outcome. *American Journal of Psychiatry*, **152**, 1500–3.

Nixon, R. D., Sweeney, L., Erickson, D. B. & Touyz, S. W. (2003). Parent–child inter-action therapy: a comparison of stand-ard and abbreviated treatments for oppositional defiant preschoolers. *Journal of Consulting & Clinical Psychology*, **71**, 251–60.

Norton, C. R., Cox, B. J. & Malan, J. (1992). Nonclinical panickers: a critical review. *Clinical Psychology Review*, **12**, 121–39.

Nosé, M., Cipriani, A., Biancosino, B., Grassi, L. & Barbui, C. (2006). Efficacy of pharmacotherapy against core traits of borderline personality disorder: meta-analysis of randomized controlled trials. *International Journal of Clinical Psychopharmacology*, **21**, 345–53.

Novaco, R. W. (1976). The functions and regulation of the arousal of anger. *American Journal of Psychiatry*, **133**, 1124–8.

Nowinski, J., Baker, S. & Carroll, K. (1992). *Twelve Step Facilitation Therapy Manual: A Clinical Research Guide for Therapists Treating Individuals with Alcohol Abuse and Dependence (DHHS Publication No. ADM 92–1893)*. Rockville, MD: US Department of Health and Human Services.

Nowinski, J., Baker, S. & Carroll, K. (1994). *Twelve Step Facilitation Therapy Manual* (Project Match Monograph Series, Vol. 1; NIH Publication No. 94–3722). Rockville, MD: National Institute on Alcohol Abuse and Alcoholism.

Nunes, E. V. & Levin, F. R. (2004). Treatment of depression in patients with alcohol or other drug dependence: a meta-analysis. *Journal of the American Medical Association*, **291**, 1887–96.

O'Connor, P. G. & Kosten, T. R. (1998). Rapid and ultrarapid opioid detoxification techniques. *Journal of the American Medical Association*, **279**, 229–34.

O'Connor, T. G., Bredenkamp, D. & Rutter, M., The English and Romanian Adoptees (ERA) Study Team (1999). Attachment disturbances and disorders in children exposed to early severe dep-rivation. *Infant Mental Health Journal*, **20**, 10–29.

O'Farrell, T. J. & Fals-Stewart, W. (2000). Behavioral couples therapy for alcohol-ism and drug abuse. *Journal of Substance Abuse Treatment*, **18**, 51–4.

O'Herlihy, A., Worrall, A., Lelliott, P., Jaffa, T., Hill, P. & Banerjee, S. (2003). Distribution and characteristics of inpatient child and adolescent mental health services in England and Wales.

British Journal of Psychiatry, **183**, 847–51.

O'Malley, J. E., Anderson, W. H. & Lazare, A. (1972). Failure of outpatient treatment of drug abuse. I. Heroin. *American Journal of Psychiatry*, **128**, 865–8.

O'Neill, R. E., Horner, R. H., Albin, R. W. et al. (1997). *Functional Analysis of Problem Behavior: A Practical Assessment Guide*, 2nd edn. Pacific Grove, CA: Brooks/Cole.

Oden, S. & Asher, S. R. (1977). Coaching children in social skills for friendship making. *Child Development*, **48**, 495–506.

Olatunji, B. O., Deacon, B. J. & Abramowitz, J. S. (2009). Is hypochondriasis an anxiety disorder? *British Journal of Psychiatry*, **194**, 481–2.

Oldham, J., Phillips, K., Gabbard, G. et al. (2001). Practice guideline for the treatment of patients with borderline personality disorder. American Psychiatric Association. American Journal of Psychiatry, **158**, 1–52.

Oliver-Africano, P., Murphy, D. & Tyrer, P. (2009). Aggressive behavior in adults with intellectual disability: defining the role of drug treatment. *CNS Drugs*, **23**, 903–13.

Oliveto, A. H., Feingold, A., Schottenfeld, R., Jatlow, P. & Kosten, T. R. (1999). Desipramine in opioid-dependent cocaine abusers maintained on buprenorphine vs. methadone. *Archives of General Psychiatry*, **56**, 812–20.

Olmsted, M. P., Davis, R., Rockert, W., Irvine, M. J., Eagle, M. & Garner, D. M. (1991). Efficacy of a brief group psychoeducational intervention for bulimia nervosa. *Behavior Research Therapy*, **29**(1), 71–83.

Olmsted, M. P., Daneman, D., Rydall, A. C., Lawson, M. L. & Rodin, G. (2002). The effects of psychoeducation on disturbed eating attitudes and behavior in young women with type 1 diabetes mellitus. *International Journal of Eating Disorders*, **32**, 230–9.

Olweus, D., Limber, S. & Mihalic, S. (2000). *Blueprints for Violence Prevention: Bullying Prevention Program*. Boulder, CO: Center for Study and Prevention of Violence.

Orgogozo, J.-M., Rigaud, A.-S., Stöffler, A., Möbius, H.-J. & Forette, F. (2002). Efficacy and safety of memantine in patients with mild to moderate vascular dementia: a randomized, placebo-controlled trial (MMM 300). *Stroke*, **33**, 1834–9.

Öst, L. G. & Sterner, U. (1987). Applied tension: a specific behavioral method for treatment of blood phobia. *Behaviour Research and Therapy*, **25**(1), 25–9.

Öst, L., Salkovskis, P. & Hellstrom, K. et al. (1991). One-session therapist-directed exposure vs. self-exposure in the treatment of spider phobia. *Behavior Therapy*, **22**, 407–22.

Öst, L. G., Brandberg, M. & Alm, T. (1997). One versus five sessions of exposure in the treatment of flying phobia. *Behaviour Research and Therapy*, **35** (11), 987–96.

Öst, L. G., Svensson, L., Hellstrom, K. & Lindwall, R. (2001). One-session treatment of specific phobias in youths: a randomized clinical trial. *Journal of Consulting Clinical Psychology*, **69**(5), 814–24.

Ostafin, B. D. (2008). Surfing the urge: experiential acceptance moderates the relation between automatic alcohol motivation and hazardous drinking. *Journal of Social and Clinical Psychology*, **27**, 404–18.

Otto, M. W., Pollack, M. H., Sachs, G. S., Reiter, S. R., Meltzer-Brody, S. & Rosenbaum, J. F. (1993). Discontinuation of benzodiazepine treatment: efficacy of cognitive behavioural therapy for patients with panic disorder. *American Journal of Psychiatry*, **150**, 1485–90.

Otto, M. W., Pollack, M. H., Gould, R. A., Worthington, J. J., McArdle, E. T. & Rosenbaum, J. F. (2000). A comparison of the efficacy of clonazepam and cognitive-behavioral group therapy for the treatment of social phobia. *Journal of Anxiety Disorders*, **14**, 345–58.

Otto, M. W., Tuby, K. S., Gould, R. A., McLean, R. Y. & Pollack, M. H. (2001). An effect-size analysis of the relative efficacy and tolerability of serotonin selective reuptake inhibitors for panic disorder. *American Journal of Psychiatry*, **158**(12), 1989–92.

Ottolini, M. C., Hamburger, E. K., Loprieato, J. O. et al. (2001). Complementary and alternative medicine use among children in the Washington, DC area. *Ambulatory Pediatrics*, **1**, 122–5.

Oude-Voshaar, R. C., Gorgels, W. J. & Mol, A. J. J. (2003). Tapering off long-term benzodiazepine use with or without group cognitive-behavioural therapy: three-condition, randomised controlled trial. *British Journal of Psychiatry*, **182**, 498–504.

Oude-Voshaar, R. C., Gorgels, W. J., Mol, A. J. et al. (2006a). Long-term outcome of two forms of randomised benzodiazepine discontinuation. *British Journal of Psychiatry*, **188**, 188–9.

Oude-Voshaar, R. C., Couvée, J. E., van Balkom, A. J. L. M., Mulder, P. G. H. & Zitman, F. G. (2006b). Strategies for discontinuing long-term benzodiazepine use: meta-analysis. *British Journal of Psychiatry*, **189**, 213–20.

Ouimette, P. C., Finney, J. W. & Moos, R. H. (1997). Twelve-step and cognitive behavioral treatment for substance abuse: a comparison of treatment effectiveness. *Journal of Consulting and Clinical Psychology*, **65**, 230–40.

Overshott, R., Vernon, M., Morris, J. & Burns, A. (2010). Rivastigmine in the treatment of delirium in older people: a pilot study. *International Psychogeriatrics*, **22**, 812–8.

Owen, P. L., Slaymaker, V., Tonigan, J. S. et al. (2003). Participation in Alcoholics Anonymous: intended and unintended change mechanisms. *Alcoholism: Clinical and Experimental Research*, **27**, 524–32.

Owen, R., Sikich, L., Marcus, R. N. et al. (2009). Aripiprazole in the treatment of irritability in children and adolescents with autistic disorder. *Pediatrics*, **124**, 1533–40.

Oyebode, F. (2004). Invited commentary on The rediscovery of recovery. *Advances in Psychiatric Treatment*, **10**, 48–9.

Palinkas, L. A., Atkins, C. J., Miller, C. & Ferreira, D. (1996). Social skills training for drug prevention in high-risk female adolescents. *Preventative Medicine*, **25**, 692–701.

Palmer, R. L., Birchall, H., McGrain, L. & Sullivan, V. (2002). Self-help for bulimi disorders: a randomized controlled tria comparing minimal guidance with face-to-face or telephone guidance. *British Journal of Psychiatry*, **181**, 230–5.

Pande, A. C., Davidson, J. R, Jefferson, J. W. et al. (1999). Treatment of social phobia with gabapentin: a placebo-controlled study. *Journal of Clinical Psychopharmacology*, **19**, 341–8.

Pande, A. C., Feltner, D. E., Jefferson, J. W. et al. (2004). Efficacy of the novel anxiolytic pregabalin in social anxiety disorder: a placebo-controlled, multicenter study. *Journal of Clinical Psychopharmacology*, **24**, 141–9.

Parellada, E., Baeza, I., de Pablo, J. et al. (2004). Risperidone in the treatment of patients with delirium. *Journal of Clinical Psychiatry*, **65**, 348–53.

Parker, G. (2002). Differential effectiveness of newer and older antidepressants appears mediated by an age effect on the phenotypic expression of depression. *Acta Psychiatrica Scandinavica*, **106**(3), 168–70.

Parker, G., Parker, K. et al. (2003). Gender differences in response to differing antidepressant drug classes: two negative studies. *Psychological Medicine*, **33**(8), 1473–7.

Parkinson Study Group (1999). Low-dose clozapine for the treatment of drug-induced psychosis in Parkinson's disease. *New England Journal of Medicine*, **340**, 757–63.

Parr, J. M., Kavanagh, D. J., Cahill, L., Mitchell, G. & Young, R. (2008). Effectiveness of current treatment approaches for benzodiazepine discontinuation: a meta-analysis. *Addiction*, **104**, 13–24.

Paton, C. (2008). Prescribing in pregnancy. *British Journal of Psychiatry*, **192**, 321–22.

Patterson, G. R. & Gullion, M. E. (1968). *Living With Children: New Methods for Parents and Teachers*. Champaign, IL: Research Press.

Peck Peterson, S. M., Caniglia, C., Royster A. J., Macfarlane, E., Plowman, K., Baird, S. J. & Wu, N. (2005). Blending functional communication training and choice making to improve task engagement and decrease problem behaviour. *Educational Psychology*, **25**, 257–74.

Pediatric OCD Treatment Study (POTS) Team (2004). Cognitive-behavior therapy, sertraline, and their combination for children and adolescents with obsessive-compulsive disorder: the pediatric OCD treatment study (POTS) randomised controlled trial. *Journal of the American Medical Association*, **292** (16), 1969–76.

Pekkala, E. & Merinder, L. (2002). Psychoeducation for schizophrenia. *The Cochrane Database of Systematic Reviews*, **2**, CD002831. doi: 10.1002/14651858.CD002831. Oxford: Update Software Ltd.

Pelham, W. E., Vodde-Hamiliton, M., Murphy, D. A., Greenstein, J. & Vallano, G. (1991). The effects of methylphenidate on ADHD adolescents in recreational, peer group and classroom settings. *Journal of Clinical Child Psychology*, **20**, 293–300.

Pendleton, V. R., Goodrick, G. K., Poston, W. S., Reeves, R. & Foreyt, J. P. (2002). Exercise augments the effects of cognitive-behavioral therapy in the treatment of binge-eating. *International Journal of Eating Disorders*, **31**(2), 172–84.

Perimentis, P., Gyftopoulos, K., Giannitsas, K. et al. (2004). A comparative, crossover study of the efficacy and safety of sildenafil and apomorphine in men with evidence of arteriogenic erectile dysfunction. *International Journal of Impotency Research*, **16**, 2–7.

Perry, J.C., Banon, E. & Ianni, F. (1999). Effectiveness of psychotherapy for personality disorder. *American Journal of Psychiatry*, **156**, 1312–21.

Perry, P.J., Stambaugh, R.L., Tsuang, M.T. & Smith, R.E. (1981). Sedative-hypnotic tolerance testing and withdrawal comparing diazepam to barbiturates. *Journal of Clinical Psychopharmacology*, **1**, 289–96.

Pertschuk, M.J., Forster, J., Buzby, G. & Mullen, J.L. (1981). The treatment of anorexia nervosa with total parenteral nutrition. *Biological Psychiatry*, **16**(6), 539–50.

Pesenti, F., Mavrotheris, S., Serra, C., Lucchio, P. & Pucciarelli, S. (1999). Use of percutaneous endoscopic gastrostomy in anorexia nervosa: case report. *Rivista Italiana di Nutrizione Parenterale ed Enterale*, **17**(1), 24–7.

Peskind, E.R., Tsuang, D.W., Bonner, L.T. et al. (2005). Propranolol for disruptive behaviours in nursing home residents with probable or possible Alzheimer disease: a placebo-controlled study. *Alzheimer's Disease and Associated Disorders*, **19**, 23–8.

Petitjean, S., Stohler, R., Deglon, J. et al. (2001). Double-blind randomized trial of buprenorphine and methadone in opiate dependence. *Drug and Alcohol Dependence*, **62**, 97–104.

Petrakis, I., Carroll, K., Nich, C. et al. (2000). Disulfiram treatment for cocaine dependence in methadone-maintained opioid addicts. *Addiction*, **95**, 219–28.

Petry, N. (2006). Contingency management treatments: a uniquely American approach, or perhaps even better suited for European drug abuse treatment? *British Journal of Psychiatry*, **189**, 97–8.

Petry, N., Tedford, J., Austin, M., Nich, C., Carroll, K.C. & Rounsaville, B.J. (2004). Prize reinforcement contingency management for treating cocaine users: how long can we go, and with whom. *Addiction*, **99**, 349–60.

Petry, N.M., Peirce, J.M., Stitzer, M.L. et al. (2005). Effect of prize-based incentives on outcomes in stimulant abusers in outpatient psychosocial treatment programs: A National Drug Abuse Treatment Clinical Trials Network study. *Archives of General Psychiatry*, **62**, 1148–56.

Pharoah, F.M., Rathbone, J., Mari, J.J. & Streiner, D. (2003). Family intervention for schizophrenia. *The Cochrane Database of Systematic Reviews*, **3** CD000088. doi: 10.1002/14651858 CD000088. Oxford: Update Software Ltd.

Pigott, T.A. & Seay, S.M. (1999). A review of the efficacy of selective serotonin reuptake inhibitors in obsessive compulsive disorder. *Journal of Clinical Psychiatry*, **60**, 101–6.

Pike, K.M., Walsh, B.T., Vitousek, K. Wilson, G.T. & Bauer, J. (2003) Cognitive behaviour therapy in the post hospitalization treatment of anorexi nervosa. *American Journal of Psychiatry*, **160**, 2046–9.

Pilling, D., Bebbington, P., Kuipers, E. et al. (2002a). Psychological treatments in schizophrenia II: meta-analyses of randomized controlled trials of social skills training and cognitive remediation. *Psychological Medicine*, **32**, 783–91.

Pilling, D., Bebbington, P., Kuipers, E. et al. (2002b). Psychological treatments in schizophrenia: I. Meta-analysis of family intervention and cognitive behaviour therapy. *Psychological Medicine*, **32**, 763–82.

Pollack, M. H., Allgulander, C., Bandelow, B. et al. (2003). WCA recommendations for the long-term treatment of panic disorder. *CNS Spectrums*, **8**(8) Suppl. 1, 17–30.

Pollak, P., Tison, F., Rascol, O. et al. (2004). Clozapine in drug induced psychosis in Parkinson's disease: a randomized, placebo controlled study with open follow up. *Journal of Neurology, Neurosurgery and Psychiatry*, **75**, 689–95.

Pollock, B. G., Mulsant, B. H., Rosen, J. et al. (2002). Comparison of citalopram, perphenazine, and placebo for the acute treatment of psychosis and behavioral disturbances in hospitalized demented patients. *American Journal of Psychiatry*, **159**, 460–5.

Pomeranz, B. (1989). Acupuncture research related to pain, drug addiction and nerve regeneration. In: B. Pomeranz, G. Stux, eds. *Scientific Bases of Acupuncture*. Berlin, Germany: Springer-Verlag, pp. 35–52.

Porst, H. (1989). Prostaglandin E in erectile dysfunction (German language article). *Urologe A*, **28**, 94–8.

Powers, P. S. & Santana, C. A. (2002). Eating disorders: a guide for the primary care physician. *Primary Care*, **29**, 81–98.

Powers, P. S. & Bannon, Y. (2004). Medical co-morbidity of anorexia nervosa, bulimia nervosa, and binge eating disorder. In: T. Brewerton ed. *Clinical Handbook of Eating Disorders: An Integrated Approach (Medical Psychiatry 26)*. Marcel Dekker. New York:

Pratt, B. M. & Woolfenden, S. R. (2002). Interventions for preventing eating disorders in children and adolescents. *Cochrane Database of Systematic Reviews*, **2**, CD002891.

Price, J., Cole, V. & Goodwin, G. M. (2009). Emotional side-effects of selective serotonin reuptake inhibitors: qualitative study. *British Journal of Psychiatry*, **195**, 211–17.

Prochazka, A. V., Weaver, M. J., Keller, R. T., Fryer, G. E., Licari, P. A. & Lofaso, D. (1998). A randomized trial of nortriptyline for smoking cessation. *Archives of Internal Medicine*, **158**, 2035–9.

Project Match Research Group (1997). Matching alcoholism treatments to client heterogeneity: Project MATCH post-treatment drinking outcomes. *Journal of Studies on Alcoholism*, **58**, 7–29.

Project MATCH Research Group (1998). Matching alcoholism treatments to client heterogeneity: Project MATCH three year drinking outcomes. *Alcoholism: Clinical and Experimental Research*, **22**, 1300–11.

Pull, C. B. (2006). Current status of virtual reality therapy in anxiety disorders. *Current Opinion in Psychiatry*, **18**, 7–14.

Pusey, H. (2000). Dementia care: interventions with people with dementia and their informal caregivers. *Mental and Health Care*, **3**, 204-7.

Rabey, J. M., Prokhorov, T., Miniovitz, A., Dobronevsky, E. & Klein, C. (2007). Quetiapine for agitation or psychosis in patients with dementia and parkinsonism. *Movement Disorders*, **22**, 313-18.

Rabkin, J. G., Wagner, G. J. & Rabkin, R. (1999). Testosterone therapy for human immunodeficiency virus-positive men with and without hypogonadism. *Journal of Clinical Psychopharmacology*, **19**(1), 19-27.

Rabkin, J. G., Wagner, G. J. & Rabkin, R. (2000). A double-blind, placebo-controlled trial of testosterone therapy for HIV-positive men with hypogonadal symptoms. *Archives of General Psychiatry*, **57**(2), 141-7; discussion 155-6.

Raine, A., Mellingen, K., Liu, J., Venables, P. & Mednick, S. A. (2003). Effects of environmental enrichment at ages 3-5 years on schizotypal personality and antisocial behavior at ages 17 and 23. *American Journal of Psychiatry*, **196**, 1627-35.

Raistrick, D., Hodgson, R. & Ritson, B. (1999). *Tackling Alcohol Together*. London: Free Association Books.

Rakic, Z., Starcevic, V., Maric, J. & Kelin, K. (1996). The outcome of sex reassignment surgery in Belgrade: 32 patients of both sexes. *Archives of Sexual Behavior*, **25**(5), 515-25.

Rangecroft, M. E. H., Tyrer, S. P. & Berney, T. P. (1997). The use of seclusion and emergency medication in a hospital for people with learning disability. *British Journal of Psychiatry*, **170**, 273-7.

Ranger, M., Tyrer, P., Milošeska, K., Fourie, H., Khaleel, I., North, B. & Barrett, B. (2009). Cost-effectiveness of nidotherapy for comorbid personality disorder and severe mental illness: randomized controlled trial. *Epidemiologia e Psichiatria Sociale*, **18**, 128-36.

Ravndal, E. (2001). An outcome study of a therapeutic community based in the community: a five-year prospective study of drug abusers in Norway. In: B. Rawlings & R. Yates, eds. *Therapeutic Communities*, 4th edn. Philadelphia: Jessica Kingsley Publishers, pp. 224-40.

Rawson, R. A., Huber, A., McCann, M. J. et al. (2002). A comparison of contingency management and cognitive-behavioral approaches during methadone maintenance for cocaine dependence. *Archives of General Psychiatry*, **59**, 817-24.

Rawson, R. A., Marinelli-Casey, P., Anglin, M. D. et al. & Methamphetamine Treatment Project Corporate Authors (2004). A multi-site comparison of psychosocial approaches for the treatment of methamphetamine dependence. *Addiction*, **99**, 708-17.

Reas, D. L. & Grilo, C. M. (2008). Review and meta-analysis of pharmacotherapy for binge-eating disorder. *Obesity (Silver Spring)*, **16**, 2024-38.

Reau, N. R., Senturia, Y. D., Lebailly, S. A. & Christoffel, K. K. (1996). Infant and toddler feeding patterns and problems: normative data and a new direction. *Developmental and Behavioral Pediatrics*, **17**, 149-53.

Rehman, J., Lazer, S., Benet, A. E., Schaefer, L. C. & Melman, A. (1999). The reported sex and surgery satisfactions of 28 postoperative male-to-female transsexual patients. *Archives of Sexual Behavior*, **28**, 71–89.

Reich, D. B., Winternitz, S., Hennen, J., Watts, T. & Stanculescu, C. (2004). A preliminary study of risperidone in the treatment of posttraumatic stress disorder related to childhood abuse in women. *Journal of Clinical Psychiatry*, **65**, 1601–6.

Reichow, B. & Wolery, M. (2009). Comprehensive synthesis of early intensive behavioral interventions for young children with autism based on the UCLA young autism project model. *Journal of Autism and Developmental Disorders*, **39**, 23–41.

Reid, M. J., Webster-Stratton, C. & Hammond, M. (2003). Follow-up of children who received the *Incredible Years* intervention for Oppositional-Defiant Disorder: maintenance and prediction of 2-year outcome. *Behavior Therapy*, **34**, 471–91.

Reinecke, M. A., Ryan, N. E. & DuBois, D. L. (1998). Cognitive-behavioral therapy of depression and depressive symptoms during adolescence: a review and meta-analysis. *Journal of the American Academy of Child and Adolescent Psychiatry*, **37**, 26–34.

Research Unit on Paediatric Psychopharmacology Anxiety Study Group (RUPPS) (2001). Fluvoxamine for the treatment of anxiety disorders in children and adolescents. *New England Journal of Medicine*, **344**, 1279–85.

Resick, P. A., Nishith, P., Weaver, T. L., Astin, M. C. & Feuer, C. A. (2002). A comparison of cognitive-processing therapy with prolonged exposure and a waiting condition for the treatment of chronic posttraumatic stress disorder in female rape victims. *Journal of Consulting Clinical Psychology*, **70**, 867–79.

Resnick, S. G., Rosenheck, R. A. & Lehman, A. F. (2004). An exploratory analysis of correlates of recovery. *Psychiatric Services*, **55**, 540–7.

Resnick, S. G., Fontana, A., Lehman, A. F. & Rosenheck, R. A. (2005). An empirical conceptualization of the recovery orientation. *Schizophrenia Research*, **75**, 119–28.

Ressler, K. J., Rothbaum, B. O., Tannenbaum, L. et al. (2004). Cognitive enhancers as adjuncts to psychotherapy: use of D-cycloserine in phobic individuals to facilitate extinction of fear. *Archives in General Psychiatry*, **61**(11), 1136–44.

Ricca, V., Mannucci, E., Mezzani, B. et al. (1997). Cognitive-behavioral therapy versus combined treatment with group psychoeducation and fluoxetine in bulimic outpatients. *Eating Weight Disorders*, **2**(2), 94–9.

Richters, J. E., Arnold, L. E., Jensen, P. S. et al. (1995). NIMH Collaborative Multisite Multimodal Treatment Study of Children with ADHD: background and rationale. *Journal of the American Academy of Child and Adolescent Psychiatry*, **34**, 987–1000.

Rickels, K., Schweizer, E., Case, W. G. & Greenblatt, D. J. (1990). Long-term therapeutic use of benzodiazepines.

I. Effects of abrupt discontinuation. *Archives of General Psychiatry*, **47**, 899–907.

Rickels, K., Schweizer, E., Weiss, S. Zavodnick, S. (1993). Maintenance drug treatment for panic disorder. II. Short- and long-term outcome after drug taper. *Archives of General Psychiatry*, **50**, 61–8.

Rigotti, N. A. (2002). Treatment of tobacco use and dependence. *New England Journal of Medicine*, **346**, 506–12.

Riper, H., Kramer, J., Smit, F., Conijn, B., Schippers, G. & Cuijpers, P. (2008). Web-based self-help for problem drinkers: a pragmatic randomized trial. *Addiction*, **103**, 218–27.

Risse, S. C., Whitters, A., Burke, J., Chen, S., Scurfield, R. M. & Raskind, M. A. (1990). Severe withdrawal symptoms after discontinuation of alprazolam in eight patients with combat-induced posttraumatic stress disorder. *Journal of Clinical Psychiatry*, **51**, 206–9.

Ritchie, C. W., Ames, D., Clayton, T. & Lai, R. (2004). Metaanalysis of randomized trials of the efficacy and safety of donepezil, galantamine, and rivastigmine for the treatment of Alzheimer disease. *American Journal of Geriatric Psychiatry*, **12**(4), 358–69.

Robb, A. S., Silber, T. J., Orrell-Valente, J. K. et al. (2002). Supplemental nocturnal nasogastric refeeding for better short term outcome in hospitalized adolescent girls with anorexia nervosa. *The American Journal of Psychiatry*, **159**(8), 1347–53.

Roberts, G. & Wolfson, P. (2004). The rediscovery of recovery: open to all. *Advances in Psychiatric Treatment*, **10**, 37–48.

Robertson, B., Karlsson, I., Eriksson, L. et al. (1996). An atypical neuroleptic drug in the treatment of behavioural disturbances and psychotic symptoms in elderly people. *Dementia*, **7**, 142–6.

Robin, A. L., Gilroy, M. & Dennis, A. B. (1998). Treatment of eating disorders in children and adolescents. *Clinical and Psychological Reviews*, **18**, 421–6.

Robin, A. L., Siegel, P. T., Moye, A. W., Gilroy, M., Dennis, A. B. & Sikand, A. (1999). A controlled comparison of family versus individual therapy for adolescents with anorexia nervosa. *Journal of the American Academy of Child and Adolescent Psychiatry*, **38**, 1482–9.

Robinson, G. M., Sellers, E. M. & Janacek, E. (1981). Barbiturate and hypnosedative withdrawal by a multiple oral Phenobarbital loading dose technique. *Clinical and Pharmacological Therapy*, **30**, 71–6.

Rodebaugh, T. L., Holaway, R. M. & Heimberg, R. G. (2004). The treatment of social anxiety disorder. *Clinical Psychology Review*, **24**, 883–908.

Roerig, J. L., Mitchell, J. E., deZwaan, M et al. (2003). The eating disorders medicine cabinet revisited: A clinician's guide to appetite suppressants and diuretics. *International Journal Of Eating Disorders*, **33**, 443–57.

Rogers, S. L., Doody, R. S., Mohs, R. C. Friedhoff, L. T. & the Donepezil Study Group (1998a). Donepezil improves cognition and global function in Alzheimer disease: a 15-week, double blind, placebo-controlled study

Archives of Internal Medicine, **158**, 1021–31.

Rogers, S. L., Farlow, M. R., Doody, R. S., Mohs, R., Friedhoff, L. T. & the Donepezil Study Group (1998b). A 24-week, double-blind, placebo-controlled trial of donepezil in patients with Alzheimer's disease. *Neurology*, **50**, 136–45.

Rohde, L. A., Barbosa, G., Polanczyk, G. et al. (2001). Factor and latent class analysis of DSM-IV ADHD symptoms in a school sample of Brazilian adolescents. *Journal of the American Academy of Child and Adolescent Psychiatry*, **40**, 711–18.

Romeo, R., Knapp, M., Tyrer, P., Crawford, M. & Oliver-Africano, P. (2009). The treatment of challenging behaviour in intellectual disabilities: cost-effectiveness analysis. *Journal of Intellectual Disabilities Research*, **53**, 633–43.

Roozen, H. G., Boulogne, J. J., van Tulder, M. W., van den Brink, W., De Jong, C. A. & Kerkhof, A. J. (2004). A systematic review of the effectiveness of the community reinforcement approach in alcohol, cocaine and opioid addiction. *Drug and Alcohol Dependence*, **74**, 1–13.

Rose, S., Bisson, J. & Wessely, S. (2003). A systematic review of single-session psychological interventions ('debriefing') following trauma. *Psychotherapy and Psychosomatics*, **72**, 176–84.

Rosen, G. M., Lilienfeld, S. O., Frueh, C., McHugh, P. R. & Spitzer, R. L. (2010). Reflections on PTSD's future in DSM-V. *British Journal of Psychiatry*, **197**, 343–4.

Rosenberg, P. B., Drye, L. T., Martin, B. K., et al.; DIADS-2 Research Group (2010). Sertraline for the treatment of depression in Alzheimer disease. *American Journal of Geriatric Psychiatry*, **18**, 136–45.

Rosenvinge, J. H. & Klusmeier, A. K. (2000). Treatment for eating disorders from a patient satisfaction perspective: a Norwegian replication of a British study. *European Eating Disorders Review*, **8**, 293–300.

Ross, M. W. & Need, J. A. (1989). Effects of adequacy of gender reassignment surgery on psychological adjustment: a follow-up of fourteen male-to-female patients. *Archives of Sexual Behavior*, **18**, 145–53.

Rosselló, J. & Bernal, G. (1999). The efficacy of cognitive-behavioral and interpersonal treatments for depression in Puerto Rican adolescents. *Journal of Consulting & Clinical Psychology*, **67**, 734–45.

Rothbaum, B. O., Astin, M. C. & Marsteller, F. (2005). Prolonged exposure therapy versus Eye Movement Desensitization and Reprocessing (EMDR) for PTSD rape victims. *Journal of Traumatic Stress*, **18**, 607–16.

Rotunda, R. J., O'Farrell, T. J., Murphy, M. & Babey, S. H. (2008). Behavioral couples therapy for comorbid substance use disorders and combat-related post-traumatic stress disorder among male veterans: an initial evaluation. *Addictive Behaviors*, **33**, 180–7.

Rounsaville, B. J. & Carroll, K. M. (1997). Individual psychotherapy. In: J. H. Lowinsohn, P. Ruiz & R. B. Millman, eds. *Comprehensive Textbook of Substance Abuse*, 3rd edn. New York: Williams and Wilkins, pp. 430–9.

Royal College of Psychiatrists (2005). *Third Report of the Royal College of Psychiatrists' Special Committee on ECT*. London: Royal College of Psychiatrists.

Roy-Byrne, P. P. & Cowley, D. (2002). Pharmacologic treatments for panic disorder, generalized anxiety disorder, specific phobia and social anxiety disorders. In: P. E. Nathan & J. Gorman, eds. *A Guide to Treatments That Work*. New York: Oxford University Press, pp. 337–65.

Rubin, E. H., Drevets, W. C. & Burke, W. J. et al. (1988). The nature of psychotic symptoms in senile dementia of the Alzheimer type. *Journal of Geriatric Psychiatry and Neurology*, **1**, 16–20.

Rubio, G., Manzanares, J., Lopez-Munoz, F. et al. (2002). Naltrexone improves outcome of a controlled drinking program. *Journal of Substance Abuse Treatment*, **23**, 361–6.

Rudnick, A. (2001). Ethics of ECT for children. *Journal of the American Academy of Child and Adolescence Psychiatry*, **40**, 387.

Ruggiero, G.M., Laini, V, Mauri, M.C., et al (2001). A single blind comparison of amisulpride, fluoxetine and clomipramine in the treatment of restricting anorectis. *Progress in Neuropsychopharmaclolgy & Biological Psychiatry*, **25**, 1049–59

Ruma, P. R., Burke, R. V. & Thompson, R. W. (1996). Group parent training: is it effective for children of all ages? *Behavior Therapy*, **27**, 159–69.

Rund, B. R. (1994). The relationship between psychosocial and cognitive functioning in schizophrenic patients and expressed emotion and communication deviance in their parents. *Acta Psychiatrica Scandinavica*, **90**,133–40.

Rush, A. J., Marangell, L. B., Sackeim, H. A. et al. (2005). Vagus nerve stimulation for treatment-resistant depression: a randomized, controlled acute phase trial. *Biological Psychiatry*, **58**, 347–54.

Rush, A. J., Trivedi, M. H., Wisniewski, S. R. et al. (2006a). Bupropion-Sr, sertraline, or venlafaxine-XR after failure of SSRIs for depression. *New England Journal of Medicine*, **354**(12), 1231–42.

Rush, A. J., Trivedi, M. H., Wisniewski, S. R. A. A. et al. (2006b). Acute and longer-term outcomes in depressed outpatients requiring one or several treatment steps: a STAR*D report. *American Journal of Psychiatry*, 2006, **163**, 1905–17.

Russell, G. F., Szmukler, G. L., Dare, C. & Eisler, I. (1987). An evaluation of family therapy in anorexia nervosa and bulimia nervosa. *Archives of General Psychiatry*, **44**, 1047–56.

Ruttenber, A. J., Lawler-Heavner, J., Yin, M., Wetli, C. V., Hearn, W. L. & Mash, D. C. (1997). Fatal excited delirium following cocaine use: epidemiologic findings provide new evidence for mechanisms of cocaine toxicity. *Journal of Forensic Science* **42**, 25–31.

Rutter, M. & Sonuga-Barke, E. J. (2010) Overview of findings from the ERA study, inferences, and research implications. *Monographs of the Society fo Research in Child Development*, **75** 212–29.

Rutter, M. and the English and Romanian Adoptees (ERA) study team (1998) Developmental catch-up, and defici following adoption after severe globa early privation. *Journal of Child Psychology and Psychiatry*, **39**, 465–76.

Rynn, M. A., Siqueland, L. & Rickels, K. (2001). Placebo-controlled trial of sertraline in the treatment of children with generalized anxiety disorder. *The American Journal of Psychiatry*, **158**, 2008–14.

Sachdev, P. S., McBride, R., Loo, C. K. et al. (2001). Right versus left prefrontal transcranial magnetic stimulation for obsessive-compulsive disorder: a preliminary investigation. *Journal of Clinical Psychiatry*, **62**, 981–4.

Sackeim, H. A., Rush, A. J., George, M. S. et al. (2001). Vagus nerve stimulation (VNS) for treatment-resistant depression: efficacy, side effects, and predictors of outcome. *Neuropsychopharmacology*, **25** (5), 713–28.

Sajaniemi, N., Mäkelä, J., Salokorpi, T., von Wendt, L., Hämäläinen, T. & Hakamies-Blomqvist, L. (2001). Cognitive performance and attachment patterns at four years of age in extremely low birth weight infants after early intervention. *European Child and Adolescent Psychiatry*, **10**, 122–9.

Salzer, M. S., Bickman, L. & Lambert, E. W. (1999). Dose–effect relationship in children's psychotherapy services. *Journal of Consulting and Clinical Psychology*, **67**, 228–38.

SAMHSA, National Survey On Drug Use And Health (2002). [Computer file]. 2nd ICPSR version. 2004, Research Triangle Institute [producer]. Ann Arbor, MI: Inter-university Consortium for Political and Social Research [distributor]: Research Triangle Park, NC.

SAMHSA (2003). *SAMHSA Report to Congress on the Prevention and Treatment of Co-occurring Substance Abuse Disorders and Mental Disorders.* Washington DC: US Department of Health and Human Services.

Sanchez-Craig, M., Cappell, H., Busto, U. & Kay, G. (1987). Cognitive-behavioural treatment for benzodiazepine dependence: a comparison of gradual versus abrupt cessation of drug intake. *British Journal of Addiction*, **82**, 1317–27.

Sanders, M. R., Markie-Dadds, C., Tully, L. A. & Bor, W. (2000). The Triple P-Positive Parenting Program: a comparison of enhanced, standard, and self-directed behavioral family intervention for parents of children with early onset conduct problems. *Journal of Consulting and Clinical Psychology*, **68**, 624–40.

Sano, M., Ernesto, C., Thomas, R. G., Klauber, M. R. et al. (1997). A controlled trial of selegiline, alpha-tocopherol, or both as treatment for Alzheimer's disease: The Alzheimer's Disease Cooperative Study. *New England Journal of Medicine*, **336**, 1216–22.

Satel, S. L. & Edell, W. S. (1991). Cocaine-induced paranoia and psychosis proneness. *American Journal of Psychiatry*, **148**, 1708–11.

Satterfield, J. H., Satterfield, B. & Cantwell, D. P. (1981). Three-year multi-modality study of 100 hyperactive boys. *Journal of Pediatrics*, **98**, 650–5.

Saunders, B., Wilkinson, C. & Phillips, M. (1995). The impact of a brief motivational intervention with opiate users attending a methadone programme. *Addiction*, **90**, 415–24.

Schachar, R., Tannock, R., Cunningham, C. & Corkum, P. (1997). Behavioral, situational, and temporal effects of treatment of ADHD with methylphenidate. *Journal of the American Academy of Child and Adolescent Psychiatry*, **36**, 754–63.

Schachter, H. M., Pham, B., King, J., Langford, S. & Moher, D. (2001). How efficacious and safe is short-acting methylphenidate for the treatment of attention-deficit disorder in children and adolescents? A meta-analysis. *Canadian Medical Association Journal*, **165**, 1475–88.

Schaeffer, C. M. & Borduin, C. M. (2005). Long-term follow-up to a randomized clinical trial of multisystemic therapy with serious and violent juvenile offenders. *Journal of Consulting & Clinical Psychology*, **73**, 445–53.

Schmidt, P. J., Nieman, L., Danaceau, M. A. et al. (2000). Estrogen replacement in perimenopause-related depression: a preliminary report. *American Journal of Obstetrics & Gynecology*, **183**(2), 414–20.

Schmidt, U., Lee, S., Beecham, J. et al. (2007). A randomized controlled trial of family therapy and cognitive behavior therapy guided self-care for adolescents with bulimia nervosa and related conditions. *American Journal of Psychiatry*, **164**, 591–8.

Schmidt, U., Andiappan, M., Gover, M. et al. (2008). Randomised controlled trial of CD-ROM-based cognitive-behavioural self-care for bulimia nervosa. *British Journal of Psychiatry*, **193**, 493–500.

Schneider, L. S. & Dagerman, K. S. (2004). Psychosis of Alzheimer's disease: clinical characteristics and history. *Journal of Psychiatric Research*, **38**, 105–11.

Schneider, L. S., Pollock, V. E. & Lyness, S. A. (1990). A meta-analysis of controlled trials of neuroleptic treatment in dementia. *Journal of the American Geriatrics Society*, **38**, 553–63.

Schneider, N. G., Olmstead, R., Mody, F. V. et al. (1995). Efficacy of a nicotine nasal spray in smoking cessation: a placebo-controlled, double-blind trial. *Addiction*, **90**, 1671–82.

Schneider, N. G., Olmstead, R., Nilsson, F., Mody, F. V., Franzon, M. & Doan, K. (1996). Efficacy of a nicotine inhaler in smoking cessation: a double-blind, placebo controlled trial. *Addiction*, **91**, 1293–306.

Schneider, W. N., Drew-Cates, J., Wong, T. M. et al. (1999). Cognitive and behavioural efficacy of amantadine in acute traumatic brain injury: an initial double-blind placebo-controlled study. *Brain Injury*, **13**, 863–72.

Schopler, E. (1997). Implementation of TEACCH philosophy. In: D. J. Cohen & F. R. Volkmar, eds. *Handbook of Autism and Pervasive Developmental Disorders*, 2nd edn. New York: John Wiley, pp. 767–98.

Schottenfeld, R. S., Pakes, J. R., Oliveto, A. Ziedonis, D. & Kosten, T. R. (1997). Buprenorphine vs. methadone maintenance treatment for concurrent opioid dependence and cocaine abuse. *Archives in General Psychiatry*, **54** 713–20.

Schover, L. R. & Leiblum, S. R. (1994). Commentary: the stagnation of se therapy. *Journal of Psychology and Human Sexuality*, **6**, 5–30.

Schwartz, T. L. & Masand, P. D. (2000). Treatment of delirium with quetiapine. Primary Care Companion. *Journal of Clinical Psychiatry*, **2**, 10–12.

Schweizer, E., Rickels, K., Case, W. G. & Greenblatt, D. J. (1991). Carbamazepine treatment in patients discontinuing long-term benzodiazepine therapy: effects on withdrawal severity and outcome. *Archives of General Psychiatry*, **48**, 448–52.

Scott, J. & Clare, L. (2003). Do people with dementia benefit from psychological interventions offered on a group basis? *Clinical Psychology and Psychotherapy*, **10**, 186–96.

Scott, S., Spender, Q., Doolan, M., Jacobs, B. & Aspland, H. (2001). Multicentre controlled trial of parenting groups for childhood antisocial behaviour in clinical practice. *British Medical Journal*, **323**, 1–7.

Scotti, J. R., Evans, I. M., Meyer, L. H. et al. (1991). A meta-analysis of intervention research with problem behavior: treatment validity and standards of practice. *American Journal on Mental Retardation*, **93**, 233–56.

Scottish Intercollegiate Guidelines Network (2003). *The Management of Harmful Drinking and Alcohol Dependence in Primary Care, a National Clinical Guideline*. Edinburgh: Royal College of Physicians.

Segal, R. (2001). Hypnosis in the treatment of an eating disorder. *Australian Journal of Clinical & Experimental Hypnosis*, **29** (1), 26–36.

Segal, Z. V., Williams, J. M. G. & Teasdale, J. D. (2002). *Mindfulness-Based Cognitive Therapy for Depression*. New York: Guilford Press.

Seida, J. K., Ospina, M. B., Karkhaneh, M., Hartling, L., Smith, V. & Clark, B. (2009). Systematic reviews of psychosocial interventions for autism: an umbrella review. *Developmental Medicine and Child Neurology*, **51**, 95–104.

Seidman, S. N., Spatz, E., Rizzo, C. & Roose, S. P. (2001). Testosterone replacement therapy for hypogonadal men with major depressive disorder: a randomized, placebo-controlled clinical trial. *Journal of Clinical Psychiatry*, **62** (6), 406–12.

Seifer, R., Sameroff, A. J., Baldwin, C. P. & Baldwin, A. L. (1992). Child and family factors that ameliorate risk between 4 and 13 years of age. *Journal of the American Academy of Child & Adolescent Psychiatry*, **31**, 893–903.

Seivewright, H., Green, J., Salkovskis, P., Barrett, B., Nur, U. & Tyrer, P. (2008). Randomised controlled trial of cognitive behaviour therapy in the treatment of health anxiety in a genitourinary medicine clinic. *British Journal of Psychiatry*, **192**, 332–7.

Selvini-Palazzoli, M. (1974). *Self Starvation: From the Intrapsychic to the Transpersonal Approach to Anorexia Nervosa*. London: Chaucer Publishing.

Serfaty, M. & McCluskey, S. (1998). Compulsory treatment of anorexia nervosa and the moribund patient. *European Eating Disorders Review*, **6**(1), 27–37.

Serfaty, M. A., Turkington, D., Heap, M., Ledsham, L. & Jolley, E. (1999).

Cognitive therapy versus dietary counseling in the outpatient treatment of anorexia nervosa: effects of the treatment phase. *European Eating Disorders Review*, **7**, 334–50.

Shaner, A., Eckman, T., Roberts, L. & Fuller, T. (2003). Feasibility of a skills training approach to reduce substance dependence among individuals with schizophrenia. *Psychiatric Services*, **54**, 1287–9.

Shanti, C. M. & Lucas, C. E. (2003). Cocaine and the critical care challenge. *Critical Care Medicine*, **31**, 1851–9.

Shapiro, D. A., Barkham, M., Rees, A., Hardy, G. E., Reynolds, S. & Startup, M. (1994). Effects of treatment duration and severity of depression on the effectiveness of cognitive-behavioral and psychodynamic-interpersonal psychotherapy. *Journal of Consulting and Clinical Psychology*, **62**(3), 522–34.

Shapiro, J. R., Berkman, N. D., Brownley, K. A. et al. (2007). Bulimia nervosa treatment: a systematic review of randomized controlled trials. *International Journal of Eating Disorders*, **40**, 321–36.

Shaw, P., Sporn, A., Gogtay, N. et al. (2006). Childhood-onset schizophrenia: a double-blind, randomized clozapine-olanzapine comparison. *Archives of General Psychiatry*, **63**, 721–30.

Shea, S., Turgay, A., Carroll, A. et al. (2004). Risperidone in the treatment of disruptive behavioural symptoms in children with autistic and other pervasive developmental disorders. *Pediatrics*, **114**, 634–41.

Sheehan, D. V., Ballenger, J. & Jacobsen, G. (1980). Treatment of endogenous anxiety with phobic, hysterical, and hypochondriacal symptoms. *Archives of General Psychiatry*, **37**, 51–9.

Shelton, R. C., Williamson, D. J., Corya, S. A. et al. (2005). Olanzapine/Fluoxetine combination for treatment-resistant depression: a controlled study of SSRI and nortriptyline resistance. *Journal of Clinical Psychiatry*, **66**, 1289–97.

Shiffman, S., Dresler, C. M., Hajek, P., Gilburt, S. J. A., Targett, D. A. & Strahs, K. R. (2002). Efficacy of a nicotine lozenge for smoking cessation. *Archives of Internal Medicine*, **162**, 1267.

Shifren, J. L. (2004). The role of androgens in female sexual dysfunction. *Mayo Clinic Proceedings*, **79** (4 Suppl), S19–24.

Shifren, J. L., Braunstein, G. D., Simon, J. A. et al. (2000). Transdermal testosterone treatment in women with impaired sexual function after oophorectomy. *New England Journal of Medicine*, **434**, 682–8.

Shirk, S. R. (2001). Development and cognitive therapy. *Journal of Cognitive Psychotherapy*, **15**, 155–63.

Sikich, L., Frazier, J., McClellan, J. et al. (2008). Findings from the Treatment of Early-Onset Schizophrenia Spectrum Disorders (TEOSS) study. *American Journal of Psychiatry*, **165**, 1420–31.

Silagy, C., Mant, D., Fowler, G. & Lodge, M. (1994). Meta-analysis on efficacy of nicotine replacement therapies in smoking cessation. *Lancet*, **343**, 139–42.

Silagy, C., Lancaster, T., Stead, L., Mant, D. & Fowler, G. (2002). Nicotine replacement for smoking cessation. *Cochrane Database of Systematic Reviews*. Oxford: Update Software Ltd.

Silk, K. R. & Jibson, M. D. (2010). Personality disorders. In: A. J. Rothschild, ed. *The Evidence-Based Guide to Antipsychotic*

Medications. Washington, DC: American Psychiatric Publishing, Inc., pp. 101-24.

Silva, R. R., Dinohra, M. D., Munoz, M. D. & Alpert, M. (1996). Carbamazepine use in children and adolescents with features of attention-deficit hyperactivity disorder: a meta-analysis. *Journal of the American Academy of Child and Adolescent Psychiatry*, **35**, 352-8.

Silverman, K., Higgins, S. T., Brooner, R. K. et al. (1996). Sustained cocaine abstinence in methadone maintenance patients through voucher-based reinforcement therapy. *Archives of General Psychiatry*, **53**, 409-15.

Simons, A. D., Murphy, G. E., Levine, J. L. & Wetzel, R. D. (1986). Cognitive therapy and pharmacotherapy for depression. *Archives of General Psychiatry*, **43**, 43-8.

Sienaert, P. (2011). What we have learned about electroconvulsive therapy and its relevance for the practising psychiatrist. *Canadian Journal of Psychiatry*, **56**, 5-12.

Sipahimalani, A. & Masand, P. S. (1998). Olanzapine in the treatment of delirium. *Psychosomatics*, **39**, 422-30.

Slattery, J., Chick, J., Cochrane, M. et al. (2003). *Prevention of Relapse in Alcohol Dependence. Health Technology Assessment Report 3.* Glasgow: Health Technology Board for Scotland.

Small, J. G., Klapper, M. H., Kellams, J. J. et al. (1988). Electroconvulsive treatment compared with lithium in the management of manic states. *Archives in General Psychology*, **45**, 727-32.

Smelson, D. A., Dixon, L., Craig, T., Remolina, S., Batki, S., Niv, N. & Owen, R. (2008). Pharmacological treatment of schizophrenia and co-occurring substance use disorders. *CNS Drugs*, **22**, 903-16.

Smelson, D., Kalman, D., Losonczy, M. F. et al. (2010). A brief treatment engagement intervention for individuals with co-occurring mental illness and substance use disorders: results of a randomized clinical trial. Community Mental Health Journal. DOI:10.1007/s10297-010-9346-9

Smith, B. H., Waschbusch, D. A., Willoughby, M. T. & Evans, S. (2000). The efficacy, safety, and practicality of treatments for adolescents with attention-deficit/hyperactivity disorder (ADHD). *Clinical Child and Family Psychology Review*, **3**, 243-67.

Smith, D. E. & Wesson, D. R. (1971). A phenobarbital technique for the withdrawal of barbiturate abuse. *Archives of General Psychiatry*, **24**, 56-60.

Smith, D. E. & Wesson, D. R. (1985). Benzodiazepine dependence syndromes. In: D. E. Smith & D. R. Wesson, eds. *The Benzodiazepines: Current Standards for Medical Practice.* Lancaster, UK: MTP Press, pp. 235-48.

Smith, G. J., Amner, G., Johnsson, P. & Franck, A. (1997). Alexithymia in patients with eating disorders: an investigation using a new projective technique. *Perceptual and Motor Skills*, **85**, 247-56.

Smits, J., Conall, M. & Otto, M. W. (2006). Combining cognitive-behavioral therapy and pharmacotherapy for the treatment of panic disorder. *Journal of Cognitive Psychotherapy*, **20**(1), 75-84.

So, C. C. & Wong, K. F. (2002). *The Brain and the Inner World: An Introduction to*

Neuroscience of Subjective Experience. London: Karnac Press.

Soares, B. F. O., Lima, M. S., Reisse, R. A. A. P. & Farrell M. (2002). Dopamine agonists for cocaine dependence (Cochrane Review). In: *The Cochrane Library*, **2**. Oxford: Update Software.

Soares, C. N., Almeida, O. P., Joffe, H. & Cohen, L. S. (2001). Efficacy of estradiol for the treatment of depressive disorders in perimenopausal women: a double-blind, randomized, placebo-controlled trial. *Archives of General Psychiatry*, **58** (6), 529–34.

Sobell, M. B. & Sobell, L. C. (2000). Stepped care as a heuristic approach to the treatment of alcohol problems. *Journal of Consulting and Clinical Psychology*, **68**, 573–9.

Sofuoglu, M. & Kosten, T. R. (2006). Emerging pharmacological strategies in the fight against cocaine addiction. *Expert Opinion on Emerging Drugs*, **11** (1), 91–8.

Sofuoglu, M., Dudish-Poulsen, S., Brown, S. B. & Hatsukami, D. K. (2003). Association of cocaine withdrawal symptoms with more severe dependence and enhanced subjective response to cocaine. *Drug and Alcohol Dependence*, **69**, 273–82.

Sokolski, K. N., Conney, J. C. et al. (2004). Once-daily high-dose pindolol for SSRI-refractory depression. *Psychiatry Research*, **125**(2), 81–6.

Solomon, S. M. & Kirby, D. F. (1990). The refeeding syndrome: a review. *Journal of Parenteral and Enteral Nutrition*, **14**, 90–7.

Sorenson, J. L. & Copeland, A. L. (2000). Drug abuse treatment as an HIV prevention strategy: a review. *Drug and Alcohol Dependence*, **59**, 17–31.

Spector, A., Orrell, M., Davies, S. & Woods, R. T. (2000). Reminiscence therapy for dementia. *Cochrane Database of Systematic Reviews*, **2**, CD001120.

Spector, A., Orrell, M., Davies, S. & Woods, R. (2003). Reminiscence therapy for dementia. *Cochrane Database of Systematic Reviews*, 3. Oxford: Update Softward Ltd.

Spence, S. H., Donovan, C. & Brechman-Toussaint, M. (2000). The treatment of childhood social phobia: the effectiveness of a social skills training-based cognitive-behavioural intervention, with and without parental involvement. *Journal of Child Psychology and Psychiatry, and Allied Disciplines*, **41**, 713–26.

Spencer, S.-J., Rutter, D. & Tyrer, P. (2010). Integration of nidotherapy into the management of mental illness and anti-social personality: a qualitative study. *International Journal of Social Psychiatry*, **56**, 50–9.

Spencer, T., Biederman, J., Wilens, T. Harding, M., O'Donnell, D. & Griffin, S. (1996). Pharmacotherapy of attention deficit hyperactivity disorder across the life cycle. *Journal of the American Academy of Child and Adolescent Psychiatry*, **35**, 409–32.

Spencer, T., Heiligenstein, J. H. Biederman, J. et al. (2002). Results from 2 proof-of-concept, placebo-controlled studies of atomoxetine in children with attention-deficit/hyperactivity disorder. *Journal of Clinical Psychiatry*, **63**, 1140–7.

Spiegel, D. A., Bruce, T. J., Gregg, S. F. & Nuzzarello, A. (1994). Does cognitive behaviour therapy assist slow-taper alprazolam discontinuation in panic disorder? *American Journal of Psychiatry*, **151**, 876–81.

Spivak, K., Sanchez-Craig, M. & Davila, R. (1994). Assisting problem drinkers to change on their own: effect of specific and non-specific advice. *Addiction*, **89**, 1135–42.

Srisurapanont, M. & Jarusuraisin, N. (2003). Opioid antagonists for alcohol dependence. In: *The Cochrane Library*. Chichester: John Wiley & Sons Ltd.

Srisurapanont, M., Jarusuraisin, N. & Kittirattanapaiboon, P. (2002). Treatment for amphetamine dependence and abuse (Cochrane Review). In: *The Cochrane Library*, 2. Oxford: Update Software.

Stams, G.-J. J. M., Juffer, F., van Ijzendoorn, M. H. & Hoksbergen, R. A. C. (2001). Attachment-based intervention in adoptive families in infancy and children's development at age 7: two follow-up studies. *British Journal of Developmental Psychology*, **19**, 159–80.

Stangier, U., Heidenreich, T., Peitz, M., Lauterbach, W. & Clark, D. M. (2003). Cognitive therapy for social phobia: individual versus group treatment. *Behaviour Research & Therapy*, **41**, 991–1007.

Stanislav, S. W., Fabre, T., Crismon, M. L. et al. (1994). Buspirone's efficacy in organic-induced aggression. *Journal of Clinical Psychopharmacology*, **14**, 126–30.

Staring, A. B. P., Van der Gaag, M., Koopmans, G. T et al. (2010). Treatment adherence therapy in people with psychotic disorders: randomised controlled trial. *British Journal of Psychiatry*, **197**, December issue.

Stefano, S. C., Bacaltchuk, J., Blay, S. L. & Appolinario, J. C. (2008). Antidepressants in short-term treatment of binge eating disorder: systematic review and meta-analysis. *Eating Behavior*, **9**, 129–36.

Stein, M. B. & Kean, Y. M. (2000). Disability and quality of life in social phobia: epidemiologic findings. *American Journal of Psychiatry*, **157**, 1606–13.

Stein, B. D., Jaycox, L., Kataoka, S. et al. (2003). A mental health intervention for schoolchildren exposed to violence: a randomised controlled trial. *Journal of the American Medical Association*, **290**, 603–11.

Stein, D. J., Cameron, A., Amrein, R., Montgomery, S. A. & Moclobemide Social Phobia Clinical Study Group (2002). Moclobemide is effective and well tolerated in the long-term pharmacotherapy of social anxiety disorder with or without comorbid anxiety disorder. *International Clinical Psychopharmacology*, **17**, 161–70.

Stein, D. J., Westenberg, H. G., Yang, H., Li, D. & Barbato, L. M. (2003). Fluvoxamine CR in the long-term treatment of social anxiety disorder: the 12- to 24-week extension phase of a multi-centre, randomized, placebo-controlled trial. *International Journal of Neuropsychopharmacology*, **6**, 317–23.

Stein, M., Tiefer, L. & Melman, A. (1990). Follow-up observations of operated male-to-female transsexuals. *Journal of Urology*, **143**, 1188–92.

Stein, M. B., Norton, G. R., Walker, J. R., Chartier, M. J. & Graham, R. (2000). Do SSRIs enhance the efficacy of very brief cognitive behavioral therapy for panic disorder? A pilot study. *Psychiatry Research*, **94**, 191–200.

Stein, M. B., Pollack, M. H., Brystritsky, A., Kelsey, J. E. & Mangano, R. M. (2005). Efficacy of low and higher dose extended-release venlafaxine in generalized social anxiety disorder: a 6-month randomized controlled trial. *Psychopharmacology (Berlin)*, **177**, 280–8.

Stephens, R. S., Roffman, R. A. & Curtin, L. (2000). Comparison of extended versus brief treatments for marijuana use. *Journal of Consulting and Clinical Psychology*, **68**, 898–908.

Stewart, R. (2002). The interface between cerebrovascular disease, depression and dementia. In: E. Chiu, D. Ames & C. Katona, eds. *Vascular Disease and Affective Disorders*. London: Martin Dunitz Publishing.

Stice, E. & Shaw, H. (2004). Eating disorder prevention programs: a meta-analytic review. *Psychology Bulletin*, **130**, 206–07.

Stirman, S. W., DeRubeis, R. J., Crits-Christoph, P. & Brody, P. E. (2003). Are samples in randomized controlled trials of psychotherapy representative of community outpatients? A new methodology and initial findings. *Journal of Consulting and Clinical Psychology*, **71**, 963–72.

Stoffers, J., Vollm, B. A., Rucker, G., Timmer, A., Huband, N. & Lieb, K. (2010). Pharmacological interventions for borderline personality disorder. *Cochrane Database of Systematic Reviews*, **6**, CD005653.

Strawn, J. R., Keeshin, B. R., DelBello, M. P. et al. (2010). Psychopharmacologic treatment of post traumatic stress disorder in children and adolescents: a review. *Journal of Clinical Psychiatry*, **71**, 932–41.

Street, J. S., Clark, W. S., Gannon, K. S. et al. (2000). Olanzapine treatment of psychotic and behavioral symptoms in patients with Alzheimer disease in nursing care facilities: a double-blind, randomized, placebo-controlled trial. The HGEU Study Group. *Archives of General Psychiatry*, **57**, 968–76.

Striegel-Moore, R. H., Leslie, D., Petrill, S. A., Garvin, V. & Rosenheck, R. A. (2000). One-year use and cost of inpatient and outpatient services among female and male patients with an eating disorder: evidence from a national database of health insurance claims. *International Journal of Eating Disorders*, **27**, 381–9.

Substance Abuse and Mental Health Services Administration (SAMHSA) (2008). Results from the 2007 National Survey on Drug Use and Health national findings. Rockville, MD: Department of Health and Human Services, Substance Abuse and Mental Health Services Administration.

Sultzer, D. L., Gray, K. F., Gunay, I., Berisford, M. A. & Mahler, M. E. (1997). A double-blind comparison of trazodone and haloperidol for treatment of agitation in patients with dementia. *American Journal of Geriatric Psychiatry*, **5**, 60–9.

Sumathipala, A., Siribaddana, S., Abeysingha, M. R., et al. (2008). Cognitive-behavioural therapy v. structured care for medically unexplained symptoms: randomised controlled trial. *British Journal of Psychiatry*, **193**, 51-9.

Sundgot-Borgen, J., Rosenvinge, J. H., Bahr, R. & Schneider, L. S. (2002). The effect of exercise, cognitive therapy, and nutritional counseling in treating bulimia nervosa. *Medicine & Science in Sports & Exercise*, **34**(2), 190-5.

Susser, E., Valencia, E., Conover, S., Felix, A., Wei-Yann, T. & Wyatt, R. (1997). Preventing recurrent homelessness among mentally ill men: a "critical time" intervention after discharge from a shelter. *American Journal of Public Health*, **87**, 256.

Swinson, R., Cox, B. & Woszczyna, C. (1992). Use of medical services and treatment for panic disorder with agoraphobia and for social phobia. *Canadian Medical Association Journal*, **147**, 878-83.

Szabo, C. P. & Green, K. (2002). Hospitalized anorexics and resistance training: impact on body composition and psychological well-being: a preliminary study. *Eating and Weight Disorders*, **7**(4), 293-7.

Szekely, C. A., Thorne, J. E., Zandi, P. P. et al. (2004). Nonsteroidal anti-inflammatory drugs for the prevention of Alzheimer's disease: a systematic review. *Neuroepidemiology*, **23**, 159-69.

Taieb, O., Cohen, D., Mazet, P. et al. (2000). Adolescents' experience with ECT. *Journal of the American Academy of Child and Adolescence Psychiatry*, **39**, 943-4.

Tam, S. W., Worcel, M. & Wyllie, M. (2001). Yohimbine: a clinical review. *Pharmacology and Therapeutics*, **91**, 215-43.

Taragano, F. E., Lysketos, C. G., Mangone, C. A. et al. (1997). A double-blind, randomized, fixed-dose trial of fluoxetine vs. amitryptiline in the treatment of major depression complicating Alzheimer's disease. *Psychosomatics*, **38**, 246-52.

Tariot, P. N., Erb, R., Leibovici, A. et al. (1994). Carbamazepine treatment of agitation in nursing home patients with dementia: a preliminary study. *Journal of the American Geriatrics Society*, **42**, 1160-6.

Tariot, P. N., Erb, R., Podgorski, C. A. et al. (1998). Efficacy and tolerability of carbamazepine therapy followed by further carbamazepine treatment in patients with dementia. *Journal of Clinical Psychiatry*, **60**, 684-9.

Tariot, P. N., Cummings, J. L., Katz, I. R. et al. (2001). A randomized, double-blind, placebo-controlled study of the efficacy and safety of donepezil in patients with Alzheimer's disease in the nursing home setting. *Journal of the American Geriatrics Society*, **49**, 1590-9.

Tasca, G. A., Flynn, C. & Bissada, H. (2002). Comparison of group climate in an eating disorders partial hospital group and a psychiatric partial hospital group. *International Journal of Group Psychotherapy*, **52**, 409-17.

Taub, E., Steiner, S. S., Weingarten, E. & Walton, K. G. (1994). Effectiveness of broad spectrum approaches to relapse prevention in severe alcoholism: a long-term, randomized, controlled trial of Transcendental Meditation, EMG biofeedback and electronic neurotherapy. *Alcoholism Treatment Quarterly*, 11, 187-220.

Tauscher, J., Tauscher-Wisniewski, D. & Kasper, S. (2000). Treatment of patients with delirium. *American Journal of Psychiatry*, 157, 1711.

Taylor, E., Dopfner, M., Sergeant, J. et al. (2004). European clinical guidelines for hyperkinetic disorder - first upgrade. *European Child and Adolescent Psychiatry*, 13 (Suppl. 1), 17-30.

Taylor, J. L., Novaco, R. W., Gillmer, B. & Thorne, I. (2002). Cognitive-behavioural treatment of anger intensity among offenders with intellectual disabilities. *Journal of Applied Research in Intellectual Disabilities*, 15, 151-65.

Teasdale, J. D., Segal, Z. V., Williams, J. M. G., Ridgeway, V. A., Sousby, J. M. & Lau, M. A. (2000). Prevention of relapse/recurrence in major depression by mindfulness-based cognitive therapy. *Journal of Consulting and Clinical Psychology*, 68(4), 615-23.

Tenneij, N. H., van Megen, H. J., Denys, D. A. & Westenberg, H. G. (2005). Behavior therapy augments response of patients with obsessive-compulsive disorder responding to drug treatment. *Journal of Clinical Psychiatry*, 66, 1169-75.

Terman, J. S., Terman, M., Lo, E. S. & Cooper, T. B. (2001). Circadian time of morning light administration and therapeutic response in winter depression. *Archives of General Psychiatry*, 58(1), 69-75.

Terman, M., Terman, J. S., Quitkin, F. M., McGrath, P. J., Stewart, J. W. &

Rafferty, B. (1989). Light therapy for seasonal affective disorder: a review of efficacy. *Neuropsychopharmacology*, 2(1), 1-22.

Terman, M., Amira, L., Terman, J. S. & Ross, D. C. (1996). Predictors of response and nonresponse to light treatment for winter depression. *American Journal of Psychiatry*, 153(11), 1423-9.

Thase, M. E., Entsuah, A. R. & Rudolph, R. L. (2001). Remission rates during treatment with venlafaxine or selective serotonin reuptake inhibitors. *British Journal of Psychiatry*, 178, 234-41.

The TADS Team (2007). The treatment for adolescents with depression study (TADS): Long-term effectiveness and safety outcomes. *Archives of General Psychiatry*, 64, 1132-44.

Thompson, A., Shaw, M., Harrison, G., Verne, J., Ho, D. & Gunnell, D. (2004). Patterns of hospital admission for adult psychiatric illness in England: analysis of Hospital Episode Statistics data. *British Journal of Psychiatry*, 185, 334-41.

Thomsen, P. H. (1998). Obsessive-compulsive disorder in children and adolescents: clinical guidelines. *European Child and Adolescent Psychiatry* 7, 1-11.

Thorén, P., Asberg, M., Cronholm, B., Jörnestedt, L. & Träskman, L. (1980). Clomipramine treatment of obsessive compulsive disorder. I. A controlled clinical trial. *Archives of General Psychiatry*, 37, 1281-5.

Tiihonen, J., Lonnqvist, J., Wahlbeck, K. et al. (2009). 11-year follow-up of mortality in patients with schizophrenia:

population-based cohort study (FIN11 study). *Lancet*, **374**, 620–7.

Titov, N., Andrews, G., Choi, I., Schwencke, G. & Mahoney, A. (2008). Shyness 3: randomized controlled trial of guided versus unguided Internet-based CBT for social phobia. *Australian and New Zealand Journal of Psychiatry*, **42**, 1030–40.

Tohen, M., Kryzhanovskaya, L., Carlson, G. et al. (2007). Olanzapine versus placebo in the treatment of adolescents with bipolar mania. *American Journal of Psychiatry*, **164**, 1547–56.

Tolin, D. F., Maltby, N., Diefenbach, G. J., Hannan, S. E. & Worhunsky, P. (2004). Cognitive-behavioral therapy for medication nonresponders with obsessive-compulsive disorder: a wait-list-controlled open trial. *Journal of Clinical Psychiatry*, **65**, 922–31.

Tollefson, G. D., Birkett, M., Koran, L. Genduso, L. (1994). Continuation treatment of OCD: double-blind and open-label experience with fluoxetine. *Journal of Clinical Psychiatry*, **55** (Suppl), 69–76.

Tonigan, J. S., Toscova, R. & Miller, W. R. (2002). Meta-analysis of the literature on Alcoholics Anonymous: sample and study characteristics moderate findings. *Journal of Studies on Alcohol*, **57**, 65–72.

Touyz, S. W., Beumont, P. J. V., Glaun, D., Phillips, T. & Cowie, I. (1984). A comparison of lenient and strict operant conditioning programmes in refeeding patients with anorexia nervosa. *British Journal of Psychiatry*, **144**, 517–20.

Touyz, S. W., Garner, D. M. & Beumont, P. J. V. (1995). The inpatient management of the adolescent patient with anorexia nervosa. In: H-Ch. Steinhausen, ed. *Anorexia and Bulimia Nervosa: Eating Disorders in Adolescence.* Berlin, New York: Walter de Gruyter, pp. 247–70.

Treasure, J. L., Todd, G., Brolly, M., Tiller, J., Nehmed, A. & Denman, F. (1995). A pilot study of a randomized trial of cognitive analytical therapy vs. educational behavioural therapy for adult anorexia nervosa. *Behaviour Research and Therapy*, **33**, 363–7.

Treasure, J., Angélica, M., Claudino, A. M. & Zucker, N. (2010). Eating disorders. *Lancet*, **375**, 583–93.

Treatment for Adolescents with Depression Study (TADS) Team (2004). Fluoxetine, cognitive-behavioral therapy, and their combination for adolescents with depression: Treatment for Adolescents with Depression Study (TADS) randomized controlled trial. *Journal of the American Medical Association*, **292**, 807–20.

Trigazis, L., Tennankore, D., Vohra, S. & Katzman, D. K. (2004). The use of herbal remedies by adolescents with eating disorders. *International Journal of Eating Disorders*, **35**, 223–8.

Trivedi, M. H., Rush, A. J., Wisniewski, S. R. et al. (2006). Evaluation of outcomes with citalopram for depression using measurement-based care in STAR*D: implications for clinical practice. *American Journal of Psychiatry*, **163** (1), 28–40.

Trumpler, F., Oez, S., Stahli, P., Brenner, H. D. & Juni, P. (2003). Acupuncture for alcohol withdrawal: a randomized, controlled trial. *Alcohol and Alcoholism*, **38**, 369–75.

Tsoi, W. F. (1993). Follow-up study of transsexuals after sex-reassignment surgery. *Singapore Medical Journal*, **34**, 515–7.

Tsoi, W. F., Kok, L. P., Yeo, K. L. & Ratnam, S. S. (1995). Follow-up study of female transsexuals. *Annals of the Academy of Medicine, Singapore*, **24**, 664–7.

Tumur, I., Kaltenthaler, E., Ferriter, M., Beverley, C. & Parry, G. (2007). Computerised cognitive behaviour therapy for obsessive-compulsive disorder: a systematic review. *Psychotherapy and Psychosomatics*, **76**, 196–202.

Tyrer, P. (1986). *How to Stop Taking Tranquillisers*. London: Sheldon Press.

Tyrer, P. (2007). Personality diatheses: a superior explanation than disorder. *Psychological Medicine*, **37**, 1521–5.

Tyrer, P. (2009). *Harmonising the Environment with the Patient*. London: RCPsych Press.

Tyrer, P. & Baldwin, D. (2006). Generalised anxiety disorder. *Lancet*, **368**, 2156–66.

Tyrer, P. & Kendall, T. (2009). The spurious advance of antipsychotic drug therapy. *Lancet*, **373**, 4–5.

Tyrer, P. J. & Lader, M. H. (1973). Effects of beta-blockade with sotalol in chronic anxiety. *Clinical Pharmacology and Therapeutics*, **14**, 418–26.

Tyrer, P. & Lader, M. H. (1974). Response to propranolol and diazepam in somatic and psychic anxiety. *British Medical Journal*, **2**, 14–16.

Tyrer, P., Rutherford, D. & Huggett, T. (1981). Benzodiazepine withdrawal symptoms and propranolol. *Lancet*, **i**, 520–2.

Tyrer, P., Owen, R. & Dawling, S. (1983). Gradual withdrawal of diazepam after long-term therapy. *Lancet*, **i**, 1402–6.

Tyrer, P., Murphy, S., Oates, G. & Kingdon, D. (1985). Psychological treatment for benzodiazepine dependence. *Lancet*, **1**, 1042–3.

Tyrer, P., Seivewright, N., Murphy, S. et al. (1988). The Nottingham study of neurotic disorder: comparison of drug and psychological treatments. *Lancet*, **ii**, 235–40.

Tyrer, P., Murphy, S. & Riley, P. (1990). The Benzodiazepine Withdrawal Symptom Questionnaire. *Journal of Affective Disorders*, **19**, 53–61.

Tyrer, P., Mitchard, S., Methuen, C. & Ranger, M. (2003a). Treatment-rejecting and treatment-seeking personality disorders: Type R and Type S. *Journal of Personality Disorders*, **17**, 265–70.

Tyrer, P., Sensky, T. & Mitchard, S. (2003b). The principles of nidotherapy in the treatment of persistent mental and personality disorders. *Psychotherapy and Psychosomatics*, **72**, 350–6.

Tyrer, P., Oliver-Africano, P. C., Ahmed, Z. et al. (2008). Risperidone, haloperidol and placebo in the treatment of aggressive challenging behaviour in intellectual disability: randomised controlled trial. *Lancet*, **371**, 55–61.

Tyrer, P., Miloŝeska, K., Whittington, C. et al. (2011). Nidotherapy in the treatment of substance misuse, psychosis and personality disorder: secondary analysis of a controlled trial. *The Psychiatrist*, **35**, 9–14.

Tyrer, S. P., Walsh, A., Edwards, D. E. et al. (1984). Factors associated with a good response to lithium in aggressive mentally handicapped subjects. *Progress in Neuropsychopharmacology and Biological Psychiatry*, **8**, 751–5.

Uehara, T., Kawashima, Y., Goto, M., Tasaki, S. I. & Someya, T. (2001). Psychoeducation for the families of patients with eating disorders and changes in expressed emotion: a preliminary study. *Comprehensive Psychiatry*, **42**(2), 132–8.

Uher, R., Perroud, N., Ng, M. Y. et al. (2010). Genome-wide pharmacogenetics of antidepressant response in the GENDEP project. *American Journal of Psychiatry*, **167**, 555–64.

UK Alcohol Forum (2001). *Guidelines for the Management of Alcohol Problems in Primary Care and General Psychiatry*. High Wycombe, Bucks: Tangent Medical Education.

United Nations Office for Drug Control and Crime Prevention (2000). *World Drug Report 2000*. Oxford: Oxford University Press.

US Department of Health and Human Services (1999). *TIP 32: Treatment of Adolescents with Substance Use Disorders* (DHHS Publication No. SMA 99-3283). Rockville, MD: Author.

US Department of Health and Human Services (2003). *Helping Patients with Alcohol Problems: A Health Practitioner's Guide*. National Institute of Health, National Institute on Alcohol and Alcoholism.

Üstün, T. B., Ayuso-Mateos, J. L., Chatterji, S., Mathers, C. Murray, CJL (2004). Global burden of depressive disorders in the year 2000. *British Journal of Psychiatry*, **184**, 386–92.

van den Boom, D. C. (1994). The influence of temperament and mothering on attachment and exploration: an experimental manipulation of sensitive responsiveness among lower-class mothers with irritable infants. *Child Development*, **65**, 1457–77.

van den Boom, D. C. (1995). Do first-year intervention effects endure? Follow-up during toddlerhood of a sample of Dutch irritable infants. *Child Development*, **66**, 1798–816.

Van den Borre, R., Vermote, R., Buttiens, M. et al. (1993). Risperidone as add-on therapy in behavioral disturbances in mental-retardation: a double-blind placebo-controlled cross-over study. *Acta Psychiatrica Scandinavica*, **87**, 167–71.

Van den Hout, M. & Barlow, D. (2000). Attention, arousal and expectancies in anxiety and sexual disorders. *Journal of Affective Disorders*, **61**, 241–56.

Van der Windt, F., Dohle, G. R., van der Tak, J. & Slob, A. K. (2002). Intracavernosal injection therapy with and without sexological counselling in men with erectile dysfunction. *BJU International*, **89**, 901–4.

Van Kesteren, P. J., Asscheman, H. Megens, J. A. & Gooren, L. J. (1997). Mortality and morbidity in transsexual subjects treated with cross-sex hormones. *Clinical Endocrinology*, **47**, 337–42.

Van Lankveld, J. J. D. M. (1998). Bibliotherapy in the treatment of sexual dysfunctions: a meta-analysis. *Journal of*

Consulting and Clinical Psychology, **66**, 702–8.

Van Putten, T. & Fawzy, F. I. (1976). Sex conversion surgery in a man with severe gender dysphoria: a tragic outcome. *Archives of General Psychiatry*, **33**(6), 751–3.

Van Reekum, R., Clarke, D., Conn, D. et al. (2002). A randomized placebo-controlled trial of the discontinuation of long-term anti-psychotics in dementia. *International Psychogeriatrics*, **14**, 197–210.

Vandereycken, W. & Pieters, G. (1978). Short-term weight restoration in anorexia nervosa through operant conditioning. *Scandinavian Journal of Behaviour Therapy*, **7**, 221–36.

Vandereycken, W. (2003). The place of inpatient care in the treatment of anorexia nervosa: questions to be answered. *International Journal of Eating Disorders*, **34**, 409–22.

Vandrey, R. G. & Haney, M. (2009). Pharmacotherapy for cannabis dependence: how close are we? *CNS Drugs*, **23**, 543–53.

Vandrey, R. G., Budney, A. J., Moore, B. A. & Hughes, J. R. (2005). A cross-study comparison of cannabis and tobacco withdrawal. *American Journal on Addictions*, **14**, 54–63.

Vasilaki, E. I., Hosier, S. G. & Cox, W. M. (2006). The efficacy of motivational interviewing as a brief intervention for excessive drinking: a meta-analytic review. *Alcohol and Alcoholism*, **41**, 328–35.

Vataja, R., Pohjasvaara, T., Leppavuori, A. & Erkinjutti, T. (2002). Post stroke depression. In E. Chiu, D. Ames & C. Katona, eds. *Vascular Disease and Affective Disorders*. London: Martin Dunitz Publishing.

Vaughn, C. E. & Leff, J. P. (1976). The influence of family and social factors on the course of psychiatric illness: a comparison of schizophrenic and depressed neurotic patients. *British Journal of Psychiatry*, **129**, 125–37.

Verheul, R., Van Den Bosch, L. M., Koeter, M. W., De Ridder, M. A., Stijnen, T. & Van Den Brink, W. (2003). Dialectical behaviour therapy for women with borderline personality disorder: 12-month, randomised clinical trial in The Netherlands. *British Journal of Psychiatry*, **182**, 135–40.

Versiani, M., Nardi, A. E., Mundim, F. D., Alves, A. B., Liebowitz, M. R. & Amrein, R. (1992). Pharmacotherapy of social phobia: a controlled study with moclobemide and phenelzine. *British Journal of Psychiatry*, **161**, 353–60.

Vieten, C., Astin, J. A., Buscemi, R. & Galloway, G. P. (2010). Development of an acceptance-based coping intervention for alcohol dependence relapse prevention. *Substance Abuse*, **31**, 108–16.

Vinks, A. A. & Walson, P. D. (2003). Pharmacokinetics 1: developmental principles. In: A. Martin, L. Scahill, D. S. Charney & J. F. Leckman, eds. *Pediatric Psychopharmacology: Principles and Practice*. Oxford: Oxford University Press.

Virtué-Ortega, J. (2010). Applied behavior analytic intervention for autism in early childhood: meta-analysis, meta-regression and dose-response meta-analysis of multiple outcomes. *Clinical Psychology Review*, **30**, 387-99.

Vocks, S., Tuschen-Caffier, B., Pietrowsky, R., Rustenbach, S. J., Kersting, A. & Herpertz, S. (2010). Meta-analysis of the effectiveness of psychological and pharmacological treatments for binge eating disorder. *International Journal of Eating Disorders*, **43**, 205-17.

Volpicelli, J. R., Rhines, K. C., Rhines, J. S. et al. (1997). Naltrexone and alcohol dependence: role of subject compliance. *Archives of General Psychiatry*, **54**, 737-42.

Von Keitz, A. T., Stroberg, P., Bukofzer, S., Mallard, N. & Hibberd, M. (2002). A European multicentre study to evaluate the tolerability of apomorphine sublingual administered in a forced dose-escalation regimen in patients with erectile dysfunction. *BJU International*, **89**, 409-15.

Wagner, K. D., Ambrosini, P., Rynn, M. et al. (2003). Efficacy of sertraline in the treatment of children and adolescents with major depressive disorder: two randomized controlled trials. *Journal of the American Medical Association*, **290**, 1033-41.

Wagner, K. D., Kowatch, R. A., Emslie, G. J. et al. (2006). A double-blind, randomized, placebo-controlled trial of oxcarbazepine in the treatment of bipolar disorder in children and adolescents. *American Journal of Psychiatry*, **163**, 1179-86.

Wagner, K. D., Robb, A. S., Findling, R. L., Jin, J., Gutierrez, M. M. & Heydorn, W. E. (2004). A randomized, placebo-controlled trial of citalopram for the treatment of major depression in children and adolescents. *American Journal of Psychiatry*, **161**, 1079-83.

Wagner, K. D., Redden, L., Kowatch, R. A. et al. (2009). A double-blind, randomized, placebo-controlled trial of divalproex extended-release in the treatment of bipolar disorder in children and adolescents. *Journal of the American Academy of Child and Adolescent Psychiatry*, **48**, 519-32.

Waldinger, M. D., Hengeveld, M. W., Zwinderman, A. H. & Olivier, B. (2001). Effect of SSRI antidepressants on ejaculation: a double-blind randomized, placebo-controlled study with fluoxetine, fluvoxamine, paroxetine and sertraline. *Journal of Clinical Psychopharmacology*, **21**(2), 241-2.

Walitzer, K. S. & O'Connors, G. J. (1999). Treating problem drinking. *Alcohol Research and Health*, **23**, 138-43.

Walkup, J. T., Albano, A. M., Piacentini, J. et al. (2008). Cognitive behavioural therapy, sertraline or a combination in childhood anxiety. *New England Journal of Medicine*, **359**, 2753-66.

Wallace, P., Cutler, S. & Haines, A. (1988). Randomised controlled trial of general practitioner intervention in patients with excessive alcohol consumption. *British Medical Journal*, **297**, 663-8.

Waller, D. & Fairburn, C. G. (2004). Eating disorders. In D. Waller & A. McPherson, eds. *Women's Health*, 5th edn. Oxford: Oxford University Press, pp. 519-51.

Waller, D., Fairburn, C. G., McPherson, A., Kay, R., Lee, A. & Nowell, T. (1996). Treating bulimia nervosa in primary care: a pilot study. *International Journal of Eating Disorders*, **19**, 99–103.

Walsh, B. T., Fairburn, C. G., Mickley, D., Sysko, R. & Parides, M. K. (2004). Treatment of bulimia nervosa in a primary care setting. *American Journal of Psychiatry*, **161**, 556–61.

Walter, G. & Rey, J. M. (2003). How fixed are child psychiatrists' views about ECT in the young? *The Journal of ECT*, **19**, 88–92.

Walsh, B. T., Seidman, S. N. et al. (2002). Placebo response in studies of major depression: variable, substantial, and growing. *Journal of the American Medical Association*, **287**(14), 1840–7.

Walsh, R. & Shapiro, S. L. (2006). The meeting of meditative disciplines and Western psychology: a mutually enriching dialogue. *American Psychologist*, **61**, 227–39.

Walter, G., Rey, J. M. & Mitchell, P. B. (1999). Practitioner review: electroconvulsive therapy in adolescents. *Journal of Child Psychology and Psychiatry*, **40**, 325–34.

Washington Post (2006). Article 3 October. http://www.washingtonpost.com/wp-dyn/content/article/2006/10/02/AR2006100201378.html

Webster-Stratton, C. (1981). Modification of mothers' behaviors and attitudes through a videotape modeling group discussion program. *Behavior Therapy*, **12**, 634–42.

Webster-Stratton, C. & Reid, M. J. (2004). Strengthening social and emotional competence in young children: the foundation for early school readiness and success incredible years classroom social skills and problem-solving curriculum. *Infants and Young Children*, **17**, 96–113.

Webster-Stratton, C., Reid, M. J. & Hammond, M. (2004). Treating children with early-onset conduct problems: intervention outcomes for parent, child, and teacher training. *Journal of Clinical Child and Adolescent Psychology*, **33**, 105–24.

Webster-Stratton, C. Reid, M. J. & Stoolmiller, M. (2008). Preventing conduct problems and improving school readiness: Evaluation of the Incredible Years teacher and child training programs in high-risk schools. *Journal of Child Psychology and Psychiatry*, **49**, 471–88.

Weinmann, S., Roll, S., Schwarzbach, C., Vauth, C. & Willich, S. N. (2010). Effects of *Ginkgo biloba* in dementia: systematic review and meta-analysis. *BMC Geriatrics*, **10**, 14.

Weisner, C., Greenfield, T. & Room, R. (1995). Trends in the treatment of alcohol problems in the U.S. general population, 1979 through 1990. *American Journal of Public Health*, **85**, 55–60.

Weiss, B., Catron, T., Harris, V. & Phung, T. M. (1999). The effectiveness of traditional child psychotherapy. *Journal of Consulting and Clinical Psychology*, **67**, 82–94.

Weissman, M. M. (1979). The psychological treatment of depression: evidence for the efficacy of psychotherapy alone, in comparison with, and in combination with pharmacotherapy. *Archives of General Psychiatry*, **36**, 1261–9.

Weisz, J. R., Weiss, B., Alicke, M. D. & Klotz, M. L. (1987). Effectiveness of psychotherapy with children and adolescents: a meta-analysis for clinicians. *Journal of Consulting and Clinical Psychology*, **55**, 542–9.

Weisz, J. R., Weiss, B., Han, S. S., Granger, D. A. & Morton, T. (1995). Effects of psychotherapy with children and adolescents revisited: a meta-analysis of treatment outcome studies. *Psychological Bulletin*, **117**, 450–68.

Weisz, J. R., Hawley, K. M. & Doss, A. J. (2004). Empirically tested psychotherapies for youth internalizing and externalizing problems and disorders. *Child and Adolescent Psychiatric Clinics of North America*, **13**, 729–815.

Wells, K. C. (2004). Treatment of ADHD in children and adolescents. In: P. M. Barrett & T. H. Ollendick, eds. *Handbook of Interventions that Work with Children and Adolescents: Prevention and Treatment*. Chichester, UK: John Wiley & Sons, Ltd, pp. 343–68.

Wells, K. C., Epstein, J. N., Hinshaw, S. P. et al. (2000). Parenting and family stress treatment outcomes in attention-deficit/hyperactivity disorder (ADHD): an empirical analysis in the MTA Study. *Journal of Abnormal Child Psychology*, **28**, 543–53.

Wells-Parker, E., Bangert-Drowns, R., McMillen, R. & Williams, M. (1995). Final results from a meta-analysis of remedial interventions with drink/drive offenders. *Addiction*, **90**, 907–26.

West, R., Hajek, P., Foulds, J., Nilsson, F., May, S. & Meadows, A. (2000). A comparison of the abuse liability and dependence potential of nicotine patch, gum, spray and inhaler. *Psychopharmacologia*, **149**, 198–202.

West, S. L., O'Neal, K. K. & Graham, C. W. (2000). A meta-analysis comparing the effectiveness of buprenorphine and methadone. *Journal of Substance Abuse*, **12**, 405–14.

Westermeyer, J., Weiss, R. & Ziedonis, D. (2003). *Integrated Treatment for Mood and Substance Use Disorders*. Baltimore, Maryland: The Johns Hopkins University Press.

Whalen, C. K., Henker, B. & Granger, D. A. (1990). Social judgment processes in hyperactive boys: effects of methylphenidate and comparisons with normal peers. *Journal of Abnormal Child Psychology*, **18**, 297–316.

Whitaker-Azmitia, P. M., Druse, M., Walker, P. et al. (1996). Serotonin as a developmental signal. *Behaviour Brain Research*, **73**, 19–29.

Whittington, C. J., Kendall, T., Fonagy, P., Cottrell, D., Cotgrove, A. & Boddington, E. (2004). Selective serotonin reuptake inhibitors in childhood depression: systematic review of published versus unpublished data. *Lancet*, **363**, 1341–5.

Whitworth, A. B., Fischer, F., Lesch, O. M. et al. (1996). Comparison of acamprosate and placebo in long-term treatment of alcohol dependence. *Lancet*, **347**, 1438–42.

WHO Collaborating Centre for Research and Training for Mental Health (2004). *WHO Guide to Mental and Neurological Health in Primary Care*. London: RSM Press.

Wilberg, T., Friis, S., Karterud, S. Mehlum, L., Urnes, O. & Vaglum, P. (1998). Outpatient group psychotherapy: a valuable continuation treatment for patients with borderline personality disorder treated in a day hospital? A 3-year follow-up study. *Nordic Journal of Psychiatry*, **52**, 213–22.

Wilcock, G. K., Ballard, C. G., Cooper, J. A. & Loft, H. (2008). Memantine for agitation/aggression and psychosis in moderately severe to severe Alzheimer's disease: a pooled analysis of 3 studies. *Journal of Clinical Psychiatry*, **69**, 341–8.

Wilfley, D. E., Welch, R. R., Stein, R. I. et al. (2002). A randomized comparison of group cognitive-behavioral therapy and group interpersonal psychotherapy for the treatment of overweight individuals with binge-eating disorder. *Archives of General Psychiatry*, **59**(8), 713–21.

Wilfley, D. E., Crow, S. J., Hudson, J. I. et al. (2008). Efficacy of sibutramine for the treatment of binge eating disorder: a randomized multicenter placebo-controlled double-blind study. *American Journal of Psychiatry*, **165**, 51–8.

Wilk, A. I., Jensen, N. M. & Havighurst, T. C. (1997). Meta analysis of randomized control trials addressing brief interventions in heavy alcohol drinkers. *Journal of General Internal Medicine*, **12**, 274–83.

Willer, M. G., Thuras, P. & Crow, S. J. (2005). Implications of the changing use of hospitalization to treat anorexia nervosa. *American Journal of Psychiatry*, **162**, 2374–6.

Williams, M. A., Campbell, E. B., Raynor, W. J. et al. (1985). Reducing acute confusional states in elderly patients with hip fractures. *Research in Nursing and Health*, **8**, 329–37.

Williams, S. K., Scahill, L., Vitiello, B. et al. (2006). Risperidone and adaptive behavior in children with autism. *Journal of the American Academy of Child and Adolescent Psychiatry*, **45**, 431–9.

Williamson, D. A., Thaw, J. M. & Varnado-Sullivan, P. J. (2001). Cost-effectiveness analysis of a hospital-based cognitive-behavioral treatment program for eating disorders. *Behavior Therapy*, **32**, 459–77.

Willner, P., Jones, J., Tams, R. & Green, G. (2002). A randomised controlled trial of the efficacy of a cognitive-behavioural anger management group for adults with learning disabilities. *Journal of Applied Research in Intellectual Disabilities*, **15**, 224–35.

Wilson, G. T. & Fairburn, C. G. (2002). Eating disorders. In: P. E. Nathan & J. M. Gorman, eds. *Treatments that Work*, 2nd edn. New York: Oxford University Press, pp. 559–92.

Wilson, G. T., Wilfley, D. E., Agras, W. S. & Bryson, S. W. (2010). Psychological treatments of Binge Eating Disorder *Archives of General Psychiatry*, **67** 94–101.

Winblad, B., Engedal, K., Soininen, H et al. & the Donepezil Nordic Study Group (2001). A 1-year, randomized placebo-controlled study of donepezil in patients with mild to moderate AD *Neurology*, **57**, 489–95.

Winblad, B., Black, S. E., Homma, A et al. (2009). Donepezil treatment in severe Alzheimer's disease: a pooled analysis of three clinical trials *Current Medical Research Opinion*, **25** 2577–87.

Winston, A. & Webster, P. (2003). Inpatient treatment. In: J. Treasure, U. Schmidt &

E. van Furth, eds. *Handbook of Eating Disorders*, 2nd edn. Chichester: John Wiley and Sons.

Winters, N. C. (2003). Feeding problems in infancy and early childhood. *Primary Psychiatry*, **10**(6), 30–4.

Wiseman, C. V., Sunday, S. R., Klapper, F., Harris, W. A. & Halmi, K. A. (2001). Changing patterns of hospitalization in eating disorder patients. *International Journal of Eating Disorders*, **30**, 69–74.

Wong, I. C., Camilleri-Novak, D., Stephens, P. et al. (2003). Rise in psychotropic drug prescribing in children in the UK: an urgent public health issue. *Drug Safety*, **26**, 1117–8.

Woods, B., Spector, A., Jones, C., Orrell, M. & Davies, S. (2005). Reminiscence therapy for dementia. *Cochrane Database of Systematic Reviews*, **2**, CD001120.

Woodside, D. B. & Kaplan, A. S. (1994). Day hospital treatment in males with eating disorders: response and comparison to females. *Journal of Psychosomatic Research*, **38**, 471–5.

Woody, G. E., Luborsky, L., McLellan, A. T. et al. (1983). Psychotherapy for opiate addicts. Does it help? *Archives in General Psychiatry*, **40**(6), 639–45.

Woolfenden, S. R., Williams, K. & Peat, J. K. (2002). Family and parenting interventions for conduct disorder and delinquency: a meta-analysis of randomised controlled trials. *Archives of Disease in Childhood*, **86**, 251–6.

Wykes, T. & Huddy, V. (2009). Cognitive remediation for schizophrenia: it is even more complicated. *Current Opinion in Psychiatry*, **22**(2), 161–7.

Wynne, L. C., Ryckoff, I. M., Day, J. & Hirsch, S. (1958). Pseudomutuality in the family relations of schizophrenics. *Psychiatry*, **21**(2), 205–20.

Yagcioglu, A. E., Kivircik, A., Turgut, T. I. et al. (2005). A double-blind controlled study of adjunctive treatment with risperidone in schizophrenic patients partially responsive to clozapine: efficacy and safety. *Journal of Clinical Psychiatry*, **66**, 63–72.

Yager, J., Siegfreid, S. L. & DiMatteo, T. L. (1999). Use of alternative remedies by psychiatric patients: illustrative vignettes and a discussion of the issues. *American Journal of Psychiatry*, **156**, 1432–8.

Yamda, N., Martin-Iverson, M. T., Daimon, K., Tsujimoto, T. & Takashashi, S. (1995). Clinical and chronobiological effects of light therapy on non-seasonal affective disorders. *Biological Psychiatry*, **37**, 866–73.

Yanos, P., Rosenfield, S. & Horwitz, A. (2001). Negative and supportive social interactions and quality of life among persons diagnosed with severe mental illness. *Community Mental Health Journal*, **37**, 405.

Yaryura-Tobias, J. A. & Neziroglu, F. A. (1996). Venlafaxine in obsessive-compulsive disorder. *Archives of General Psychiatry*, **53**, 653–4.

Yatham, L. N. (2003). Acute and maintenance treatment of bipolar mania: the role of atypical antipsychotics. *Bipolar Disorders*, **5** (Suppl. 2), 7–19.

Yoder, P. J. & Stone, W. L. (2006). Randomized comparison of two communication interventions for preschoolers with autism spectrum disorders. *Journal of Consulting and Clinical Psychology*, **74**, 426-35.

Young, J. E. (1990). *Cognitive Therapy for Personality Disorders: A Schema-Focused Approach*. Sarasota, Florida: Professional Resource Exchange.

Zanarini, M. C., Frankenburg, F. R., Hennen, J. & Silk, K. R. (2004). Mental Health Service utilization by borderline personality disorder patients and Axis II comparison subjects followed prospectively for 6 years. *Journal of Clinical Psychiatry*, **65**, 28-36.

Zeanah, C. H., Smyke, A. T. & Dumitrescu, A. (2002). Attachment disturbances in young children: II. Indiscriminate behaviour and institutional care. *Journal of the American Academy of Child and Adolescent Psychiatry*, **41**, 983-9.

Zecevic, N. & Verney, C. (1995). Development of the catecholamine neurons in human embryos and fetuses, with special emphasis on the innervation of the cerebral cortex. *Journal of Comparative Neurology*, **351**, 509-35.

Zgierska, A., Rabago, D., Zuelsdorff, M., Coe, C., Miller, M. & Fleming, M. (2008). Mindfulness meditation for alcohol relapse prevention: a feasibility pilot study. *Journal of Addiction Medicine*, **2**, 165-73.

Zgierska, A., Rabago, D., Chawla, N., Kushner, K., Koehler, R. & Marlatt, A. (2009). Mindfulness meditation for substance use disorders: a systematic review. *Substance Abuse*, **30**, 266-94.

Zhu, S., Melcer, T., Sun, J., Rosbrook, B. & Pierce, J. (2000). Smoking cessation with and without assistance: a population-based analysis. *American Journal of Preventive Medicine*, **18**, 305-11.

Ziedonis, D. M. & Stern, R. (2001). Dual recovery therapy for schizophrenia and substance abuse. *Psychiatric Annals*, **31**, 255-64.

Ziedonis, D., Smelson, D., Rosenthal, R. et al. (2005). Improving the care of individuals with schizophrenia and substance abuse disorders. *Journal of Psychiatric Practice*, **11**, 1-25.

Zipfel, S., Reas, D. L., Thornton, C. et al. (2002). Day hospitalization programs for eating disorders: a systematic review of the literature. *International Journal of Eating Disorders*, **31**, 105-17.

Zitman, F. G. & Couvée, J. E. (2001). Chronic benzodiazepine use in general practice patients with depression: an evaluation of controlled treatment and taper-off. Report on behalf of the Dutch Chronic Benzodiazepine Working Group. *British Journal of Psychiatry*, **178**, 317-24.

Zito, J. M., Safer, D. J. & dosReis, S. (2000). Trends in the prescribing of psychotropic medications to preschoolers. *Journal of the American Medical Association*, **283**, 1025-30.

Zito, J. M., Safer, D. J., dosReis, S. et al. (2003). Psychotropic practice pattern for youth: a 10-year perspective. *Archives of Pediatric and Adolescent Medicine*, **157**, 17-25.

Zito, J. M., Safer, D. J., dosReis, S., Gardner, J. F., Boles, M. & Lynch, F. (2000). Trends in the prescribing of psychotropic medications to preschoolers. *Journal of the American Medical Association*, **283**, 1025-30.

Zuercher, J.N., Cumella, E.J., Woods, B.K., Eberly, M. & Carr, J.K. (2003). Efficacy of voluntary tube feeding in female inpatients with anorexia nervosa. *Journal of Parenteral and Enteral Nutrition*, **27**, 268–76.

Zweifel, J.E. & O'Brien, W.H. (1997). A meta-analysis of the effect of hormone replacement therapy upon depressed mood. *Psychoneuroendocrinology*, **22** (3), 189–212.

Zwerling, C., Sprince, N.L., Wallace, R.B., Davis, C.S., Whitten, P.S. & Heeringa, S.G. (1996). Alcohol and occupational injuries among older workers. *Accident Analysis and Prevention*, **28**, 371–6.

Index